Directory of Internet Sources for Health Professionals

Directory of Internet Sources for Health Professionals

Attrices Dean Griffin

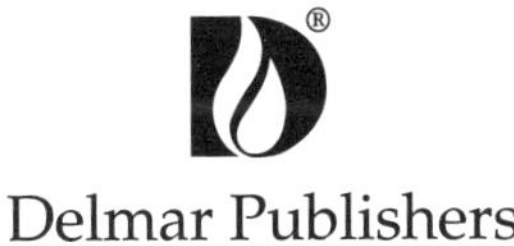

Delmar Publishers

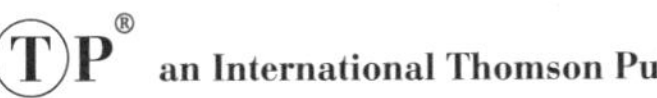

an International Thomson Publishing company

Albany • Bonn • Boston • Cincinnati • Detroit • London • Madrid
Melbourne • Mexico City • New York • Pacific Grove • Paris • San Francisco
Singapore • Tokyo • Toronto • Washington

NOTICE TO THE READER

Publisher does not warrant or guarantee any of the products described herein or perform any independent analysis in connection with any of the product information contained herein. Publisher does not assume, and expressly disclaims, any obligation to obtain and include information other than that provided to it by the manufacturer.

The reader is expressly warned to consider and adopt all safety precautions that might be indicated by the activities herein and to avoid all potential hazards. By following the instructions contained herein, the reader willingly assumes all risks in connection with such instructions.

The Publisher makes no representation or warranties of any kind, including but not limited to, the warranties of fitness for particular purpose or merchantability, nor are any such representations implied with respect to the material set forth herein, and the publisher takes no responsibility with respect to such material. The publisher shall not be liable for any special, consequential, or exemplary damages resulting, in whole or part, from the readersí use of, or reliance upon, this material.

Delmar Staff:
Publisher: Susan Simpfenderfer
Acquisitions Editor: Marlene McHugh Pratt
Developmental Editor: Debra Flis
Project Editor: William Trudell
Cover Design: Publisher's Studio
Art and Design Coordinator: Rich Killar
Marketing Manager: Darryl L. Caron
Production Services: Publisher's Studio, a division of Stratford Publishing Services

Printed in Canada
2 3 4 5 6 7 8 9 10 XXX 04 03 02 01 00 99

For more information, contact Delmar, 3 Columbia Circle, PO Box 15015, Albany, NY 12212-0515; or find us on the World Wide Web at http://www.delmar.com

International Division List

Japan:
Thomson Learning
Palaceside Building 5F
1-1-1 Hitotsubashi, Chiyoda-ku
Tokyo 100 0003 Japan
Tel: 813 5218 6544
Fax: 813 5218 6551

Australia/New Zealand
Nelson/Thomson Learning
102 Dodds Street
South Melbourne, Victoria 3205
Australia
Tel: 61 39 685 4111
Fax: 61 39 685 4199

UK/Europe/Middle East:
Thomson Learning
Berkshire House
168-173 High Holborn
London
WC1V 7AA United Kingdom
Tel: 44 171 497 1422
Fax: 44 171 497 1426

Latin America:
Thomson Learning
Seneca, 53
Colonia Polanco
11560 Mexico D.F. Mexico
Tel: 525-281-2906
Fax: 525-281-2656

Canada:
Nelson/Thomson Learning
1120 Birchmount Road
Scarborough, Ontario
Canada M1K 5G4
Tel: 416-752-9100
Fax: 416-752-810

Asia:
Thomson Learning
60 Albert Street, #15-01
Albert Complex
Singapore 189969
Tel: 65 336 6411
Fax: 65 336 7411

Spain:
Thomson Learning
Calle Magallanes, 25
28015-MADRID
ESPANA
Tel: 34 91 446 33 50
Fax: 34 91 445 62 18

Library of Congress Cataloging-in-Publication Data:
Griffin, Attrices Dean.
Directory of Internet sources for health professionals / Attrices Dean Griffin.
p. cm.
Includes bibliographical references and index.
ISBN 0-7668-0485-2
1. Medicine—Computer network resources—Directories. 2. Internet (Computer network)—Directories. I. Title
[DNLM: 1. Computer Communication Networks directories. 2. Health Services directories. 3. Databases directories. 4. Online Systems directories. W 22.1G851d 1998]
R859.7D36G75 1998
025.06'61—dc21 98-30169
DNLM/DLC for Library of Congress CIP

Contents

Alternative Medicine

Cancer

Cardiovascular Medicine

Dental Health

Dermatology

Emergency Medicine

Gastroenterology

General Medicine

Health Funding Policy

HIV/AIDS

Legal Medicine

Medical Informatics

Medical Specialties

Anesthesiology

Endocrinology

Forensic Medicine

Genetics

Pathology

Radiography

Telemedicine

Urology

Mental Health

Musculoskeletal Health

Neurology

Nursing and Home Health Care

Nutrition

Occupational Health

Ophthalmology

Otolaryngology

Pediatrics

Pharmacology

Preventive Health

Radiology

Rehabilitative Medicine

Reproductive Health

Respiratory Health

Substance Abuse

Veterinary Medicine

About the Author

Attrices Dean Griffin, author of the *Directory of Internet Sources for Health Professionals*, is a freelance social science writer-researcher. Ms. Griffin graduated from Morgan State University with a BA in English. Following graduation, Ms. Griffin taught in the Baltimore Public Schools for several years. Later she was awarded a Master's degree in counseling and psychology from Loyola College. Her highly mobile background includes several management and consultant positions in health services and development programs. As founder and former owner of a writing and research contracting business, her firm performed numerous contracts for the Departments of Health and Human Services, Defense, Labor, EPA, National Institute of Mental Health, and numerous other federal agencies. She was also a former co-owner of a mental health center specializing in family as well as adolescent services.

Ms. Griffin's recent publication credits include a number of books and articles for national and international health, business, and other reference publishers. She co-authored the reference, *Test Preparation for the GRE Sociology Test* (Research & Education Association, 1995). For the *Encyclopedia of American Industries* (Gale Publishers, Inc., 1994) and the *Encyclopedia of Global Industries* (Gale, 1996), her writing contributions consisted of a series of essays on international hospitals, skilled care nursing homes, flat glass, glass containers, herbals and medicinals, flour and grains, and legal services, to name a few. As a former columnist for the *Med-Online News*, a German publication, Ms. Griffin authored "Nibbles n' Bytes," a monthly column for physicians covering Internet medicine. Her articles on ship repair appeared in the *Motor Ship* publication. Her expertise also includes item writing for various publishers, such as CTB-McGraw-Hill. Attrices Dean Griffin resides in New York City.

Preface

The reference, *Directory of Internet Sources for Health Professionals*, is a primary source for identifying and accessing relevant Internet medical-health data. The *Directory* facilitates information essential to physicians, medical practitioners, researchers, allied health professionals, health providers, planners, organizations, students, writers, publishers, suppliers, consumers, and a growing host of Internet users. The Internet, unlike any other source, offers an infinitely timely database of medical data. For many users, however, the potential of Internet benefits frequently dissipate with the futile, time-consuming efforts to pinpoint relevant data. Alleviating this obstacle basically established the rationale for developing this unique reference to enable medical professionals to access precise Internet data more quickly and easily. Using the *Directory*, users will discover innumerable benefits for Internet medical data searchers:

- Comprehensive list of medical online data sources organized according to major medical categories
- Annotated entries accompanied by specific Internet URLs, primary topic, sponsor, site type and description, access requirements, supplementary links to more than 1,500 related sites, plus tips and keywords
- Quickie tools for Internet data searches according to keyword, category, or topic
- Data peer-reviewed by medical and health professionals
- Updates of new Internet sites provided quarterly online through Delmar Publishers' web site: http://www.delmaralliedhealth.com

Acknowledgments

The *Directory of Internet Sources for Health Professionals* is a unique reference developed in response to my personal writing and research needs. As a writer-researcher, I find the Internet to be a valuable research source. Despite voluminous information sources, identifying direct data links can be a time-consuming task. Consequently, the futility of constantly reorganizing piles of Web notes forced me to devise more structured approaches that allowed quicker identification and retrieval of medical and social science research data. So emerged the basic concept for the *Directory of Internet Sources for Health Professionals*, a reference created by a professional medical and social science data user for other such professionals.

While my simple organizational approach for Internet medical research proved personally satisfactory, only a professional health publisher such as Delmar Publishers could add the refinements required to disseminate this reference to a broader audience of medical and allied health professionals. I am extremely grateful for the assistance of Dawn Gerrain, Acquisitions Editor, Delmar Publishers, who expertly guided the start-up phase of this publication. To Debra Flis, Developmental Editor, Delmar Publishers, I offer a world of thanks for her expert assistance throughout each phase of the reference development. I appreciated the professionalism she brought to the task. Many thanks Debra. And finally, for Delmar Publishers, thank you for publishing the reference, the *Directory of Internet Sources for Health Professionals.*

Along with Delmar Publishers, I wish to thank the following individuals for reviewing the manuscript and providing valuable feedback:

Marie H. Ahrens, MS, RN
Community Health Faculty
University of Tulsa
School of Nursing
Tulsa, Oklahoma

Angela Deally, RRT
Instructor
Passaic County Community College
Respiratory Therapy Department
Paterson, New Jersey

Gena Duncan, RN, MSEd, MS in Community Health Nursing
Assistant Professor
Lutheran College of Health Professions
Fort Wayne, Indiana

Amelia Kassel, MLS
Information Broker Mentor Program
Sebastopol, California

Barbara J. Smith, BB, RT®
Instructor, Radiologic Technology
Portland Community College
Portland, Oregon

Introduction

Purpose

The primary goal of this reference, the *Directory of Internet Sources for Health Professionals*, is to enable medical professionals to identify and retrieve Internet medical and health data. To achieve this goal, the *Directory* design addressed specific objectives of content, organization, and format. The *Directory* **content** accomplishes the objective of addressing the informational, educational, and research needs of physicians, medical practitioners, researchers, allied health professionals, health providers, planners, organizations, students, writers, publishers, suppliers, and consumers. The *Directory* **organization** accomplishes the objective of expediting access to relevant Internet medical data by providing annotated entries covering a broad range of health subjects. The *Directory* **format** accomplishes the objective of providing a desktop library, complete with quickie tools, for retrieving Internet data. The *Directory of Internet Sources for Health Professionals* is an essential reference for all medical professionals, including beginners or experienced Internet users.

Directory Organization

The organization of the *Directory of Internet Sources for Health Professionals* includes the following sections:

- Introduction
- Table of contents
- Main body of *Directory* entries
- Appendices
- Index

More than a preview, this detailed Introduction serves as a mini-tutorial to optimize *Directory* benefits for both new and experienced Internet users.

Directory Entries

The *Directory* entry format adheres to the following (see Figure 1):

A **Category:** *Directory* categories reflect a unique combination of established medical disciplines and functional designations of health topics. An example is *Medical Informatics*, a nondistinct but functional medical category, featuring references, databases, organizations, and other data sources utilized by medical practitioners.

B **Primary topic:** The *Directory* uses the primary topic as another novel approach for precisely pinpointing Internet data. The primary topic qualifies the main idea of a specific data site, index, or sponsor site. The *Directory* includes a diverse range of topics appealing to variable segments of medical users. Instances of repetitious primary topics feature significant or perhaps contrasting perspectives on the same topic. The primary topic for the entry, MedWeb pediatric Internet resources (Pediatrics category) guides users to hundreds of MedWeb hyperlinked databases, research, support groups, tutorials, institutions...

C **URL (Uniform Resource Locator):** URLs open the Internet door. Although Web sites can be accessed by other methods, the URL is *the key*, only if it fits! Key the *right* URL, bingo, up pops the right Internet site. Check the listed URL for the entry, "Medical/scientific statements," located on the entry for the American Heart Association (AHA):

http://www.americanheart.org/pubs/scipub/statements/

New Internet users, take heed! Enter exactly the above URL. Experienced users probably find quicker access by (1) using "American Heart Association" as the search term or (2) abbreviating the URL to

http://www.americanheart.org/

D **Sponsor:** The site sponsor is the organization, institution, or individuals primarily responsible for developing the site content. Although site design and maintenance may be handled by external organizations, the sponsor generally maintains responsibility for the substantive data aspects. Generally, the sponsor designation is on the homepage as indicated by copyright or other identifier. As cited in Figure 1, the primary sponsor is the

American Heart Association (AHA)

E **Description:** The description is a key feature highlighting the primary entry data. For this specific AHA entry, users expect to find the following information:

Monthly statements, 1995–1997 including mouth-to-mouth ventilation by bystanders; imaging in transient ischemic attacks; pediatric Utstein style.

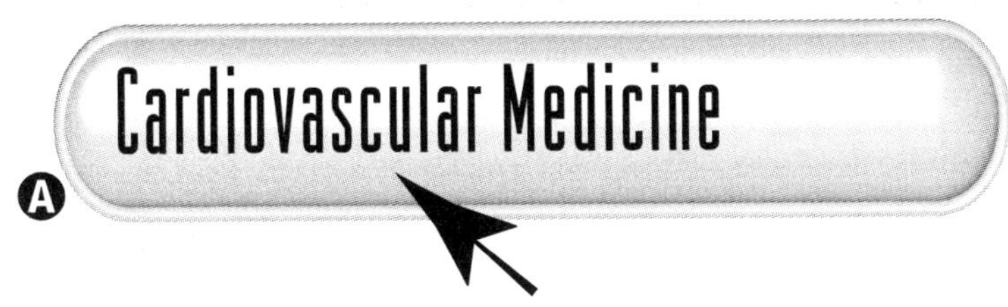

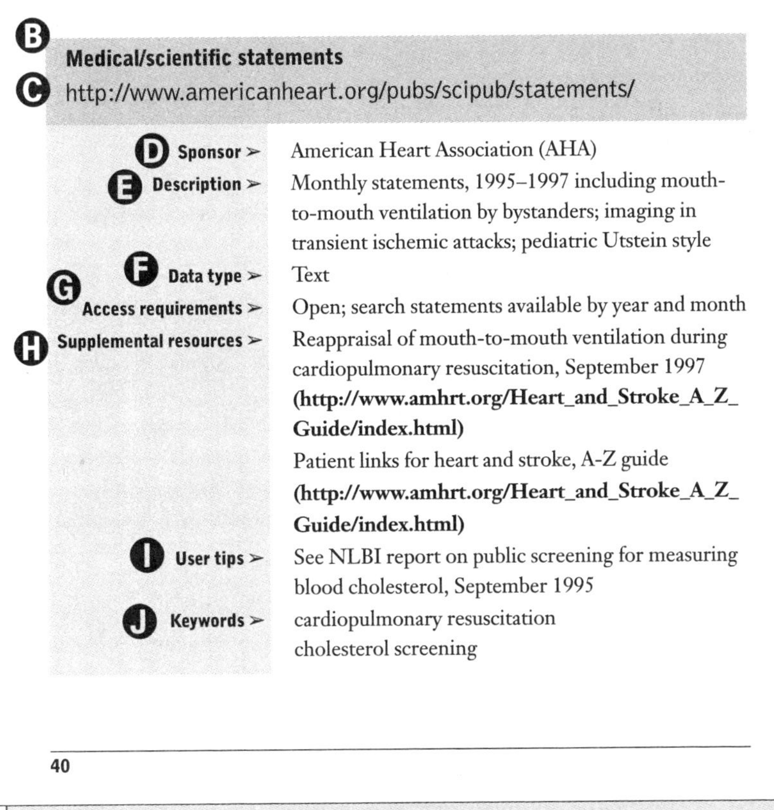

B **Medical/scientific statements**

C http://www.americanheart.org/pubs/scipub/statements/

D **Sponsor ➢** American Heart Association (AHA)

E **Description ➢** Monthly statements, 1995–1997 including mouth-to-mouth ventilation by bystanders; imaging in transient ischemic attacks; pediatric Utstein style

F **Data type ➢** Text

G **Access requirements ➢** Open; search statements available by year and month

H **Supplemental resources ➢** Reappraisal of mouth-to-mouth ventilation during cardiopulmonary resuscitation, September 1997 **(http://www.amhrt.org/Heart_and_Stroke_A_Z_Guide/index.html)**
Patient links for heart and stroke, A-Z guide **(http://www.amhrt.org/Heart_and_Stroke_A_Z_Guide/index.html)**

I **User tips ➢** See NLBI report on public screening for measuring blood cholesterol, September 1995

J **Keywords ➢** cardiopulmonary resuscitation
cholesterol screening

40

Figure 1: Sample *Directory* entry

F **Data type:** Internet data types consist of text, audio, visual, movies, animation, or a mixture or multimedia formats, all of which are represented in the *Directory*. User's computer capacity determines the type, quality, and speed of retrieving multimedia data. Most variable multimedia formats are also accompanied by a basic text format adaptable for any computer type.

G **Access requirements:** The Internet is universally open to all users with the appropriate computer hardware capacity, software, and modem. Access to all Internet sites however, is not universal. Some sites exist to serve the informational needs of selected professional or special interest groups and thereby exclude public use by requiring user registration, fees, or a password for site access. Profit making explains one motive, but sponsors also use these mechanisms to monitor site use, exchange feedback, or develop mailing lists. Similar to the **AHA** entry, the *Directory*'s entry selections consist predominantly of *free* sites with *free* registration with *no* solicitation strings attached. Sites such as the Comprehensive Epidemiologic Data Resource (CEDR) under the **Epidemiology** category maintain public access files, but some are restricted to registered CEDR investigators.

H **Supplemental resources:** The *Directory*'s supplemental resources cite additional topics and URLs that supplement primary entry data. Sources may include the sponsor homepage URL, related organizations, supplementary data, or related Internet links. Note the two supplemental resources cited under the AHA entry:

Supplemental resources ➢	Reappraisal of mouth-to-mouth ventilation during cardiopulmonary resuscitation, September 1997 **(http://www.americanheart.org/pubs/scipub/statements)** Patient links for heart and stroke, A–Z guide **(http://www.amhrt.org/Heart_and_Stroke_A_Z_Guide/index.html)**

I **User tips:** Pay attention to User tips. User tips reflect another unique benefit of the *Directory*. Time-saving tips, toll free sponsor or information numbers, and Internet assistance are samples designed to expedite Internet medical searches. **AHA user tips**, for example, suggest checking the NHLBI report on public screening for measuring blood cholesterol.

J **Keywords:** Each entry page includes one or more keywords for searching the keyword index—another technique for quicker data retrieval.

Appendix: Sponsor Representation According to Type

The **Sponsor** appendix categorizes *Directory* entries according to sponsor type. Entry sponsors represented in the *Directory* are U.S. government or related agencies/organizations; state, university, hospital, academic, or related institutions; health organizations, publishers, and conferences; foreign government or related groups; and private sector or commercial sponsors. Sponsor validation is a key element for assessing the integrity and reliability of Internet data. Where applicable, the *Directory* features peer-reviewed data. Government sponsors typically produce the most reliable data, followed by accredited institutions, professional trade associations, and prominent health organizations. User judgment and analysis represent the most significant determinants in assessing Internet data integrity.

Indexes

The *Directory* contains two indexes to assist the reader in locating information.

Quickie Search Spreadsheet Index: *Directory* entries are alphabetically listed according to category and are accompanied by the primary topic and the URL. To quickly obtain a URL, simply search the **spreadsheet** category or primary topic.

Primary Topic	URL	Page
Aging		
Aging bibliographic and database reference system	http://www.ageinfo.org/bibinfo.html	1
Alcohol and aging	http://www.drug.indiana.edu/pubs/alerts/alert2.html	2

Keyword Index: Allows the reader to locate the specific entry page by searching with a keyword.

Selection Criteria for *Directory* Entries

Entry Selection Criteria

The *Directory of Internet Sources for Health Professionals* presents a comprehensive selection essential for medical and health practitioners. Preselection entry criteria initially qualified Web sites according to the information needs of potential *Directory* users. The final selected entries adhered to the following criteria:

- **Sponsors** cover a range of government, institutions, professional associations, health organizations and facilities (national and international), publishers, and private sector groups or individuals by providing *free* Internet Web data. Official government sites normally include "gov" as part of the URL.
- **Site content** features a global data diversity related to clinical diagnosis and treatment, information management, medical education, consumerism, research, legislation, news, bulletins, conference reports, employment, and future trends, to name a few.
- **Data type** highlights variable formats of text, reports, databases, software, textbooks, audiovisuals, movies, images, and multimedia.
- **Final deselection of thousands of noteworthy medical sites** was not easy. Placement of radiography, genetics, and several other categories under the

Medical Specialties category reflects primarily an arrangement based on editorial focus. The final entry selections are those with maximum advantage to the larger group of *Directory* audience of health researchers, allied health professionals, physicians, and other potential users.

Power Boosters for Power Medical Data Searches

- **Bury hokey-pokey modems—with dignity!** Until the arrival of 128 baud modems, the slower 2600 baud modems served well. Persistent use of these modems, however, dooms users to an infinitely slower process of data retrieval, frequently a difference of up to one hour. Forget images, photographs, or multimedia with slower modems. Before investing in faster modems or any computer hardware accessories, check with a reliable computer dealer.
- **Evaporating data.** Internet data exist in a state of flux with frequent site updates, changes, and inevitable appearances and disappearances. Publication, news, and some government sites are updated daily or monthly. Sponsors sometimes include an archive bin to store past data sites.
- **Disappearing URLs.** Change of sponsors, obsolete sites or data—all explain the mystery of disappearing URLs. Before despairing, recheck the accuracy of the URL. Return to the sponsor's homepage for additional information. Many sites include a note with a direct link to the new URL.
- **Copyright statements.** Unless classified or restricted, Internet government data exist as public domain property permitting unrestricted reproduction, dissemination, and other uses without prior permission. Copyright statements by other organizations may indicate restrictions of reproduction or dissemination of text, images, or multimedia by requiring prior written permission. Read carefully the sponsor's copyright statement as a guide for data utility.
- **Guarding your personal secrets.** Similar to other electronic transfers, transmitting or revealing personal data such as software passwords, credit card numbers, or your Social Security number are Internet taboo. Because the *Directory* entries primarily exclude promotion or advertisement sites, requests for name or e-mail address presumably facilitate sponsors forwarding updates or other pertinent correspondence to users.
- **Organize searches**. Except for speed, organizing Internet searches varies very little from old-fashioned, manual card catalog searches. Outlining relevant topics, subtopics, prospective sources, along with keywords, remain top priority items for Internet searches. If searching for cardiovascular diseases, "cardiology" as a search term retrieves hundreds of unrelated sites of suppliers, hospitals, organizations, and personal homepages. Specify "cardiovascular diseases" (perhaps a specific disease) and retrieve more relevant sites for cardiovascular research.

The *Directory of Internet Sources for Health Professionals* is an essential source for medical professionals to quickly access Internet medical and health data.

Aging

Aging bibliographic and database reference system

http://www.ageinfo.org/bibinfo.html

Sponsor ➢	National Aging Information Center (NAIC), Administration on Aging, U.S. Department of Health and Human Services (DHHS)
Description ➢	Bibliographic database for policy and program materials for providers, researchers; eldercare locator database
Data type ➢	Text; search enabled
Access requirements ➢	Open
Supplemental resources ➢	*Resource Directory for Older People* **(http://www.aoa.dhhs.gov/aoa/dir/toc.html)** Eldercare locator for search of elderly service organizations **(http://www.ageinfo.org/elderloc/elderdb.html)**
User tips ➢	Zip code search available for eldercare locator
Keywords ➢	eldercare

Alcohol and aging

http://www.drug.indiana.edu/pubs/alerts/alert2.html

Sponsor ➢	Indiana Prevention Resource Center and National Institute of Alcohol Abuse
Description ➢	Alcohol alert: alcohol abuse among the elderly
Data type ➢	Text
Access requirements ➢	Open
Supplemental resources ➢	Sixty-five plus in the United States **(http://www.census.gov/ftp/pub/socdemo/www/agebrief.html)** U.S. Senate, Special Committee on Aging **(http://www.senate.gov/~aging/jurisdic.htm)**
User tips ➢	Check U.S. Senate, Special Committee, fraud hotline
Keywords ➢	elderly, substance abuse elderly, fraud

Alzheimer's Disease Education and Referral (ADEAR) Center

http://www.cais.com/adear/

Sponsor ➢	National Institute on Aging (NIA), U.S. Department of Health and Human Services (DHHS)
Description ➢	Alzheimer database, publications, and referral data
Data type ➢	Text
Access requirements ➢	Open
Supplemental resources ➢	Alzheimer research studies **(http://www.cais.com/adear/nianews.html)** Information for health professionals **(http://www.nih.gov/nia/health/health.htm)**
User tips ➢	See NIA research news
Keywords ➢	geriatrics Alzheimer's disease

Alzheimer's disease
http://med-amsa.bu.edu/Alzheimer/home.html

Sponsor ➢	Boston University Alzheimer's Disease Center
Description ➢	Research and online information for professionals and consumers
Data type ➢	Text
Access requirements ➢	Open
Supplemental resources ➢	Alzheimer's Disease Online Learning Center **(http://med-amsa.bu.edu/Alzheimer/alzlearn.htm)** Worksheet for making the home safe **(http://med-amsa.bu.edu/Alzheimer/safehome.htm)**
User tips ➢	Check bin for caregivers
Keywords ➢	Alzheimer's disease

Alzheimer's disease Web sites for lay persons
http://www.alzforum.org/public/layperson_sites.html

Sponsor ➢	Alzheimer Research Forum
Description ➢	List of Web sites, videotapes, and materials describing Alzheimer research, organizations, and transcripts
Data type ➢	Text
Access requirements ➢	Open; for families and caregivers
Supplemental resources ➢	The Alzheimer page **(http://www.biostat.wustl.edu/alzheimer/)** The dementia web **(http://dementia.ion.ucl.ac.uk/)**
User tips ➢	Domestic and international sources cited
Keywords ➢	Alzheimer's disease dementia

Clearinghouse on Abuse and Neglect of the Elderly (CANE)

http://interinc.com/NCEA/main.html

Sponsor ➢	National Center on Elder Abuse (NCEA)
Description ➢	Clearinghouse for research and literature on elder abuse
Data type ➢	Text
Access requirements ➢	Open
Supplemental resources ➢	Types of elder abuse **(http://www.interinc.com/NCEA/Elder_Abuse/main.html)**
User tips ➢	CANE responds to public inquiries
Keywords ➢	elder abuse

Elder abuse diagnosis and services

http://www.ianet.org/nyeac/

Sponsor ➢	New York Elder Abuse Coalition
Description ➢	Resources, services for elder abuse diagnosis and assistance
Data type ➢	Text
Access requirements ➢	Open
Supplemental resources ➢	Elder abuse definitions, signs, and symptom **(http://www.ianet.org/nyeac/ea_signs.htm)** National Institutes of Health Consensus Report on depression in the elderly **(http://text.nlm.nih.gov/nih/cdc/www/86text.htm)**
User tips ➢	Find out what's happening in the legislative area
Keywords ➢	elder abuse depression, elderly

European Alzheimer Projects

http://www.alzheimer-europe.org/

Sponsor ➢	European Commission and Pfizer Pharmaceutical Group
Description ➢	Alzheimer project descriptions and information
Data type ➢	Text for professionals
Access requirements ➢	Open
Supplemental resources ➢	Dementia, Alzheimer's disease **(http://www.alzheimer-europe.org/frrbot01.html)** Early onset dementia and Alzheimer's disease **(http://www.alzheimer-europe.org/young.html)**
User tips ➢	See site index for additional topics
Keywords ➢	Alzheimer's disease dementia, early onset

Geriatric topics

http://www.mayo.edu/geriatrics-rst/2.GeriPage.html

Sponsor ➢	Mayo Clinic Rochester
Description ➢	Geriatric topics in long-term and home health care
Data type ➢	Text
Access requirements ➢	Open
Supplemental resources ➢	Dementia: Management of behavior problems **(http://www.mayo.edu/geriatrics-rst/Behav.html)** Research on long-term care, AHCPR **(http://www.ahcpr.gov/research/longtrm1.htm)**
User tips ➢	Hit bin for geriatrics pearls
Keywords ➢	dementia elderly behavior

International comparisons of care for aging
http://aspe.os.dhhs.gov/daltcp/home/internat.htm#INDICATORS

Sponsor ➢ Office of Disability, Aging, and Long-Term Care Policy (DALTCP)

Description ➢ Overview and comparative international data on aging

Data type ➢ Text

Access requirements ➢ Open

Supplemental resources ➢ DALTCP homepage
(http://aspe.os.dhhs.gov/daltcp/home.htm)
Nursing home care in five nations
(http://aspe.os.dhhs.gov/daltcp/intrnatl/nh5nates.htm)

User tips ➢ See reports of children and working age adults with disabilities

Keywords ➢ international nursing home care
long term care

Nursing home costs, hospital admissions, and hospice use
http://www.elder-law.com/elder/1996/issue344.html

Sponsor ➢ Elder Law Information

Description ➢ Statistics regarding eldercare costs

Data type ➢ Newsletter

Access requirements ➢ Open

Supplemental resources ➢ Quitclaim to children
(http://www.elder-law.com/elder/1996/issue349.html)
Nursing home selection considerations
(http://nursinghomeinfo.com/needs.html)

User tips ➢ Check Elder Law index for additional topics

Keywords ➢ nursing home costs
quitclaim to children

Services for seniors over age 50

http://www.aarp.org/

Sponsor ➢ American Association of Retired Persons (AARP)

Description ➢ Services and news for persons over age 50

Data type ➢ Text; photos

Access requirements ➢ Sites open; AARP membership restricted by age

Supplemental resources ➢ Living healthy
(http://www.aarp.org/health/home.html)
Keeping Social Security solvent
(http://www.aarp.org/focus/ssecure/part_2/solvent.htm)

User tips ➢ Check insurance and pharmaceutical services

Keywords ➢ employment, elderly
insurance

Services for the elderly

http://www.ncoa.org/

Sponsor ➢ National Council on the Aging (NCOA), U.S. Department of Health and Human Services (DHHS)

Description ➢ Health, social, and economic news for the elderly

Data type ➢ Text

Access requirements ➢ Open

Supplemental resources ➢ Independent living grants for organizations
(http://www.ncoa.org/sp_projs/inn_ind_living.htm#eligibility)
Employment of elderly workers
(http://www.ncoa.org/memonly/naowes/Default.htm)

User tips ➢ See tips for re-entering the workforce

Keywords ➢ elderly employment

Skilled nursing facilities under Medicare

http://www.hcfa.gov/medicare/snfs.htm

Sponsor ➢	Health Care Financing Administration (HCFA), U.S. Department of Health and Human Services (DHHS)
Description ➢	Definition, eligibility, standards, and services for skilled nursing facilities under Medicare
Data type ➢	Text
Access requirements ➢	Open
Supplemental resources ➢	Medigap insurance: Alternatives for Medicare beneficiaries **(http://geronet.ph.ucla.edu/GAO/medigap.txt)** U.S. General Accounting Office (GAO) publications on elderly health, long-term care **(http://geronet.ph.ucla.edu/GAO/gao.htm)**
User tips ➢	See FAQs page
Keywords ➢	Medicare skilled nursing facilities

Task force report: Long-term care reform in the States, July 1997

http://www.ncsl.org/ihpp/ltc/report.htm

Sponsor ➢ National Conference of State Legislatures

Description ➢ Report of long-term care problems; solutions; lessons learned

Data type ➢ Text

Access requirements ➢ Open

Supplemental resources ➢ Intergovernmental Health Policy Project **(http://www.ncsl.org/ihpp/index.htm)**
Long-term care: Issues and future directions [U.S. Government Accounting Office (GAO) report] **(http://linear.chsra.wisc.edu/chsra/dur/ltc.htm)**

User tips ➢ See forum net and index of audiotapes

Keywords ➢ nursing home care
long term care

III European Congress of Gerontology

http://www.nig.nl/congres/3rdeuropeancongress1995/ttp-abs.html

Sponsor ➢ Netherlands Institute of Gerontology (NIG)

Description ➢ Electronic book of conference abstracts

Data type ➢ Data for professionals

Access requirements ➢ Open

Supplemental resources ➢ How to find an abstract **(http://www.nig.nl/congres/3rdeuropeancongress1995/area.html)**
Oral diseases in the elderly **(http://www.nig.nl/congres/3rdeuropeancongress1995/abstract/077-0820.html)**

User tips ➢ See index of keynote lectures

Keywords ➢ oral diseases
gerontology

Women and aging

http://www.brandeis.edu/heller/national/index.html

Sponsor >	National Policy and Resource Center on Women and Aging
Description >	Research and online information for professionals and consumers
Data type >	Text
Access requirements >	Open
Supplemental resources >	Transcripts on Alzheimer's disease at Journal Graphics Home **(http://www.tv-radio.com/~kelsy/topics/alzheime.htm)** The Alzheimer's Association **(http://www.alz.org)**
User tips >	Check the National Institute on Aging for list of all Alzheimer's disease centers
Keywords >	geriatrics Alzheimer's disease

Allied Health

Accreditation of allied health programs for athletic training
http://www.cewl.com/cewl/jrc-at/jrcfaq.html

Sponsor ➢	Joint Review Committee—Athletic Training (JRC-AT)
Description ➢	Accreditation procedures related to athletic training
Data type ➢	Text
Access requirements ➢	Open
Supplemental resources ➢	Guide to careers for women in sports, fitness, and health **(http://www.melpomene.org/career.htm)** Joint Commission on Accreditation of Healthcare Organizations (JCAHO) and National Committee for Quality Assurance (NCQA) at a glance **(http://www.okqchomehealth.com/indepth/glance.htm)**
User tips ➢	See JRC-AT online forms for program completion certificates
Keywords ➢	athletic training accreditation

Allied health professions registration in Massachusetts

http://www.magnet.state.ma.us/reg/ah.htm

Sponsor ➢ Commonwealth of Massachusetts, Division of Registration

Description ➢ Registration qualifications for allied health professionals in Massachusetts

Data type ➢ Text

Access requirements ➢ Open

Supplemental resources ➢ Allied mental health and human services registration, MA **(http://www.magnet.state.ma.us/reg/mh.htm)**

User tips ➢ Check licensure or registration for individual states

Keywords ➢ allied health licensure

Allied health resources

http://www.delmaralliedhealth.com

Sponsor ➢ Delmar Publishers

Description ➢ Information on health care assisting resources, network opportunities, and teaching materials

Data type ➢ Variable

Access requirements ➢ Open

Supplemental resources ➢ Delmar directory of health and other publications **(http://www.delmar.com/delmar.html)**
Thomson Publishing homepage **(http://www.thomson.com)**

User tips ➢ See list of Thomson publishers specializing in health references

Keywords ➢ allied health

Allied health resources—genetic counselors

http://www.kumc.edu/GEC/prof/nsgc.html

Sponsor ➢ National Society of Genetic Counselors

Description ➢ Information on genetic counselor resources

Data type ➢ Variable

Access requirements ➢ Open

Supplemental resources ➢ Genetic testing benefits **(http://www.hospital-news.com/hosnew14.htm#1)**

User tips ➢ Genetic testing available for free or low cost at academic research centers

Keywords ➢ allied health
genetic testing

Allied health travel grants

http://www.aaaai.org/profinfo/membserv/allied/abstrav/abstravl.html

Sponsor ➢ American Academy of Allergy, Asthma and Immunology (AAAAI) Allied Health Professionals Committee

Description ➢ Application procedure for requesting travel grants

Data type ➢ Text

Access requirements ➢ Open

Supplemental resources ➢ Use of resources in allergy office **(http://www.aaaai.org/profinfo/membserv/allied/articles/resource.html)**
Asthma and Allergy Foundation of America, "the power," asthma management **(http://www.aafa.org/pbnews.html)**

User tips ➢ Abstract travel requests limited to members

Keywords ➢ allied health
asthma

Evaluation of health professions schools
http://futurehealth.ucsf.edu/ccph/exsumm.html#IV_FIND

Sponsor ➢ The Center for the Health Professions, University of California, San Francisco

Description ➢ Evaluation report—1996–1997

Data type ➢ Report

Access requirements ➢ Open

Supplemental resources ➢ The Center for the Health Professions homepage **(http://futurehealth.ucsf.edu/home.html)**
Summary of written response to report on the future of health care workforce regulation
(http://futurehealth.ucsf.edu/home.html)

User tips ➢ Review homepage for Pew Scholars Program in the biomedical sciences

Keywords ➢ health professions schools

Health care assisting resources
http://www.delmaralliedhealth.com/hca/index.html

Sponsor ➢ Delmar Publishers

Description ➢ Health care assisting training videos, books, and other resources for home health aides, medical assisting, and others

Data type ➢ Text

Access requirements ➢ Open

Supplemental resources ➢ Allied health discussion forums
(http://www.delmaralliedhealth.com/members/forums/index.html)
Health information management, Allied Health Forum
(http://forum.thomson.com/visible/h...se/topics/docNumber/increasing/d/0)

User tips ➢ Join the forums

Keywords ➢ health care assisting
allied health forums

Home health services reimbursement, Ohio

http://aopha.org/pphhr.htm

Sponsor ➢ Association of Ohio Philanthropic Home Administration (AOPHA)

Description ➢ AOPHA position paper

Data type ➢ Text

Access requirements ➢ Open

Supplemental resources ➢ Proposed background checks for home health agency employees
(http://www.aoa.dhhs.gov/pr/homehealthregs.html)
Association of Schools of Allied Health Professions
(http://www.hsc.missouri.edu/shrp/asahp/index.html)

User tips ➢ See AOPHA chart of home health payments by state

Keywords ➢ home health reimbursement
home health aides

Magnetic resonance technologist training

http://www.t2star.com/smrt/curr_guide.html

Sponsor ➢ International Society for Magnetic Resonance in Medicine (ISMRM)

Description ➢ Sample curriculum for MRI technologist training

Data type ➢ Text

Access requirements ➢ Open

Supplemental resources ➢ ISMRM homepage
(http://www.ismrm.org/)

User tips ➢ See homepage for MR-related links

Keywords ➢ magnetic resonance technologists

Medical assistants certification and licensure

http://www.aama-ntl.org/ed/certlic.html

Sponsor ➢ American Association of Medical Assistants (AAMA)

Description ➢ Medical assistant certification and licensure facts

Data type ➢ Text

Access requirements ➢ Open

Supplemental resources ➢ AAMA homepage
(http://www.aama-ntl.org/)
AAMA reference and study aids for certification examination
(http://www.aama-ntl.org/ed/refstudy.html)

User tips ➢ See bin for related occupations

Keywords ➢ medical assistant certification

Medical technologists

http://www.amt1.com/mt.html

Sponsor ➢ American Medical Technologists (AMT)

Description ➢ AMT certification of medical technologists, phlebotomy technicians, office laboratory technicians

Data type ➢ Text

Access requirements ➢ Open

Supplemental resources ➢ Brochure on medical technologist requirements
(http://www.amt1.com/mt.html)
Medical sonography, ultrasound technologists
(http://www.ardms.org/frmain.htm)

User tips ➢ See homepage for AMT annual meeting

Keywords ➢ medical technologists
sonographers

Medical transcription careers

http://www.aamt.org/aamt/carfaq.htm

Sponsor ➢	American Association for Medical Transcription (AAMT)
Description ➢	Questions and answers about medical transcription careers
Data type ➢	Text
Access requirements ➢	Open
Supplemental resources ➢	AAMT homepage **(http://www.aamt.org/aamt/)** Evaluating medical transcription advertising **(http://www.aamt.org/aamt/student.htm)**
User tips ➢	See AAMT training recommendations for medical transcription
Keywords ➢	medical transcription

National Health Care Skill Standards Project (NHCSSP)

http://www.fwl.org/nhcssp/health.htm

Sponsor ➢	Far West Laboratory for Educational Research and Development and Southwest Regional Laboratory
Description ➢	Collaborative project of health, industry, labor, and educational organizations to develop skill standards for health care workers
Data type ➢	Text
Access requirements ➢	Open
Supplemental resources ➢	How NHCSSP works **(http://www.fwl.org/nhcssp/nhcss0a.htm)**
User tips ➢	Check skills standards homepage
Keywords ➢	allied health skills

Ophthalmic medical assisting
http://www.jcahpo.com/index.html#top

Sponsor ➢	Joint Commission on Allied Health Personnel in Ophthalmology (JCAHPO)
Description ➢	Ophthalmic medical assisting certification
Data type ➢	Text
Access requirements ➢	Open
Supplemental resources ➢	What is JCAHPO? **(http://www.jcahpo.com/index.html#top)** Tutorial: Examination and management of the injured eye **(http://www.cewl.com/cewl/cewlol/articles/20001.html)**
User tips ➢	Check JCAHPO homepage for continuing education (CE) program listing
Keywords ➢	ophthalmic medical assisting medical education

Physician assistants (PAs) and emergency medicine
http://www.aapa.org/gandp/emerg.htm

Sponsor ➢	American Academy of Physician Assistants (AAPA)
Description ➢	Report on practice credentials; hospital issues; cost effectiveness of PAs in emergency medicine
Data type ➢	Report
Access requirements ➢	Open
Supplemental resources ➢	AAPA homepage **(http://www.aapa.org/)** Society of Emergency Medicine physician assistants national homepage **(http://www.sempa.org/)**
User tips ➢	See link for employment opportunities
Keywords ➢	physician assistants

Profiles of allied health top industry employers
http://www.healthopps.com/healthopps/health3.html

Sponsor ➢	Health Opps
Description ➢	Profiles of hospitals, private sector, and other top health care employers
Data type ➢	Text; graphics
Access requirements ➢	Open
Supplemental resources ➢	Links to U.S. *Bureau of Labor Statistics Occupational Outlook Handbook* **(http://www.healthopps.com/healthopps/health18.html)**
User tips ➢	Browse employer profiles before initiating allied health job search
Keywords ➢	allied health employment

Psychiatric technicians
http://www.aapt.com/whatis.htm

Sponsor ➢	American Association of Psychiatric Technicians, Inc. (AAPT)
Description ➢	What is a psychiatric technician?
Data type ➢	Text
Access requirements ➢	Open
Supplemental resources ➢	AAPT homepage **(http://www.aapt.com/index.html)**
User tips ➢	Check for updated site after renovation
Keywords ➢	psychiatric technician

Radiologic technologists
http://www.asrt.org/

Sponsor ➢ American Society of Radiologic Technologists (ASRT)

Description ➢ Continuing education, home study, and references for radiologic technicians

Data type ➢ Text

Access requirements ➢ Open

Supplemental resources ➢ Homepage for Joint Review Committee on Education in Radiologic Technology (JRCERT) **(http://hudson.idt.net/~jrcert/main.html)**

User tips ➢ See ASRT site for home study references

Keywords ➢ radiologic technologist

Rural physicians and physician assistants education loan repayment program
http://hlunix.hl.state.ut.us/primary_care/elrp.html

Sponsor ➢ Bureau of Primary Care and Rural Health Systems, Utah Department of Health

Description ➢ Education loan repayment program for qualified physicians and physician assistants

Data type ➢ Text

Access requirements ➢ Open

Supplemental resources ➢ News, physician assistant **(http://www4.usnews.com/usnews/edu/beyond/bcchot8.htm)**
Allied health scholarship programs, Health Resources and Services Administration (HRSA) **(http://www.hrsa.dhhs.gov/bhpr/dsa/allschol.HTM)**

User tips ➢ Program restricted to State of Utah rural, licensed physicians and physician assistants

Keywords ➢ rural health
educational funding

Standards for hair removal
http://www.isdt.org/p19.htm

Sponsor ➢ International Society of Dermal Therapists

Description ➢ Permanent hair removal standards for practice operations

Data type ➢ Text

Access requirements ➢ Open

Supplemental resources ➢ Dermal therapists homepage **(http://www.isdt.org/)**
Photodynamic therapy **(http://www.isdt.org/p54.htm)**

User tips ➢ See homepage for data about unwanted hair and its removal

Keywords ➢ hair removal
dermal therapists

Vision 2006
http://www.ahima.org/vision/vision.overview.html

Sponsor ➢ American Health Information Management Association (AHIMA)

Description ➢ AHIMA's planning strategy for future health information management professions

Data type ➢ Text

Access requirements ➢ Open

Supplemental resources ➢ AHIMA homepage **(http://www.ahima.org/)**
Cinahl database access through AHIMA **(http://www.ahima.org/library/online.access.html)**

User tips ➢ Cinahl is a subscription online database

Keywords ➢ health information management

Alternative Medicine

Adverse events of some Chinese herbal medicines
http://www.Acupuncture.com/Herbology/Toxic.htm

Sponsor ➢	Acupuncture.com
Description ➢	Review of English language literature of adverse events involving Chinese herbs
Data type ➢	Article; some graphics
Access requirements ➢	Open
Supplemental resources ➢	Acupuncture treatment for substance abuse **(http://www.Acupuncture.com/Acup/Addict.htm)** List of acupuncture insurers **(http://www.Acupuncture.com/News/Insuranc.htm)**
User tips ➢	See homepage for acupuncture statistical results
Keywords ➢	substance abuse acupuncture

Alternative medical courses at U.S. medical schools

http://cpmcnet.columbia.edu/dept/rosenthal/guide.html

Sponsor ➢ The Rosenthal Center for Complementary and Alternative Medicine

Description ➢ U.S. medical schools with alternative medical studies

Data type ➢ Text

Access requirements ➢ Open

Supplemental resources ➢ Center homepage **(http://cpmcnet.columbia.edu/dept/rosenthal/AM_Information.html)**

User tips ➢ See Rosenthal Center homepage for legal and regulatory information

Keywords ➢ medicine education, alternative
legal medicine

Alternative medicine bibliography

http://www.pitt.edu/~cbw/refe.html

Sponsor ➢ Charles B. Wessel, University of Pittsburgh

Description ➢ Bibliography of studies on use of alternative therapies

Data type ➢ Text

Access requirements ➢ Open

Supplemental resources ➢ The Alternative Medicine Homepage **(http://www.pitt.edu/~cbw/altm.html)**
Research on plant and marine products for cancer treatment **(http://oncolink.upenn.edu/pda_html/6/engl/600733.html)**

User tips ➢ Check homepage for definition of alternative medicine on homepage

Keywords ➢ alternative medicine
marine medicine

American Indian ethnobotany database

http://www.umd.umich.edu/cgi-bin/herb/

Sponsor ➢ University of Michigan–Dearborn

Description ➢ Search enabled database of foods, drugs, dyes, fibers, and plant uses by Native North American peoples

Data type ➢ Text for professionals

Access requirements ➢ Open

Supplemental resources ➢ American Indian ethnobotany **(http://www.umd.umich.edu/resources/...t2/besci/anthro/about_ethnobot.html)**

User tips ➢ See homepage for search instructions

Keywords ➢ botanical medicine

Environmental links to breast cancer

http://www.wri.org/health/slidntro.htm

Sponsor ➢ World Resource Institute

Description ➢ Slide show of environmental impact on cancer and reproductive diseases in humans, fish, and other animals

Data type ➢ Text; slides

Access requirements ➢ Open

Supplemental resources ➢ World Resources Institute homepage **(http://www.wri.org/)**
Marine medicinal products research **(http://epnws1.ncifcrf.gov:2345/dis3d/natprod/marine.html)**

User tips ➢ See Institute homepage for trends and indicators

Keywords ➢ aquatic medicinals
environmental health

Ethnobotany

http://www.gene.com/ae/RC/Ethnobotany/index.html

Sponsor ➢ Resource Center

Description ➢ Ethnobotany; classification of plants; South American medicines

Data type ➢ Text

Access requirements ➢ Open

Supplemental resources ➢ Introduction to ethnobotany **(http://www.gene.com/ae/RC/Ethnobotany/page2.html)**
Medicines that changed the world **(http://www.gene.com/ae/RC/Ethnobotany/page4.html)**

User tips ➢ Check Central and South American articles regarding medicines, foods, and tubers

Keywords ➢ ethnobotany

Garlic and pregnancy

http://www.mistral.co.uk/garlic/preg.htm

Sponsor ➢ The Garlic Information Centre

Description ➢ Garlic benefits for pregnancy complications

Data type ➢ Brief summaries; graphics

Access requirements ➢ Open

Supplemental resources ➢ Garlic Centre homepage **(http://www.mistral.co.uk/garlic/index.htm)**
Garlic and impotence **(http://www.mistral.co.uk/garlic/impotenc.htm)**

User tips ➢ See bin for garlic and cholesterol

Keywords ➢ nutrition
reproductive health

Herbage ethnobotanical monographs
http://www.herbweb.com/pix/A.htm

Sponsor ➢ Tim Johnson

Description ➢ Herbage database

Data type ➢ Text and graphics

Access requirements ➢ Open

Supplemental resources ➢ Herbal remedies: acne and its causes **(http://www.herbal-remedies.com/ailments/acne.html)**

User tips ➢ Check monographs for benefits of common plants such as carrots and many other vegetables

Keywords ➢ botanical medicine
dermatology

Homeopathy: Natural medicine for the 21st century
http://www.homeopathic.org/index1.htm

Sponsor ➢ National Center for Homeopathy

Description ➢ Homeopathy resources and training

Data type ➢ Text

Access requirements ➢ Open

Supplemental resources ➢ What is homeopathy? **(http://www.homeopathic.org/whishome.htm)**

User tips ➢ Searchable 1997 National Center for Homeopathy directory

Keywords ➢ homeopathy
natural medicine

Medical acupuncture
http://www.med.auth.gr/~karanik/english/main.htm

Sponsor ➢	International Council of Medical Acupuncture and Related Techniques (ICMART)
Description ➢	Web page of medical acupuncture basics, journals, and resources
Data type ➢	Text; search enabled
Access requirements ➢	Open
Supplemental resources ➢	Bibliography, acupuncture in ulcerative conditions **(http://www.med.auth.gr/~karanik/english/articles/ulcercon.html)** Bibliographies in acupuncture, National Library of Medicine (NLM) **(http://wwwindex.nlm.nih.gov/pubs/cbm/acupuncture.html)**
User tips ➢	ICMART acupuncture page also available in Greek; check bin for veterinary acupuncture
Keywords ➢	acupuncture

Medicinal and poisonous plant databases
http://www.inform.umd.edu/EdRes/Col..._biology/Medicinals/medicinals.html

Sponsor ➢	Michael C. Tims
Description ➢	Plant databases describing biology, folklore, historical use, and recent experiments
Data type ➢	Text; photos; search enabled
Access requirements ➢	Open
Supplemental resources ➢	Mistletoe folklore and present uses **(http://www.inform.umd.edu/EdRes/Col...t_biology/Medicinals/mistletoe.html)**
User tips ➢	Check bin for mistletoe research
Keywords ➢	botanicals poisonous plants

Medicinal biological researchers

http://walden.mo.net/~tonytork/resindex.html

Sponsor ➢ Anthony R. Torkelson, Ph.D.

Description ➢ Index of medicinal biological researchers including contact numbers

Data type ➢ Text

Access requirements ➢ Open

Supplemental resources ➢ Ethnomedicinals homepage for botany and pharmacy links **(http://walden.mo.net/~tonytork/)**

User tips ➢ Check link for medicinal plants

Keywords ➢ pharmaceutical medicine
ethnomedicinals

Medicines from the sea

http://www.columbuscenter.org/~judy/scitalk/

Sponsor ➢ Columbus Center for Marine Biotechnology

Description ➢ Report and references on medicines from the sea

Data type ➢ Text

Access requirements ➢ Open

Supplemental resources ➢ Chinese medicines and sea horses **(http://www.sddt.com/files/librarywi...7_96/DN96_07_30/DN96_07_30_1ay.html)**

User tips ➢ Glossary included

Keywords ➢ aquatic medicine

Office of Alternative Medicine (OAM) Clearinghouse

http://altmed.od.nih.gov/oam/clearinghouse/#access

Sponsor ➢	Office of Alternative Medicine (OAM), National Institutes of Health
Description ➢	Provides information regarding OAM's programs and research in complementary and alternative medicine
Data type ➢	Text; resource materials
Access requirements ➢	Open
Supplemental resources ➢	National Institutes of Health (NIH) homepage **(http://www.nih.gov/)**
User tips ➢	Clearinghouse services are free; limited numbers of copies can be requested; toll free telephone: 1-888-644-6226
Keywords ➢	alternative medicine complementary medicine

Phytochemical and ethnobotanical databases

(http://www.ars-grin.gov/~ngrisb/)

Sponsor ➢	Agriculture Research Service (ARS), U.S. Department of Agriculture (USDA)
Description ➢	Query page for ethnobotanical uses for specific plants
Data type ➢	Text
Access requirements ➢	Open
Supplemental resources ➢	Cyberbotanica: Plants and cancer treatments **(http://biotech.chem.indiana.edu/botany/)**
User tips ➢	Cyberbotanica provides free online educational resources on plants and cancer treatments
Keywords ➢	botanical medicines ethnobotany

Practitioner Reference Guide
http://www.europa.com/~itm/pract.htm

Sponsor ➢	Institute for Traditional Medicine (ITM) Online
Description ➢	Chinese medicine in the United States
Data type ➢	Text
Access requirements ➢	Open
Supplemental resources ➢	Homepage **(http://www.europa.com/~itm/index.html)**
User tips ➢	Separate bins for practitioners and patients
Keywords ➢	herbal medicine

Resources for herbalists
http://www.ronan.net/%7Ermhi/a/g.favoritwebs.html

Sponsor ➢	Rocky Mountain Herbal Institute
Description ➢	Chinese herbology online directory of sources for herbology education, databases, and discussion groups
Data type ➢	Hyperlinked directory
Access requirements ➢	Open; direct access for most sites
Supplemental resources ➢	The herb, spice, and medicinal plant digest; back copies online **(http://www.ronan.net/%7Ermhi/a/g.favoritwebs.html)**
User tips ➢	Good sources; some are inaccessible
Keywords ➢	herbal medicine

Cancer

Bone Marrow Transplants—A Book of Basics for Patients

http://www.oncolink.upenn.edu/specialty/chemo/bmt/bmt_1.html#chapter_1

Sponsor ➢	OncoLink, University of Pennsylvania Cancer Center
Description ➢	Chapter 1: Nuts and bolts of bone marrow transplant
Data type ➢	Online reference
Access requirements ➢	Open
Supplemental resources ➢	*Blood & Marrow Transplant Newsletter* **(http://www.bmtnews.org/)** Attorney referral form for assistance with insurance denials of transplants **(http://www.bmtnews.org/attorney.html)**
User tips ➢	See homepage for newsletter archives
Keywords ➢	transplants, blood marrow

Bone marrow transplant for multiple myeloma
http://www.oncolink.upenn.edu/classroom/bmtmm/intro.html

Sponsor ➢	OncoLink, University of Pennsylvania Cancer Center
Description ➢	Audio lecture on the role of bone marrow transplant in treatment of multiple myeloma
Data type ➢	Audio
Access requirements ➢	Requires RealAudio player
Supplemental resources ➢	Statistics for stem cell transplant at Children's Memorial Hospital **(http://www.childmmc.edu/cmhweb/cmhdepts/hemoncweb/stemcellweb/stats.html)**
User tips ➢	Download RealAudio player **(http://www.oncolink.upenn.edu/classroom/bmtmm/intro.html)**
Keywords ➢	bone marrow transplant stem cell transplant

Breast Cancer Information Clearinghouse
http://nysernet.org/bcic/

Sponsor ➢	NYSERNet, Inc.
Description ➢	Provides list of organizations for e-mail medical advice and online support discussions; breast cancer information and support data
Data type ➢	Text
Access requirements ➢	Open
Supplemental resources ➢	National Institutes of Health (NIH) release, high bone mass associated with breast cancer risk **(http://www.nih.gov/niams/news/bmdbreastca.htm)**
User tips ➢	E-mail for National Alliance of Breast Cancer Organizations **(NABCOinfo@aol.com)**
Keywords ➢	breast cancer women's health

Cancer research and programs

http://www.cancer.org/main.html

Sponsor ➢ American Cancer Society (ACS)

Description ➢ Summaries of research projects

Data type ➢ Text; search enabled

Access requirements ➢ Open

Supplemental resources ➢ Great American Smokeout commit to quit plan **(http://www.cancer.org/gasp/contract.html)**
American Association for Cancer Research (AACR) **(http://www.aacr.org/)**

User tips ➢ Browse bins for patient and consumer data

Keywords ➢ respiratory health
substance abuse

CCG Protocol: D9602 for low-risk rhabdomyosarcoma

http:www.nccf.org/nccf/protocol/d9602.htm

Sponsor ➢ National Childhood Cancer Foundation (NCCF)

Description ➢ Protocol hypothesis and eligibility criteria

Data type ➢ Text

Access requirements ➢ PDF protocol text files accessible to users with account and password

Supplemental resources ➢ NCCF homepage **(http://www.nccf.org/index.htm)**
Children's Cancer Group (CCG) clinical trial protocols and institutions, NCCF homepage **(http://www.nccf.org/index.htm)**

User tips ➢ Contact number: 1-800-458-6223

Keywords ➢ childhood cancer
clinical trial

Clinical trials information for physicians

http://cancer.med.upenn.edu/pdq_html/3/engl/303901.html

Sponsor ➢ OncoLink, University of Pennsylvania

Description ➢ NCI/PDQ description of trials (adjuvant and neoadjuvant), supportive care, prevention/early detection, and treatment referral trials

Data type ➢ Data for physicians and health care providers

Access requirements ➢ Open

Supplemental resources ➢ National Cancer Institute (NCI) physician referral form **(http://wwwicic.nci.nih.gov/proto/refform.html)**

User tips ➢ Consumer information service number for patients: 1-800-422-6237

Keywords ➢ clinical trials

Clinical trials information, National Cancer Institute (NCI)

http://cancer.med.upenn.edu/clinical_trials/

Sponsor ➢ OncoLink, University of Pennsylvania

Description ➢ NCI Cooperative Cancer Research Groups

Data type ➢ Data for patients and health care providers

Access requirements ➢ Open

Supplemental resources ➢ Gynecologic oncology group (GOG/CHTN) ovarian tissue bank **(http://www.oncolink.upenn.edu/spec...n_onc/ovarian/gog_tissue_bank.html)**
Cancer Cooperative Research groups **(http://www.oncolink.upenn.edu/resources/coop_groups/)**

User tips ➢ Providers, check NCI online referral provided by International Cancer Information Center, NCI

Keywords ➢ clinical trials
cancer, ovarian

Ethnic-oriented cancer information

http://cancernet.nci.nih.gov/ethnic/ethnic_health.htm

Sponsor ➢ CancerNet, National Cancer Institute (NCI), National Institutes of Health (NIH)

Description ➢ Peer reviewed cancer data for African Americans, Asians, Hispanics, and other groups

Data type ➢ Variable

Access requirements ➢ Open; for health practitioners, patients, and consumers

Supplemental resources ➢ CancerNet files for patients; professionals; basic researchers
(http://cancernet.nci.nih.gov/)

User tips ➢ Available in Spanish

Keywords ➢ cancer information
ethnic health

Gastrointestinal cancers

http://www.oncolink.com/disease/gastro1/

Sponsor ➢ OncoLink, University of Pennsylvania Cancer Center

Description ➢ Consumer data describing anal, colon, esophageal, liver, and other cancers

Data type ➢ Text; some graphics

Access requirements ➢ Open

Supplemental resources ➢ Cancerlit topic searches, gastrointestinal cancers
(http://cancernet.nic.nih.gov/clinpdq/canlit/gastro.html)
Additional consumer information on cancer causes, support
(http://www.oncolink.com/)

User tips ➢ Check homepage for automatic subscription to the Stomach-Onc support group

Keywords ➢ gastrointestinal cancers

Health professionals—global resources

http://cancernet.nci.nih.gov/global/glo_hp.htm

Sponsor ➢ Cancernet, National Cancer Institute (NCI), National Institutes of Health (NIH)

Description ➢ Web cancer sites, NCI-designated cancer federal agencies, and other facilities

Data type ➢ Variable

Access requirements ➢ Open

Supplemental resources ➢ Cancernet, NCI homepage
(http://cancernet.nci.nih.gov/)
Cancerlit topic searches
(http://cancernet.nci.nih.gov/canlit/canlit.htm)

User tips ➢ Loads of patient information

Keywords ➢ cancer resources

International bone marrow transplant registry

http://www.social.com/health/nhic/data/hr1400/hr1495.html

Sponsor ➢ International Bone Marrow Transplant Registry (IBMTR)

Description ➢ Statistical source for collection, organization, and dissemination of registry data

Data type ➢ Registry

Access requirements ➢ Open

Supplemental resources ➢ Bone marrow transplantation and peripheral blood stem cell publication, National Cancer Institute (NCI)
(http://cancernet.nci.nih.gov/clinpd...od_Stem_Cell_Transplantation.html#1)
National Program of Cancer Registries, CDC
(http://www.cdc.gov/nccdphp/dcpc/npcr/)

User tips ➢ Bone marrow registry does not maintain roster of potential donors

Keywords ➢ bone marrow transplants
cancer registry

Leukemia information
http://www.meds.com/leukemia/leukemia.html

Sponsor ➢ Leukemia Information Center

Description ➢ Professional information describing acute myeloid leukemia (AML)

Data type ➢ Variable

Access requirements ➢ Open

Supplemental resources ➢ Information libraries for colon and lung cancers **(http://www.meds.com/)**

User tips ➢ Patient data include adult AML, cancer screening, radiotherapy, and other topics

Keywords ➢ acute myeloid leukemia (AML)
cancer libraries

National Action Plan on Breast Cancer (NAPBC)
http://www.napbc.org/

Sponsor ➢ National Action Plan on Breast Cancer (NAPBC)

Description ➢ Clinical trials and other data related to breast cancer

Data type ➢ Variable

Access requirements ➢ Open

Supplemental resources ➢ See hot topics bin
Gateway to resources
(http://www.napbc.org/)

User tips ➢ Available in Spanish

Keywords ➢ breast cancer
clinical trial

NCI/PDQ treatment and prevention statements

http://www.oncolink.upenn.edu/pdq_html/

Sponsor ➢ OncoLink, University of Pennsylvania Cancer Center

Description ➢ PDQ treatment summaries and news for health professionals and patients as related to treatment, prevention, and investigations of newly approved drugs

Data type ➢ Text for health professionals and researchers

Access requirements ➢ Open

Supplemental resources ➢ PDQ statements for surgery for renal cell carcinoma: Single center experience with 100 patients
(http://oncolink.upenn.edu/pdq_html/cites/03/03386.html)
OncoLink homepage
(http://www.oncolink.upenn.edu/index.html)

User tips ➢ Available in Spanish; PDQ search tools available through Grateful Med and other servers

Keywords ➢ cancer treatment, prevention

Nonsteroidal antiandrogens in treatment of advanced prostate cancer

http://www.comed.com/Prostate/advanced/antiandrogens.html

Sponsor ➢ CoMed Communications Internet Health Forum (CCIHF)

Description ➢ Report, treatment of advanced prostate disease

Data type ➢ Text

Access requirements ➢ Open

Supplemental resources ➢ CCIHF homepage **(http://comed.com/index.spml)**
Internet Grateful Med **(http://igm.nlm.nih.gov/)**

User tips ➢ Grateful Med maintains several databases of cancer information

Keywords ➢ prostate cancer
nonsteroidal antiandrogens

Online medical dictionary—cancer

http://www.graylab.ac.uk/omd/index.html

Sponsor ➢ CancerWeb

Description ➢ Search enabled medical dictionary

Data type ➢ Dictionary

Access requirements ➢ Open

Supplemental resources ➢ Oncology trainee forum in the United Kingdom, with curriculum **(http://www.graylab.ac.uk/cancerweb/trainees.html)**
Curriculum for specialist training in medical oncology **(http://www.graylab.ac.uk/cancerweb/trainees/doc/curric.html)**

User tips ➢ Check structured training discussion developed by United Kingdom Royal Colleges

Keywords ➢ oncology training
medical education

Oral cancer

http://www.oralcancer.org/

Sponsor ➢ Oral Cancer Information Center, Oral Health Education Foundation, Inc.

Description ➢ Oral cancer resources

Data type ➢ Text

Access requirements ➢ Open

Supplemental resources ➢ Support for people with oral, head, and neck cancer **(http://www.spohnc.org)**
American Society for Clinical Oncology (ASCO) **(http://www.asco.org/)**

User tips ➢ Browse bins for additional information

Keywords ➢ oral cancer
otolaryngology

START oncology reference

http://www.oncoweb.com/

Sponsor ➢ OncoWeb, European School of Oncology, and Greenwich Medical Online

Description ➢ Full text oncology reference describing pathology, diagnosis, staging, prognosis, and other aspects of cancer

Data type ➢ Online reference for oncologists and medical professionals

Access requirements ➢ Open; downloadable and search enabled by chapter or subtopic; registration preferred

Supplemental resources ➢ START chapter index **(http://www.oncoweb.com/START/extra.htm)**
Osteosarcoma chapter **(http://www.oncoweb.com/START/chapt-08/chapt-08.htm)**

User tips ➢ Site under construction; chapters on human tumors available

Keywords ➢ cancer
osteosarcoma

Supercomputers in medical diagnosis

http://www.tc.cornell.edu/er96/ff03summer/ff04lungs.html

Sponsor ➢ Cornell Theory Center, Cornell University Medical College

Description ➢ Report, computer assistance in diagnosing lung cancer

Data type ➢ Text

Access requirements ➢ Open

Supplemental resources ➢ *Forefronts*, Cornell Theory Center publications **(http://www.tc.cornell.edu/er96/ff03summer/index.html)**

User tips ➢ See Cornell University site for other medical studies

Keywords ➢ medical computers
lung cancer

Surveillance, epidemiology, and end results (SEER)

http://www-seer.ims.nci.nih.gov/

Sponsor ➢ National Cancer Institute (NCI), National Institutes of Health (NIH)

Description ➢ Online database of cancer incidence and survival data from cancer registries

Data type ➢ Database of registries; publications; scientific systems

Access requirements ➢ Open; hyperlinked site for medical researchers

Supplemental resources ➢ U.S. population data, 1973–1994 **(http://www-seer.ims.nci.nih.gov/Data/index.html)**
Population data for SEER registries, 1973–1994 **(http://www-seer.ims.nci.nih.gov/Data/index.html)**

User tips ➢ See SEER map of the United States

Keywords ➢ cancer morbidity
demographics

Telematics for health professionals
http://telescan.nki.nl/action/action.htm

Sponsor ➢ Netherlands Cancer Institute

Description ➢ European Internet service for cancer research, treatment, and education

Data type ➢ Multimedia

Access requirements ➢ For health practitioners; links available for patients and consumers

Supplemental resources ➢ Telescan multimedia telematics
(http://telescan.nki.nl/multimedia.html)
Newsletter for the Prompt project of computer decision systems for cancer care in general practice, hospitals, and shared care
(http://telescan.nki.nl/action/issue1d.htm)

User tips ➢ Available in major European languages

Keywords ➢ telescan
telematics

Tumor Board
http://www.tumorboard.com/

Sponsor ➢ Tumor Board

Description ➢ Source of copyright-free digital cancer pathology images

Data type ➢ Images; case of the month

Access requirements ➢ Open

Supplemental resources ➢ Case of the month
(http://www.tumorboard.com/case_of_the_month/com0897.htm)
Tumor image library
(http://www.tumorboard.com/)

User tips ➢ Contributions of user images encouraged

Keywords ➢ cancer pathology

Cardiovascular Medicine

Cardiac rehabilitation and prevention information
http://www.jhbmc.jhu.edu/cardiology/rehab/profinfo.html

Sponsor ➢	Johns Hopkins Bayview Medical Center
Description ➢	Patient care topics including cardiac rehabilitation guidelines; unstable angina; heart failure exercise
Data type ➢	Text for professionals
Access requirements ➢	Open
Supplemental resources ➢	Cardiac rehabilitation, consumer's guide **(http://text.nlm.nih.gov/ftrs/tocview)** Hypertension causes, risk factors (for patients) **(http://familyinternet.com/mhc/scr/000468sc.htm#Definition:)**
User tips ➢	See Hopkins homepage links for professional conferences and seminars
Keywords ➢	rehabilitation, cardiac healthy heart

Cardiologists resources

http://139.137.56.94:8080/HOT_HART/Heart.htm

Sponsor ➢ Cleveland Clinic Heart Center

Description ➢ Sites on cardiovascular surgery, EP and pacing, transplants, pediatric, and general cardiology

Data type ➢ Text; images

Access requirements ➢ Open

Supplemental resources ➢ Clinical information, American College of Cardiology (ACC)
(http://www.acc.org/clinical/index.html)
Cardiology Compass
(http://osler.wustl.edu/~murphy/cardiology/compass.html)

User tips ➢ See ACC national cardiovascular data registry

Keywords ➢ cardiology resources
medical education

Cardiovascular information

http://www.nhlbi.nih.gov/nhlbi/cardio/cardio.htm

Sponsor ➢ National Heart, Lung, and Blood Institute (NHLBI), National Institutes of Health (NIH)

Description ➢ Sites describing high blood pressure, cholesterol, obesity, heart attack, sleep disorders, and lung information

Data type ➢ Variable, for professionals and consumers

Access requirements ➢ Open

Supplemental resources ➢ Transfusion alert for use of red blood cells, platelets, and frozen plasma, NIH
(http://www.nhlbi.nih.gov/nhlbi/blood/transf/prof/transfin.htm)
Blood information: sickle cell; blood transfusion safety
(http://www.nhlbi.nih.gov/nhlbi/blood/blood.htm)

User tips ➢ Check NHLBI homepage for complete site index

Keywords ➢ blood transfusion safety
cardiovascular disease

Congestive heart failure
http://web.bu.edu/COHIS/cardvasc/heart/chf.htm

Sponsor ➢ Community Outreach Health Information System (COHIS), Boston University Medical Center

Description ➢ Cardiovascular diseases and problems associated with heart, blood, and vessels

Data type ➢ Text; tables; images

Access requirements ➢ Open; hyperlinked

Supplemental resources ➢ COHIS homepage **(http://web.bu.edu/COHIS/cardvasc/cvd.htm)**
Sudden cardiac death **(http://web.bu.edu:80/COHIS/cardvasc/heart/scd.htm#getbetter)**

User tips ➢ See COHIS homepage for three-dimensional medical models

Keywords ➢ congestive heart failure
sudden cardiac death

Coronary artery examination
http://www.afip.mil/homes/cardio/grosub_4.htm

Sponsor ➢ Department of Cardiovascular Pathology, Armed Forces Institute of Pathology (AFIP)

Description ➢ Method, caveats, and other details for artery examination

Data type ➢ Text for cardiologists

Access requirements ➢ Open

Supplemental resources ➢ General guidelines for gross heart submission **(http://www.afip.mil/homes/cardio/cv1.htm)**
Hypertension information for patients **(http://www.genovese.com/health/heart.htm)**

User tips ➢ See link for AFIP interesting cases

Keywords ➢ coronary artery examination
cardiology

Coronary Club Heartline
http://www.heartline-news.org/

Sponsor ➢ Cleveland Clinic Foundation

Description ➢ Data for patients on heart disease, treatment, family, and lifestyle issues

Data type ➢ Text

Access requirements ➢ Open; consumers and professionals

Supplemental resources ➢ Heartline index of newspaper articles
(http://www.heartline-news.org/HL03/03.htm)
Coronary Club
(http://www.heartline-news.org/)

User tips ➢ See homepage for other heart links

Keywords ➢ heart disease, children
healthy heart

Electrocardiographic rhythms
http://www.med-edu.com/patient/arrhythmia/rhythms-5.html#S_ARREST

Sponsor ➢ Internet Medical Education, Inc.

Description ➢ Latest edition of *Marriott's Practical Electrocardiography*, covering parasystole, sinus tachycardia, arrhythmia, and other topics

Data type ➢ Text

Access requirements ➢ Open

Supplemental resources ➢ Medical Education homepage
(http://www.med-edu.com/patient/arrhythmia/rhythms.html)
Subject reviews in cardiovascular diseases
(http://www.med-edu.com/patient/)

User tips ➢ Click the Internet's nursing index

Keywords ➢ electrocardiographic rhythms
cardiovascular diseases

Facts about heart/lung transplants

gopher://fido.nhlbi.nih.gov:70/00/educprog/other/gppubs/hrtlung.txt

Sponsor ➢ National Heart, Blood, Lung Institute (NHBLI), National Institutes of Health (NIH)

Description ➢ Discussion of heart/lung transplantation background, availability, barriers, and surgery

Data type ➢ Text

Access requirements ➢ Open

Supplemental resources ➢ NHBLI new technology **(http://www.nhbli.nih.gov/nhlbi/ttrans/hot.htm)**
TransWeb, transplantation and donation information site **(http://139.137.56.94:8080/HOT_HART/transplt/transplt.htm)**

User tips ➢ Check United Network for Organ Sharing (UNOS) site for additional information

Keywords ➢ transplants

Heart attack survival calculator

http://www.mediqual.com/library/amicalc/heart.htm

Sponsor ➢ MediQual Systems, Inc.

Description ➢ Calculation of survival probability for heart attack patients

Data type ➢ Text; tables

Access requirements ➢ Open; hyperlinked text

Supplemental resources ➢ Best outcomes benchmarks **(http://www.mediqual.com/library/benchmk/index.htm)**
Benchmarks for severely ill patients, chronic lung disease **(http://www.medqual.com/library/benchmk/topics/ppx/4tran2.htm)**

User tips ➢ See homepage for article on what's a benchmark

Keywords ➢ outcomes benchmark
chronic illness

The human heart

http://www.sln.fi.edu/biosci/

Sponsor ➢ Franklin Institute Science Museum

Description ➢ Online exploration of heart development and structure accompanied by resource materials and glossary

Data type ➢ Text; images

Access requirements ➢ Open

Supplemental resources ➢ Heart exploration table of contents **(http://sln.fi.edu/biosci/TOC.biosci.html)**

User tips ➢ Check links for interesting data

Keywords ➢ cardiology

Hypertension in African-Americans

http://www.wramc.amedd.army.mil/de...rology/lectures.nathxhtn/index.htm

Sponsor ➢ Walter Reed Army Medical Center (WRAMC) Nephrology Service

Description ➢ Report and cases describing hypertension in African-Americans; also related end organ disease, mortality, and stroke treatment

Data type ➢ Text; images

Access requirements ➢ Open

Supplemental resources ➢ Nephrology movies series **(http://www.wramc.amedd.army.mil/de...edicine/nephro/movies/movindex.htm)**
Nephrology Service homepage **(http://www.wramc.amedd.army.mil/de...icine/nephro/nephrology/index.htm!)**

User tips ➢ See homepage for end stage renal disease clinic

Keywords ➢ hypertension
nephrology

Inherited long QT syndrome

http://www.sads.org/overview.html

Sponsor ➢ Sudden Arrhythmia Death Syndromes (SADS) Foundation

Description ➢ Information regarding SADS, QT interval drugs, and research

Data type ➢ Text; patients and professionals

Access requirements ➢ Open

Supplemental resources ➢ Drugs to avoid with long QT syndrome **(http://www.sads.org/DRUGS.HTML)**
SADS homepage **(http://www.sads.org/)**

User tips ➢ Chinese and Spanish editions in progress

Keywords ➢ sudden arrhythmia death syndrome (SADS)
cardiology

Institutional resources for congenital heart defects

http://www.ohsu.edu/cliniweb/C14/C14.240.400.html

Sponsor ➢ CliniWeb, Oregon Health Sciences University

Description ➢ Hypertext links of resources for Ebstein's anomaly, heart septal defects, levocardia, and other defects

Data type ➢ Text

Access requirements ➢ Open

Supplemental resources ➢ Clinical trials: Heart disease, according to state **(http://www.centerwatch.com/studies/CAT213.HTM)**

User tips ➢ See links for universities involved in cardiology research

Keywords ➢ congenital heart defects
clinical trials, heart disease

Introduction to expert computer systems in medicine
http://wailer.uokhsc.edu/acc95-expert-systems.html

Sponsor ➢ University of Oklahoma Health Sciences Center

Description ➢ Definition, utility, and other data regarding expert systems

Data type ➢ Data for professionals

Access requirements ➢ Open

Supplemental resources ➢ Recruitment for online ECG interpretation study **(http://wailer.uokhsc.edu/ECGstudy/htdocs/index.html)**
Cardiovascular site index **(http://wailer.uokhsc.edu/ourindex.html)**

User tips ➢ See index page for new user's guide

Keywords ➢ medical computers

Medical/scientific statements
http://www.americanheart.org/pubs/scipub/statements/

Sponsor ➢ American Heart Association (AHA)

Description ➢ Monthly statements, 1995–1997 including mouth-to-mouth ventilation by bystanders; imaging in transient ischemic attacks; pediatric Utstein style

Data type ➢ Text

Access requirements ➢ Open; search statements available by year and month

Supplemental resources ➢ Reappraisal of mouth-to-mouth ventilation during cardiopulmonary resuscitation, September 1997 **(http://www.americanheart.org/pubs/scipub/statements/)**
Patient links for heart and stroke, A–Z guide **(http://www.amhrt.org/Heart_and_Stroke_A_Z_Guide/index.html)**

User tips ➢ See NHLBI report on public screening for measuring blood cholesterol, September 1995

Keywords ➢ cardiopulmonary resuscitation
cholesterol screening

Regulations regarding physician supervision of diagnostic tests
http://www.acc.org/healthpol/supervision.html

Sponsor ➢ American College of Cardiology (ACC)

Description ➢ Health Care Financing Administration (HCFA) health policy of new definitions for Medicare payments for diagnostic tests, effective January 1, 1998

Data type ➢ Text

Access requirements ➢ Open

Supplemental resources ➢ ACC homepage
(http://www.acc.org/)
1998 Medicare fee schedule for cardiovascular specialty services
(http://www.acc.org/healthpol/1998_fee.html)

User tips ➢ See homepage for additional bins

Keywords ➢ cardiovascular service fees
Medicare payments

Standards for adult nuclear cardiology training
http://www.ccs.ca/consensus/standards/norm5/

Sponsor ➢ Canadian Cardiovascular Society (CCS)

Description ➢ Standards for adult nuclear cardiovascular training

Data type ➢ Text for medical students and professionals

Access requirements ➢ Open

Supplemental resources ➢ CCS homepage
(http://www.ccs.ca/home/main.html)
Management of postmyocardial infarction patient
(http://www.ccs.ca/consensus/reports/management/)

User tips ➢ Available in French

Keywords ➢ postmyocardial infarction
cardiology training

"White coat" hypertension in black female population
http://www.cityscape.co.uk/users/ad88/med/whitecol.htm

Sponsor ➢ General Practice On-Line (peer-reviewed medical journal)

Description ➢ Abstract of study on prevalence of white coat hypertension in black females

Data type ➢ Text

Access requirements ➢ Open

Supplemental resources ➢ *International Journal of General Practice and Primary Care* homepage **(http://www.cityscape.co.uk/users/ad88/gp.htm)**
Second Australian National Blood Pressure Study (ANBP2) **(http://www.health.adelaide.edu.au/ANBP2/index.htm)**

User tips ➢ Journal article submissions are encouraged

Keywords ➢ white coat hypertension

Dental Health

ADA Dental Newsline

http://www.ada.org/consumer/radio/radio.html

Sponsor ➢	American Dental Association (ADA)
Description ➢	60-Second radio broadcasts of dental news including dental x-rays, infection control and dentures
Data type ➢	AVI slideshows with graphics and audio messages
Access requirements ➢	Download slideshows
Supplemental resources ➢	ADA Online homepage **(http://www.ada.org/)**
User tips ➢	Check ADA library
Keywords ➢	dental health dental x-rays

Computer applications in dental training
http://cpmcnet.columbia.edu/dept/de...cs/AOFC_Course/AOFC_Objectives.html

Sponsor ➢ Columbia University
Description ➢ Curriculum for computer applications in dentistry
Data type ➢ Curriculum outline
Access requirements ➢ Open
Supplemental resources ➢ Dental informatics syllabus
(http://cpmcnet.columbia.edu/dept/de...s/AOFC_Course/AOFC_DI_Syllabus.html)
User tips ➢ Check basic computer literacy section
Keywords ➢ molars
medical computers

Computer based learning materials in dentistry
http://www.derweb.ac.uk/tm1.html

Sponsor ➢ University of Sheffield
Description ➢ Demonstration utilizing computer based learning materials for professionals
Data type ➢ Multimedia; case studies; images
Access requirements ➢ Open
Supplemental resources ➢ DERWeb homepage
(http://www.derweb.ac.uk/)
DERWeb Image Library
(http://www.derweb.ac.uk/)
User tips ➢ Check page on odontogenic tumors
Keywords ➢ dental tutorial

Curriculum guidelines for oral biology
http://www2.musc.edu/AAOB/GradOBCurr.html

Sponsor ➢ American Association of Oral Biologists (AAOB)

Description ➢ Guidelines for development of graduate oral biology studies

Data type ➢ Text

Access requirements ➢ Open

Supplemental resources ➢ AAOB homepage **(http://www2.musc.edu/AAOB/AAOB.html)**
Archives of oral biology **(http://www2.musc.edu/AAOB/AAOB.html)**

User tips ➢ Check links to other WWW dental sites

Keywords ➢ oral biology

Dental hygienist
http://www.adha.org/homepage.htm

Sponsor ➢ American Dental Hygienists' Association (ADHA)

Description ➢ Dental hygienist career information

Data type ➢ Text; images

Access requirements ➢ Open

Supplemental resources ➢ Public health dental hygiene **(http://www.adha.org/carinfo/publiche.htm)**
Dental terminology **(http://www.qualitydentistry.com/dental/terms.html)**

User tips ➢ Audio message available from ADHA president

Keywords ➢ dental hygienists

Dental legislation testimony

http://www.aads.jhu.edu/kennedy.htm

Sponsor ➢ American Association of Dental Schools (AADS)

Description ➢ AADS testimony before the Senate Committee about health professions reauthorization

Data type ➢ Text; professional use

Access requirements ➢ Open

Supplemental resources ➢ AADS legislative activities **(http://www.aads.jhu.edu/dga.html)**
AADS homepage **(http://www.aads.jhu.edu/)**

User tips ➢ Check news updates

Keywords ➢ dental legislation

Dental scholarships

http://www.colgate.com/Pro/continuing_education/scholarships.html

Sponsor ➢ Colgate-Palmolive Company

Description ➢ Scholarships and fellowships in dentistry

Data type ➢ Text

Access requirements ➢ Open

Supplemental resources ➢ Professional world of studies, practice management **(http://www.colgate.com/Pro/main.html)**

User tips ➢ Order education materials designed for young patients

Keywords ➢ educational funding

Dental Telecommunication Network (DenTelNet)
http://biz.onramp.net/Den-Tel-Net/

Sponsor ➢ Dr. Carl Stewart

Description ➢ *DenTelNet Dental News*, monthly dental specialty news pertaining to oral surgery, endodontics, pathology, and other areas

Data type ➢ Text; archives of past issues

Access requirements ➢ Open

Supplemental resources ➢ Periodontal diseases **(http://biz.onramp.net/Den-Tel-Net/Den-Tel-Net/dtn95/perio997.html)**
DenTelNet Dental News, 1994–1997 **(http://biz.onramp.net/Den-Tel-Net/)**

User tips ➢ Includes dental and medical search through Medscape

Keywords ➢ dental health
periodontal diseases

Dental Trauma Server
http://www.unige.ch/smd/orthotr.html

Sponsor ➢ University of Geneva School of Dentistry

Description ➢ Maxillofacial and dental trauma injuries

Data type ➢ Images and instructions for professionals

Access requirements ➢ Open

Supplemental resources ➢ Intrusions **(http://www.unige.ch/smd/ortintr.html)**

User tips ➢ Check what's new feature

Keywords ➢ dental trauma

Dentistry resources
http://www.pitt.edu/~cbw/dental.html

Sponsor ➢	Falk Library of the Health Sciences, University of Pittsburgh
Description ➢	Comprehensive source of dentistry Web sites
Data type ➢	Menu of direct access Web sites
Access requirements ➢	Open
Supplemental resources ➢	MedWeb Dentistry: Endodontics (megasite) **(http://www.gen.emory.edu/medweb/medweb.dentistry.html)** Medical, dental, and military and federal health links **(http://www.dencom.army.mil/interest/medden.html#milmed)**
User tips ➢	Check Falk site for links to WWW sites and Gophers for dental schools
Keywords ➢	dental resources

Detecting oral cancer
http://www.tambcd.edu/oralexam/nidroc00.htm

Sponsor ➢	National Institute of Dental Research (NIDR), National Institutes of Health (NIH), and Baylor College of Dentistry
Description ➢	Tutorial diagnostic guide for dentists
Data type ➢	Images and tutorials
Access requirements ➢	Open
Supplemental resources ➢	Perioral, soft tissue examination **(http://www.tambcd.edu/oralexam/exam02.htm)**
User tips ➢	Poster materials of Web site content available
Keywords ➢	oral diagnosis tutorial soft tissue exam

Endodontic, resident case reports

http://www.tambcd.edu/endo/index.html

Sponsor ➢	Baylor College of Dentistry
Description ➢	Resident case reports of dental therapeutics
Data type ➢	Images and instructional materials
Access requirements ➢	Open
Supplemental resources ➢	Resident case reports; non-surgical root-canal treatment **(http://www.tambcd.edu/endo/Treatment/rct_con_1.html)**
User tips ➢	Images best viewed in 16-bit or greater
Keywords ➢	dental procedures root canal

Financial aid for dental students

http://www.dencom.army.mil/recruit.dir/index.html

Sponsor ➢	U.S. Army Dental Corps
Description ➢	Scholarships and financial assistance for dentistry, oral surgery, and other health professions
Data type ➢	Text
Access requirements ➢	Open
Supplemental resources ➢	Advanced education in dentistry **(http://www.dencom.army.mil/recruit.dir/gdr.html)**
User tips ➢	Check link for joining the U.S. Army Dental Corps
Keywords ➢	education funding

Job report for dental assistants

http://www.exchangenet.com/howto/career/R0381.html

Sponsor ➢ American Dental Assistants Association (ADAA)

Description ➢ Report describing responsibilities, working conditions, and other aspects of a dental assistant career

Data type ➢ Text

Access requirements ➢ Open

Supplemental resources ➢ ADAA homepage
(http://home.fuse.net/kspradlin/feloinfo.htm)
Publications, directories, and other resources for dental assistants
(http://www.dentalsite.com/assistants/index.html)

User tips ➢ See homepage for ADAA membership application

Keywords ➢ dental assistant

National Oral Health Information Clearinghouse (NOHIC)

http://www.aerie.com/nohicweb/ohmap.html

Sponsor ➢ National Institute of Dental Research (NIDR), NIH

Description ➢ Bibliographic database of oral health for persons with genetic or systemic disorders

Data type ➢ Text; slides for professionals and consumers

Access requirements ➢ Open

Supplemental resources ➢ NIDR homepage
(http://www.nidr.nih.gov/)
Slides for health professionals, "Detecting Oral Cancer"
(http://www.aerie.com/nohicweb/ohmap.html)

User tips ➢ Check guide to oral health research at NIDR

Keywords ➢ dental health
dental diseases

Oral health booklets

http://blake.oit.unc.edu/health/english/booklets/index.html

Sponsor ➢ Cedros Network

Description ➢ Booklets on Brazilian oral health, water fluoridation, AIDS

Data type ➢ Downloadable booklets

Access requirements ➢ Open

Supplemental resources ➢ Cedros homepage **(http://blake.oit.unc.edu:80/health/english/)**
Portuguese page **(http://blake.oit.unc.edu/health/portugues/booklets/caderno2.html)**

User tips ➢ Check DOLAC, Latin American Dental Directory

Keywords ➢ oral health

Pediatric dentistry

http://www.flash.net/~dkennel/index.htm

Sponsor ➢ A Linus McAllster Memorial Web Page, Pediatric Dentistry "just for kidds"

Description ➢ Pediatric dentistry topics including baby bottle tooth decay, natal and neonatal teeth, permanent molars, and other areas

Data type ➢ Images and text

Access requirements ➢ Open

Supplemental resources ➢ Ectopic eruption of first permanent molars **(http://www.flash.net/~dkennel/ectopic.htm)**

User tips ➢ Check bin for baby bottle tooth decay

Keywords ➢ pediatric dentistry
permanent molars

Systemic antibiotic therapy in oral surgery

http://www.odont.ku.dk/antibiotics/main.html

Sponsor ➢ Anders Nattestad, DDS, PhD, University of Copenhagen, Denmark

Description ➢ Risks, indicators, and other factors associated with antibiotic therapy in oral surgery

Data type ➢ Text; diagrams; images

Access requirements ➢ Open

Supplemental resources ➢ Diagram, antibiotic drug interactions **(http://www.odont.ku.dk/antibiotics/interactions.jpg)**
Endocarditis infection prevention guidelines by the American Heart Association **(http://plsgroup.com/dg/2c3be.htm)**

User tips ➢ Check bin for dental risk patients

Keywords ➢ dental surgery
antibiotics

Tempomandibular tutorial

http://www.rad.washington.edu/Anatomy/TMJ/TMJISMAP.html

Sponsor ➢ University of Washington Department of Radiology

Description ➢ Temporomandibular joints (TMJ) anatomy, arthrography, computer tomography, MRI tutorial for professionals

Data type ➢ Movies

Access requirements ➢ Open

Supplemental resources ➢ TMJ MR **(http://www.rad.washington.edu/Anatomy/TMJ/TMJMR.html)**

User tips ➢ Select a section of the TMJ tutorial

Keywords ➢ dental health
tempomandibular tutorial

Training for oral and maxillofacial surgeons
http://www.aaoms.org/resreach.html

Sponsor ➢ American Association of Oral and Maxillofacial Surgery (AAOMS)

Description ➢ Description of oral and maxillofacial surgeon training programs

Data type ➢ Text; images

Access requirements ➢ Open

Supplemental resources ➢ Bibliography of completed projects by the Commission, FDI World Dental Federation, 1995–1998 **(http://www.worldserver.pipex.com/worldental/commiss/complete.htm)**
FDI homepage **(http://www.worldserver.pipex.com/worldental/main.htm)**

User tips ➢ Check AAOMS homepage for international volunteer opportunities for oral and maxillofacial surgeons

Keywords ➢ volunteer opportunities, dental medical education

Dermatology

Annual report, 1996: Pressure sore prevention and other topics
http://www.raft.ac.uk/reports/96ar05.htm

Sponsor ➢	Restoration of Appearance and Function Trust (RAFT)
Description ➢	Annual report describing innovations of appearance restoration
Data type ➢	Text
Access requirements ➢	Open
Supplemental resources ➢	RAFT homepage **(http://www.raft.ac.uk/reports/reports.htm)**
User tips ➢	See reports on tissue repair; skin cancer; vascular surgery
Keywords ➢	dermatologic procedures pressure sore prevention

Botulinum toxin wrinkle treatment

http://medweb.nus.sg/nsc/commskin/botox.html

Sponsor ➢ National Skin Centre (NSC), Singapore

Description ➢ Article, botulinum toxin treatment for wrinkles

Data type ➢ Text

Access requirements ➢ Open

Supplemental resources ➢ National Skin Centre homepage
(http://medweb.nus.sg/nsc/nsc.html)
Research projects at the National Skin Centre from 1993–1995
(http://medweb.nus.sg/nsc/iodsres.html)

User tips ➢ See abstracts of 1995 research at NSC

Keywords ➢ botulinum
wrinkle treatment

Cutaneous drug reaction database

gopher://gopher.Dartmouth.EDU.70/00/Research/BioSci/CDRD/README

Sponsor ➢ Jerome Z. Litt, M.D.

Description ➢ Drug reaction database

Data type ➢ Text

Access requirements ➢ Open

Supplemental resources ➢ Acetazolamide
(gopher://gopher.Darmouth.EDU:70/00/Research/BioSci/CDRD/A/ACETAZOLAMIDE)

User tips ➢ Annual updates available

Keywords ➢ pharmacology
cutaneous drug reactions

Dermatology and other medical journals

http://www.webmedlit.com/

Sponsor ➢ Silver Platter Information, Inc. and Physicians' Home Page

Description ➢ Tracks twenty-three professional medical journals

Data type ➢ Text

Access requirements ➢ Open

Supplemental resources ➢ Past issues of *Archives of Dermatology* **(http://www.ama-assn.org/public/journals/derm/dermhome.htm)**
Seborrheic keratoses **(http://www.ama-assn.org/sci-pubs/jo...hive/derm/vol_133/no_11/dst7029a.htm)**

User tips ➢ Journals updated monthly

Keywords ➢ dermatology publications

Dermatology Online Atlas (DOIA) Erlangen

http://www.derma.med.uni-erlangen.de/bilddb/diagnose/englisch/dg_c.htm

Sponsor ➢ Friedrich-Alexander-University of Erlangen-Nurnberg, School of Medicine

Description ➢ Alphabetized atlas of dermatologic conditions with code and images

Data type ➢ Images and text

Access requirements ➢ Open

Supplemental resources ➢ DermIS, Dermatology Internet Service homepage **(http://www.derma.med.uni-erlangen.de/index_e.htm)**
Systemic pathology: lecture and laboratory, Indiana University **(http://www.pathology.iupui.edu/drhood.html)**

User tips ➢ DOIA available in English and German

Keywords ➢ dermatology pathology

Derminfo-Net
http://www.derm-infonet.com/

Sponsor ➢	American Academy of Dermatology
Description ➢	Current news on treatment and management of disorders of the skin, hair, and nails
Data type ➢	Text and photos
Access requirements ➢	Open; for patients and health professionals
Supplemental resources ➢	American Academy of Dermatology homepage **(http://www.aad.org/)** Mature skin: Wrinkles **(http://tray.dermatology.uiowa.edu/PIPS/MatureSkin.html#Wrinkles Be Avoided)**
User tips ➢	Check treatments for aging skin
Keywords ➢	wrinkles

DermPath Tutor: Tutorial in diagnosis
http://tray.dermatology.uiowa.edu/DPT/DPTutor.htm

Sponsor ➢	University of Iowa College of Medicine
Description ➢	Tutorial in dermatologic pathology
Data type ➢	Multimedia
Access requirements ➢	Open
Supplemental resources ➢	Clinical skin disease images **(http://tray.dermatology.uiowa.edu/home.html)** Instructions for using DermPath tutor **(http://tray.dermatology.uiowa.edu/DPT/DPTutor.htm)**
User tips ➢	Check learning modules for continuous education
Keywords ➢	dermatologic tutorial medical education

FDA hearing on autologous cells

http://www.fda.gov/search97cgi/vtop...ResultStart%3D1%26ResultCount%3D25&

Sponsor ➢ U.S. Food and Drug Administration (FDA)

Description ➢ Report of FDA public hearing, 1995

Data type ➢ Text

Access requirements ➢ Open

Supplemental resources ➢ *Dermatology Online Journal* **(http://matrix.ucdavis.edu/DOJvol1num1/journal.html)**
Hair transplantation complications, *Dermatology Times* **(http://www.modernmedicine.com/derm/cs2884.html)**

User tips ➢ Check archive for past articles

Keywords ➢ hair transplantation

Ichthyosis references

http://www.libertynet.org/~ichthyos/referenc.htm#107

Sponsor ➢ Foundation for Ichthyosis and Related Skin Types (FIRST)

Description ➢ Bibliography of ichthyosis data

Data type ➢ Text

Access requirements ➢ Open

Supplemental resources ➢ FIRST homepage **(http://www.libertynet.org/~ichthyos/index.html)**
Bibliography for ichthyosis and related skin diseases **(http://www.libertynet.org/~ichthyos/ichinfo.htm)**

User tips ➢ Check FIRST homepage for links to related sites

Keywords ➢ skin disorders
ichthyosis

National Arthritis and Musculoskeletal and Skin Diseases Information Clearinghouse (NAMSDIC)
http://chid.nih.gov/subfile/contribs/ar.html

Sponsor ➢ Combined Health Information Database (CHID)

Description ➢ Professional, consumer resources for arthritis and musculoskeletal and skin diseases, 1978–present

Data type ➢ Text

Access requirements ➢ Open

Supplemental resources ➢ Enrollment data for National Registry for Ichthyosis and Related Disorders **(http://weber.u.washington.edu/~geoff/ichthyosis.registry/)**

User tips ➢ AMS thesaurus available: toll-free number for Registry (1-800-595-1265)

Keywords ➢ skin disorders
ichthyosis

Patient education on popular treatments
http://www.asds-net.org/poptreatments.html#Overview of Popular Treatments

Sponsor ➢ American Society for Dermatologic Surgery

Description ➢ Overview of treatments; namely, dermatologic procedures, chemical peeling, dermabrasion

Data type ➢ Text and photos

Access requirements ➢ Open

Supplemental resources ➢ American Society for Dermatologic Surgery homepage
(http://www.asds-net.org/index.html)
Skin cancer fact sheet
(http://www.asds-net.org/scfactsheet.html)

User tips ➢ Check bin for additional dermatologic surgery data

Keywords ➢ dermatologic surgery
skin cancer

Plastic surgery information service
http://www.plasticsurgery.org/

Sponsor ➢	American Society of Plastic and Reconstructive Surgeons (ASPR) and Plastic Surgery Educational Foundation (PSEF)
Description ➢	Professional information on third party payers; consumer information about plastic surgery
Data type ➢	Text and graphics
Access requirements ➢	Open
Supplemental resources ➢	How to choose a qualified plastic surgeon **(http://www.plasticsurgery.org/surgery/chooseps.htm)** Fifteen ranking cosmetic procedures, *U.S. News* **(http://www.usenews.com/usnews/issue/14clip.htm)**
User tips ➢	Hit homepage bin for plastic surgery history
Keywords ➢	dermatologic procedures plastic surgery

Psoriasis drug alert
http://www.psoriasis.org/pressrel/skin-cap.html

Sponsor ➢	National Psoriasis Foundation (NPF)
Description ➢	Release: Over-the-counter (OTC) psoriasis drug potentially harmful
Data type ➢	Text
Access requirements ➢	Open
Supplemental resources ➢	NPF homepage **(http://www.psoriasis.org/index.shtml)**
User tips ➢	Site search available
Keywords ➢	skin disorders psoriasis drug alert

Types and severity of burns

http://www.alpha-tek.com/burn/type.htm

Sponsor ➢ Burn Survivors Online

Description ➢ Descriptions of burn severity

Data type ➢ Text

Access requirements ➢ Open

Supplemental resources ➢ Microwave burn prevention
(http://www.shrinershq.org/Hospitals/BurnTips/micro.html)
The Shrine of North America homepage listing burn hospitals
(http://www.shrinershq.org/index.html)

User tips ➢ Check link for "what's new"

Keywords ➢ burns
burn hospital

Ultrasound lipoplasty

http://www.surgery.org/enhanced/media/position/update/update.html

Sponsor ➢ American Society for Aesthetic Plastic Surgery

Description ➢ Overview of conventional liposuction and ultrasound-assisted lipoplasty

Data type ➢ Text

Access requirements ➢ Open

Supplemental resources ➢ Liposuction, see homepage
(http://www.surgery.org/enhanced/main/right.html)

User tips ➢ See federal review of one hundred studies on effects of silicone breast implants

Keywords ➢ lipoplasty
liposuction

Emergency Medicine

Asian Urban Disaster Mitigation Program (AUDMP)
http://hoshi.cic.sfu.ca/adpc/audmp/audmp.html

Sponsor ➢	Asian Disaster Preparedness Center (ADPC)
Description ➢	Report of disaster programs in target countries such as Laos, India, Bangladesh, and others
Data type ➢	Text
Access requirements ➢	Open
Supplemental resources ➢	Philippine Cities Disaster Mitigation Project **(http://hoshi.cic.sfu.ca/adpc/audmp/philippines/philippines.html)** ADPC homepage **(http://hoshi.cic.sfu.ca/adpc/default.html)**
User tips ➢	Check bins for India, Laos, Sri Lanka, and other locations
Keywords ➢	disaster preparedness

Concept for the Global Health Disaster Network (GHDNet)
http://hypnos.m.ehime-u.ac.jp/GHDNet/concept

Sponsor ➢ GHDNet, Ehime University School of Medicine

Description ➢ Paper explaining the need for a global health disaster network

Data type ➢ Text

Access requirements ➢ Open

Supplemental resources ➢ Global Health Disaster Network homepage **(http://hypnos.m.ehime-u.ac.jp/GHDNet/index.html)**
Internet and transmission of disaster information **(http://hypnos.m.ehime-u.ac.jp/GHDNet/Contents/intro#02)**

User tips ➢ Available in English and Japanese

Keywords ➢ global disaster planning

Database of injury mechanisms and diagnoses
http://www.cis.upenn.edu/~traumaid/mjd/html/

Sponsor ➢ TraumAID Project, University of Pennsylvania and Allegheny University

Description ➢ Search enabled database of injury diagnosis and treatment

Data type ➢ Images; text; and demos

Access requirements ➢ Open

Supplemental resources ➢ TraumAID Project homepage **(http://www.cis.upenn.edu/~traumaid/home.html)**

User tips ➢ Check homepage for demo, E-code ICD9-code DataBase

Keywords ➢ wound diagnosis
treatment

Disaster relief services

http://www.crosssnet.org/what.html

Sponsor ➢ American Red Cross

Description ➢ Description of American Red Cross disaster relief services

Data type ➢ Text

Access requirements ➢ Open

Supplemental resources ➢ Emergency Preparedness Information Exchange (EPIX)–Canada **(http://hoshi.cic.sfu.ca/epix/)**

User tips ➢ EPIX gives information about Canada's national and provincial emergency plans

Keywords ➢ disaster safety

Doctors Without Borders USA, Inc.

http://www.dwb.org/voluntr.htm

Sponsor ➢ Doctors Without Borders USA, Inc.

Description ➢ International volunteer emergency relief organization

Data type ➢ Text; photos

Access requirements ➢ Open

Supplemental resources ➢ Employment Opportunities with International Medical Corps Online **(http://www.imc-la.com/jobs2frame.htm)**

User tips ➢ E-mail contact for Doctors Without Borders **(dwb@newyork.msf.org)**; phone: 1-888-DWB-0-DWB

Keywords ➢ medical volunteers
international relief workers

Drug dosages in medical emergencies

http://www.priory.co.uk/journals/emerg.htm

Sponsor ➢	Medicine On-Line
Description ➢	Indications and dosages for specific drugs
Data type ➢	Alphabetized list and information summary
Access requirements ➢	Open
Supplemental resources ➢	Society for Academic Emergency Medicine (SAEM) emergency medicine research database project **(http://smi.bih.harvard.edu/SAEM/EMRDB.html)** MedNets emergency medicine databases **(http://www.internets.com/mednets/emergenc.htm)**
User tips ➢	Visit drug data sites in anesthesiology and critical care bins
Keywords ➢	emergency drugs

Emergency assistance: Refugees and displaced persons

http://www.cdc.gov/nceh/programs/internat/ierh/ierh.htm

Sponsor ➢	International Emergency and Refugee Health Program, NCEH, CDC
Description ➢	CDC's emergency preparedness and response to complex emergencies
Data type ➢	Text
Access requirements ➢	Open
Supplemental resources ➢	Complex emergencies: Refugees and displaced persons **(http://www.cdc.gov/nceh/programs/internat/ierh/desc/complxem.htm#lssue)** Summary, CDC assistance during crisis in the Great Lakes Region, Central Africa **(http://www.cdc.gov/nceh/programs/internat/ierh/whatsnew/1997/p9702.htm)**
User tips ➢	Check bin for CDC International Health Program Office (IHPO)
Keywords ➢	international emergency refugees

Emergency management of spider bites
http://gema.library.ucsf.edu:8081/Originals/Tamkin/recluse.html

Sponsor ➢	*Global Emergency Medicine Archives* (GEMA)
Description ➢	Emergency management of brown recluse spider bites
Data type ➢	Text
Access requirements ➢	Open
Supplemental resources ➢	GEMA homepage **(http://gema.library.ucsf.edu:8081/)** Interactive forum page **(http://gema.library.ucsf.edu:8081/conference/ForumHome.html)**
User tips ➢	See information for authors cited on main menu
Keywords ➢	spider bite

Emergency medicine and primary care
http://www.embbs.com/

Sponsor ➢	EMBBS Emergency Medicine and Primary Care
Description ➢	Emergency medicine resources including libraries of radiology; computerized tomography scan; medical photography
Data type ➢	Images and text
Access requirements ➢	Data for professionals
Supplemental resources ➢	Treatment of stab wound to left forearm **(http://www.embbs.com/aem/armstab1.html)** Diagnosis: compartment syndrome **(http://www.embbs.com/aem/armstab1dx.html)**
User tips ➢	Check pediatric advanced life support
Keywords ➢	pediatric emergency medicine wounds

Expert witness guidelines in emergency medicine
http://www.acep.org/POLICY/P0004114.HTM

Sponsor ➢ American College of Emergency Physicians (ACEP)

Description ➢ Approved expert witness guidelines for emergency medicine, 1995

Data type ➢ Text

Access requirements ➢ Open; some links accessible exclusively by ACEP members

Supplemental resources ➢ ACEP homepage
(http://www.acep.org/)
Access to Emergency Medical Services Act of 1997
(http://www.acep.org/)

User tips ➢ Review consent form to treat

Keywords ➢ emergency legal guidelines

Global Emergency Management System (GEMS) resources
http://www.fema.gov/cgi-shl/dbml.ex...on=query&template=/gems/g_index.dbm

Sponsor ➢ Federal Emergency Management Agency (FEMA)

Description ➢ Searchable database of disaster and emergency relief resources

Data type ➢ Text

Access requirements ➢ Open

Supplemental resources ➢ FEMA Federal Response Plan (Public Law 93-288, as amended)
(http://www.fema.gov/fema/fed1.htm)
Colleges, universities offering emergency management courses
(http://fema.gov/home/emi/edu/col_lst.htm)

User tips ➢ Browse GEMS resources

Keywords ➢ emergency management
disaster relief

Guide to medical abbreviations
http://ncemi.org/tla/index.htm

Sponsor ➢ National Center for Emergency Medicine Informatics (NCEMI)

Description ➢ Medical abbreviations and jargon used on the Internet

Data type ➢ Dictionary; downloadable

Access requirements ➢ Open

Supplemental resources ➢ Clinical issues in field medical care **(http://members.aol.com/tgarigan/fieldclinical/fieldclinical.html)**
MedWeb emergency medicine (megasite) **(http://www.gen.emory.edu/medweb/medweb.emergency.html)**

User tips ➢ See lecture outline for chemical agent casualty care

Keywords ➢ medical abbreviations

Medical education software archive
http://sun3.lib.uci.edu/~sclancy/med-ed/

Sponsor ➢ University of California, Irvine

Description ➢ Clearinghouse for medical education computer software

Data type ➢ Downloadable demos

Access requirements ➢ Open; demos, free download

Supplemental resources ➢ Demos: Self tutorial for physician clinical communication for emergency medicine **(http://www.medulogic.com/)**
Medical software for emergency physicians **(http://ncemi.org/cgi-bin/hot.pl?cmd...f=hot/hi-medical_software.hot&rfj=7)**

User tips ➢ Software for DOS, Windows, and Macintosh

Keywords ➢ emergency tutorial
medical software

Oklahoma bombing: Mental health response

http://www.aaets.org/arts/art5.htm

Sponsor ➢ American Academy of Experts in Traumatic Stress

Description ➢ Article on organization of mental health response to Oklahoma City bombing

Data type ➢ Text

Access requirements ➢ Open

Supplemental resources ➢ List of articles on traumatic stress from *Trauma Response* **(http://www.aaets.org/trresp.htm)**
American Academy of Experts in Traumatic Stress homepage, **(http://www.aaets.org/trresp.htm)**

User tips ➢ Read article, TWA flight 800; disaster response

Keywords ➢ mental health

Radiological Emergency Preparedness (REP) Program

http://www.fema.gov/pte/rep/

Sponsor ➢ Federal Emergency Management Agency (FEMA)

Description ➢ Health and safety plan for citizens living around commercial nuclear power plants

Data type ➢ Text

Access requirements ➢ Open

Supplemental resources ➢ REP tabletop exercise for training **(http://www.fema.gov/pte/rep/tabletop.htm)**

User tips ➢ Check FEMA reference library

Keywords ➢ emergency preparedness
radiological emergency preparedness

Self-study course for emergency response to terrorism

http://www.usfa.fema.gov/nfa/tr_ertss.htm

Sponsor ➢ National Fire Academy, U.S. Fire Administration (USFA)

Description ➢ Home course modules, glossary, and final exam for training emergency personnel response to potential terrorist incident

Data type ➢ Downloadable course materials

Access requirements ➢ For emergency, fire, and related personnel

Supplemental resources ➢ U.S. Fire Administration (USFA) homepage **(http://www.usfa.fema.gov/)**

User tips ➢ USFA seeks input on future fire research agenda

Keywords ➢ terrorism, fire training

Wound care specialization trend
http://members.aol.com/woundnet/trend.htm

Sponsor ➢ American Academy of Wound Management

Description ➢ Description of wound care specialization

Data type ➢ Text for health professionals

Access requirements ➢ Open

Supplemental resources ➢ Wound Net homepage
(http://members.aol.com/woundnet/index.html)
Links for Web resources for wound care professionals
(http://members.aol.com/woundnet/index.html)

User tips ➢ See application procedures for wound care board certification

Keywords ➢ wound care

Wound healing using color digital image processing
http://www.smtl.co.uk/World-Wide-Wounds/1997/july/Berris/Berris.html

Sponsor ➢ *World Wide Wounds*, electronic journal of Wound Management Practice

Description ➢ State of the art in computer-assisted wound measurement

Data type ➢ Journal

Access requirements ➢ Open

Supplemental resources ➢ Wounds homepage
(http://www.smtl.co.uk/World-Wide-Wounds/)

User tips ➢ Online articles updated frequently

Keywords ➢ wound treatment
medical computers

Environmental Health

Carpet emissions and indoor air quality
http://www.carpet-rug.com/carpet.html

Sponsor ➢	Carpet and Rug Institute
Description ➢	Report on carpet safety and indoor air quality
Data type ➢	Text
Access requirements ➢	Open
Supplemental resources ➢	Summary of study on effects of new carpet emissions on indoor air quality and health (Cornell University) **(http://www.tc.cornell.edu/~hedge/carpet/AHCarpetRep.html)** Source list of studies on carpets and other applications **(http://134.67.104.12/E-DRIVE/CTC/DIR2/CTCT4.TXT)**
User tips ➢	See Center project summaries on other emissions, ink, and foam
Keywords ➢	carpet emissions

Electric and magnetic fields (EMF) research
http://www.niehs.nih.gov/emfrapid/home.htm

Sponsor ➢ Electric and Magnetic Fields Research and Public Information Dissemination (EMFRAPID) Program, Centers for Disease Control and Prevention (CDC)

Description ➢ Research update on EMF regional facilities, measurements database, information sources, 1995 report to Congress

Data type ➢ Report

Access requirements ➢ Open

Supplemental resources ➢ Questions and answers about EMF **(http://www.niehs.nih.gov/emfrapid/home.htm)**
Power lines project, New York State Department of Health
(http://www.health.state.ny.us/nysdoh/consumer/environ/homeenvi.htm?)

User tips ➢ Check EMFRAPID homepage for additional reports

Keywords ➢ electric and magnetic fields (EMF)

Environmental Health Clearinghouse
http://infoventures.com/e-hlth/about-eh.html

Sponsor ➢ National Institute of Environmental Health Sciences (NIEHS)

Description ➢ Free source of information on environmental health effects, worker exposure, hazardous waste, chemical spills, and worker justice issues

Data type ➢ Text; reports

Access requirements ➢ Open

Supplemental resources ➢ NIEHS homepage
(http://www.niehs.nih.gov/)
Review of literature on herbicides
(http://infoventures.com/e-hlth/orange/phd93.html)

User tips ➢ Online computer or phone search (toll-free number: 1-800-643-4794)

Keywords ➢ herbicides
environmental health

Glossary of environmental health terms

http://www.health.state.ny.us/nysdoh/consumer/environ/toxglos.htm

Sponsor ➢	New York State Department of Health (NYSDOH)
Description ➢	Glossary categorized according to terminology, agency, units of measure, and conversion tables
Data type ➢	Glossary for consumers
Access requirements ➢	Open
Supplemental resources ➢	NYSDOH homepage **(http://www.health.state.ny.us/nysdoh/consumer/environ/homeenvi.htm?)** U.S. Environmental Protection Agency (EPA), Office of Prevention, Pesticides, and Toxic Substances **(http://www.epa.gov/internet/oppts/)**
User tips ➢	Check NYSDOH homepage for Rx for radon describing EPA-designated high radon risk areas
Keywords ➢	radon

Hazards literature database (HazLit)

http://www.Colorado.EDU/hazards/litbase/litindex.htm

Sponsor ➢	Natural Hazards Research and Applications Information Center, University of Colorado at Boulder
Description ➢	Bibliographic access of hazards data and references for researchers
Data type ➢	Database
Access requirements ➢	Open; source for researchers and organizations
Supplemental resources ➢	Natural Hazards Center at the University of Colorado, Boulder **(http://www.Colorado.EDU/hazards/)** Natural Disaster Reference Database (NDRD) **(http://ltpwww.gsfc.nasa.gov/ndrd/)**
User tips ➢	*Disaster Research* newsletter available online
Keywords ➢	natural disasters emergency medicine

Lead screening guidelines

http://WWW.CDC.GOV/nceh/programs/lead/guide/1997/docs/backgr.htm

Sponsor ➢ National Center for Environmental Health (NCEH), Centers for Disease Control and Prevention (CDC)

Description ➢ CDC release of new guidance on lead screening for children, November 3, 1997

Data type ➢ Text; reports

Access requirements ➢ Open

Supplemental resources ➢ Prevention of fetal alcohol syndrome, CDC **(http://www.cdc.gov/nceh/programs/infants/brthdfct/prevent/fas_prev.htm)**
Air pollution and respiratory health **(http://www.cdc.gov/nceh/pubcatns/19.../brosures/airpollu.htm#surveillance)**

User tips ➢ See NCEH homepage for Healthy People 2010

Keywords ➢ lead screening
pediatrics

Medical surveillance during Operations Desert Shield/Desert Storm

http://www.gulflink.osd.mil/nfl/

Sponsor ➢ Office of the Special Assistant for Gulf War Illnesses, U.S. Department of Defense (DOD)

Description ➢ Report describing medical protocols during Operations Desert Shield/Desert Storm, November 6, 1997

Data type ➢ Text

Access requirements ➢ Open; downloadable

Supplemental resources ➢ U.S. Department of Veterans Affairs eligibility health insurance reform **(http://www.va.gov/health/elig/)**
National Gulf War Resource Center, Inc. **(http://www.gulfweb.org/org_show.cfm?ID=1)**

User tips ➢ To report new information, call DOD at 1-800-472-6719

Keywords ➢ Gulf War illnesses

Mesothelioma treatment options

http://www.mesothel.com/pages/mesopage.htm

Sponsor ➢ Roger G. Worthington, P.C.

Description ➢ Articles regarding mesothelioma treatment options, history, profiles, and protocols

Data type ➢ Articles; patient profiles

Access requirements ➢ Direct link access via table of contents

Supplemental resources ➢ Asbestos Update **(http://www.mesothel.com/)**

User tips ➢ See homepage for mesothelioma

Keywords ➢ cancer
asbestos

National Toxicology Program

http://ntp-server.niehs.nih.gov/

Sponsor ➢ Collaboration of U.S. Health and Human Services agencies

Description ➢ Provides information about potentially toxic chemicals to regulatory and research agencies and the public

Data type ➢ Text; reports

Access requirements ➢ Open

Supplemental resources ➢ Testing information and study results **(http://ntp-server.niehs.nih.gov/)**

User tips ➢ See homepage for links to animal assays for toxicity/carcinogenicity

Keywords ➢ toxicology
veterinary medicine

Pesticide Information Profiles (PIPs)

http://ace.ace/orst.edu/info/extoxnet/pips/ghindex.html

Sponsor ➢ University of California–Davis, Oregon State University, Michigan State University, and Cornell University

Description ➢ Search and browse database of pesticide data

Data type ➢ Text; reports provide trade names, regulatory status, and toxicologic effects of pesticides

Access requirements ➢ Open

Supplemental resources ➢ Aluminum phosphide **(http://ace.ace.orst.edu/info/extoxnet/pips/alumphos.txt)**
Extoxnet homepage **(http://ace.ace.orst.edu/info/extoxnet/)**

User tips ➢ Check homepage for background information about Extoxnet

Keywords ➢ pesticides

Pollution database

http://www.webdirectory.com/Pollution/

Sponsor ➢ Environfacts Warehouse, U.S. Environmental Protection Agency (EPA)

Description ➢ Databases, clearinghouses providing information on pollution topics

Data type ➢ Megasite of environmental data

Access requirements ➢ Open

Supplemental resources ➢ Environfacts Warehouse homepage **(http://www.epa.gov/enviro/html/ef_home.html)**
Institute of Occupational and Environmental Health related sites **(http://www.hsc.wvu.edu/ioeh/occlink.htm)**

User tips ➢ Use homepage to query database, generate reports, and produce maps of environmental data

Keywords ➢ environmental database

Public health assessments, 1995–1996
http://atsdr1.atsdr.cdc.gov:8080/HAC/PHA/

Sponsor ➢ Agency for Toxic Substances and Disease Registry (ATSDR)

Description ➢ Full text health assessments organized according to originating ATSDR regions

Data type ➢ Text; reports

Access requirements ➢ Open; downloadable

Supplemental resources ➢ ATSDR's Hazardous Substance Release/Health Effects Database; search enabled
(http://atsdr1.atsdr.cdc.gov:8080/hazdat.html)
ATSDR homepage
(http://atsdr1.atsdr.cdc.gov:8080/)

User tips ➢ See contents and search instructions; check site listing the top twenty hazardous substances

Keywords ➢ hazardous substances
toxic substances

Public policy challenges facing chlorine chemistry
http://www.c3.org/library/cth2.html

Sponsor ➢ Chlorine Chemistry Council (CCC)

Description ➢ Potential results of chlorine ban

Data type ➢ Report

Access requirements ➢ Open

Supplemental resources ➢ CCC homepage
(http://www.c3.org/)
Vinyl plastics: An environmental profile
(http://www.c3.org/library/enviroprfl.html)

User tips ➢ See CCC homepage for additional bleach data

Keywords ➢ chlorine
environmental health

Role of climate in selected diseases in the United States

http://www.med.harvard.edu/chge/EID/more_disease.html

Sponsor ➢	Center for Health and the Global Environment, Harvard Medical School
Description ➢	Background materials for considering the role of climate in selected diseases in the United States
Data type ➢	Report
Access requirements ➢	Open
Supplemental resources ➢	Center for Health and the Global Environment homepage **(http://www.med.harvard.edu/chge/)**
User tips ➢	See homepage for newsletter
Keywords ➢	climate and health

Smoking and health

http://ash.org/

Sponsor ➢	Action on Smoking and Health (ASH)
Description ➢	News and sources on smoking and health
Data type ➢	Articles
Access requirements ➢	Open
Supplemental resources ➢	How passive smoking causes heart disease **(http://outcast.gene.com/local-bin/pphtml/ae/WN/SU/passive_smoking.html)**
User tips ➢	The latest news about smoking
Keywords ➢	passive smoking

Strategic Plan for Health Effects of Air Pollution (1997–2000)

http://www.healtheffects.org/strategy.htm

Sponsor ➢ Health Effects Institute (HEI)

Description ➢ Update of strategic plan of research on health effects of pollutants from motor vehicles and other environmental sources

Data type ➢ Research reports

Access requirements ➢ Open; direct access via table of contents

Supplemental resources ➢ HEI homepage **(http://www.healtheffects.org/)**

User tips ➢ Check HEI's quarterly newsletter

Keywords ➢ pollution

Summary of proceedings of National Conference on Air Pollution Impacts on Body Organs

http://www.intr.net/napenet/airsum.html#Droller

Sponsor ➢ National Association of Physicians for the Environment (NAPE)

Description ➢ Summary of conference proceedings of pollution impact on body organs and systems

Data type ➢ Hyperlinked text

Access requirements ➢ Direct link access via table of contents

Supplemental resources ➢ Conference summary **(http://www.intr.net/napenet/airsum.html)**
National Association of Physicians for the Environment homepage **(http://www.intr.net/napenet/index.html)**

User tips ➢ Check proceedings section on pollution impact on special populations

Keywords ➢ pollution

Teaching resources in occupational and environmental health
http://www.med.ed.ac.uk/hew/alpha.html

Sponsor ➢	University of Edinburgh
Description ➢	Educational resources including tutorials and teaching resources for air quality, critical appraisal of environmental literature, lung disease, and other topics
Data type ➢	Hyperlinked text; tutorials
Access requirements ➢	Open; direct access via hyperlinked index
Supplemental resources ➢	Homepage and index **(http://www.med.ed.ac.uk/hew/main/homepage.htm)** Airborne environmental pollutants and asthma **(http://www.med.ed.ac.uk/hew/medical/asthma.html)**
User tips ➢	Search tool available
Keywords ➢	environmental health resources

Epidemiology

Allergy and infectious diseases funding opportunities

http://web.fie.com/htbin/wfSearch

Sponsor ➢	National Institute of Allergy and Infectious Diseases (NIAID)
Description ➢	NIAID funding guide for research investigations involving disease diagnoses, treatments, and other opportunities from the *Federal Registry*, NIH Guide, and other sources
Data type ➢	Text
Access requirements ➢	Open
Supplemental resources ➢	NIAID homepage **(http://web.fie.com/htdoc/fed/nih/ali/any/menu/any/aliindex.htm)** National Foundation for Infectious Diseases fellowships **(http://www.medscape.com/Affiliates/NFID/fellow/)**
User tips ➢	Search NIAID database
Keywords ➢	education funding

Bird flu influenza outbreak

http://www.accessv.com/~mhfung/flu.htm

Sponsor ➢	Access Excellence
Description ➢	Collection of articles and reports related to bird flu morbidity
Data type ➢	Articles
Access requirements ➢	Open
Supplemental resources ➢	Influenza surveillance activities, World Health Organization (WHO) **(http://www.who.ch/ebola/ebolahome.html)**
User tips ➢	Check current news sites
Keywords ➢	influenza ebola

The Blue Book

http://hna.ffh.vic.gov.au/phb/hprot/inf_dis/bluebook/index.htm

Sponsor ➢	Public Health Division, Department of Human Services, Victoria, Australia
Description ➢	Guidelines for control of infectious diseases such as chicken pox, cholera, amoebiasis, diphtheria, AIDS
Data type ➢	Text
Access requirements ➢	Open; requires Adobe Acrobat Reader
Supplemental resources ➢	Cytomegalovirus (CMV) infection **(http://hna.ffh.vic.gov.au/phb/hprot/inf_dis/bluebook/cytomeg.htm)** Arbovirus infections **(http://hna.ffh.vic.gov.au/phb/hprot/inf_dis/bluebook/index.htm)**
User tips ➢	Large file, 676K
Keywords ➢	infectious disease control arbovirus infections

Comprehensive Epidemiologic Data Resource (CEDR)

http://cedr.lbl.gov/catalog/catalog1.html

Sponsor ➢ Office of Environment, Safety and Health, U.S. Department of Energy (DOE)

Description ➢ Analytic working data sets and files resulting from epidemiologic studies at different DOE facilities during the past thirty years

Data type ➢ Text; statistics

Access requirements ➢ Public access to CEDR data; some data files restricted to registered CEDR investigators

Supplemental resources ➢ Instructions on obtaining errata and updates
(http://cedr.lbl.gov/)
CEDR homepage
(http://cedr.lbl.gov/)

User tips ➢ See studies of atomic bomb survivors

Keywords ➢ epidemiologic research
exposure risks

Ebola vaccine candidate

http://www.gene.com/ae/WN/SU/ebola198.html

Sponsor ➢ Access Excellence

Description ➢ Article, ebola control

Data type ➢ Text; graphics

Access requirements ➢ Open

Supplemental resources ➢ Ebola virus hemorrhagic fever
(wysiwyg://299/http://www.cdc.gov/ncidod/diseases/virlfvr/ebolainf.htm)
Virus outbreak in Zaire, World Health Organization (WHO)
(http://www.who.ch/ebola/ebolahome.html)

User tips ➢ See WHO for data regarding virus outbreak in Zaire

Keywords ➢ virus
ebola

Emerging Infectious Diseases (EID)

http://www.cdc.gov/ncidod/EID/access.htm

Sponsor ➢	National Center for Infectious Disease (NCID), CDC
Description ➢	Journal of disease articles
Data type ➢	Text; tables
Access requirements ➢	Open; available in ASCII, Adobe Acrobat, and PostScript
Supplemental resources ➢	Article, perspective on foodborne diseases **(wysiwyg://69/http://www.cdc.gov/ncidod/EID/vol3no3/cohen.htm)** Access EID Spanish version **(ftp://fcv.medvet.unlp.edu.ar)**
User tips ➢	Large file; subscribers can request individual articles
Keywords ➢	epidemiology foodborne diseases

Epi Info programs for epidemiologic analysis

http://www.cdc.gov/epo/epi/epiinfo.htm

Sponsor ➢	Epidemiology Program Office, Centers for Disease Control and Prevention (CDC)
Description ➢	Public domain microcomputer software for word processing, data management, and epidemiologic analysis
Data type ➢	Downloadable software for Epi Info, Epi Map, Do Epi, and SSS 1 for public health professionals
Access requirements ➢	Open
Supplemental resources ➢	Software download page **(http://www.cdc.gov/epo/epi/software.htm)**
User tips ➢	Free software
Keywords ➢	epidemiologic software

Eurosurveillance Weekly

http://www.eurosurv.org/

Sponsor ➢ DGV of the Commission of the European Communities

Description ➢ Report of communicable disease outbreaks and news gathered from the European Union public health centers

Data type ➢ Newsletter

Access requirements ➢ Registration required for online access and inclusion on mailing list

Supplemental resources ➢ Online registration **(http://www.eurosurv.org/regform.htm)**

User tips ➢ Free subscription; weekly updates

Keywords ➢ epidemiology

Evaluating disease management interventions

http://www.sapien.net/dmw/aud/transcripts/96_09_25.htm

Sponsor ➢ Greenstone Healthcare Solutions

Description ➢ Transcript of disease management forum

Data type ➢ Text

Access requirements ➢ Open

Supplemental resources ➢ Prior chat transcripts **(http://www.sapien.net/dmw/aud/index.htm)**

User tips ➢ Check homepage for live chats

Keywords ➢ disease management

Guidelines for epidemiology practices for drug, device, and vaccine research in the United States
http://www.hsph.harvard.edu/Organizations/DDIL/gep.html

Sponsor ➢	Drugs and Devices Information Line, Harvard School of Public Health
Description ➢	Published report of guidelines for good epidemiologic practices
Data type ➢	Text
Access requirements ➢	Open
Supplemental resources ➢	Drugs and Devices Information Line homepage **(http://www.hsph.harvard.edu/Organizations/DDIL/ddilhpge.html)**
User tips ➢	Check homepage links for pharmacoepidemiology
Keywords ➢	pharmacoepidemiology

Healthy travel
http://www.travelhealth.com/genguide.htm

Sponsor ➢	Travel Health Information and Referral Service
Description ➢	Healthy travel guidelines on water, altitude, illness, seafood poisoning, and insects
Data type ➢	Text; graphics
Access requirements ➢	Open
Supplemental resources ➢	Trypanosomiasis (Chagas' disease) **(http://www.travelhealth.com/tropdz/amtrpage.htm)** Elephantiasis **(http://www.travelhealth.com/tropdz/eleppage.htm)**
User tips ➢	Check bin for background on tropical diseases
Keywords ➢	travel information travel medicine

Hepatitis A to E
http://www.cdc.gov/ncidod/diseases/hepatitis/slideset/hep00025.htm

Sponsor ➢ Centers for Disease Control and Prevention (CDC)

Description ➢ Slides of hepatitis virus

Data type ➢ Slides; text

Access requirements ➢ Open

Supplemental resources ➢ Cirrhosis, non-A non-B hepatitis **(http://korb1.sote.hu/KKK/DESCRIPT/0004/0004383E.HTM)**

User tips ➢ Full screen slide viewing

Keywords ➢ hepatitis
health statistics

Homeowner's guide to ecology and environmental management of Lyme disease
http://www.w2.com/docs2/d5/lyme1.html

Sponsor ➢ American Lyme Disease Foundation, Inc. (ALDF)

Description ➢ Control of Lyme disease

Data type ➢ Text; graphics

Access requirements ➢ Open

Supplemental resources ➢ ALDF homepage
(http://www.w2.com/docs2/d5/lyme.html)
Specific recommendations for disease control
(http://www.w2.com/docs2/d5/lyme3.html)

User tips ➢ ALDF toll free number (800-876-LYME)

Keywords ➢ Lyme disease

Leprosy management projects

http://foundation.novartis.com/leproj.htm

Sponsor ➢ Novartis Foundation Leprosy Fund

Description ➢ Description of international leprosy programs involved in case finding, field services, mobile clinics, and social marketing

Data type ➢ Text

Access requirements ➢ Open

Supplemental resources ➢ Leprosy project in Turkey
(http://foundation.novartis.com/turkey.htm)
Netherlands Leprosy Relief Association (NSL)
(http://infolep.twinfo.nl/infolep)

User tips ➢ Free information available from Infolep for leprosy workers in endemic countries

Keywords ➢ leprosy
Hansen's disease

Parasitic diseases

http://www.mic.ki.se/Diseases/c3.html

Sponsor ➢ Karolinska Institute Library and Information Center

Description ➢ Hyperlinks to parasitic resources, research, organizations, and data on skin diseases, ectoparasitic infestations

Data type ➢ Hyperlinked files

Access requirements ➢ Open; for professionals and consumers

Supplemental resources ➢ *Parasitology Journal* links (American Society of Parasitologists)
(http://www.mic.ki.se/Diseases/c3.html)
Head lice information, Harvard School of Public Health
(http://www.hsph.harvard.edu/headlice.html)

User tips ➢ Megasite resource

Keywords ➢ parasitic diseases
parasitology resources

Rare diseases clinical research database

http://rarediseases.info.nih.gov/ord/wwwprot/index.shtml

Sponsor ➢ Office of Rare Diseases (ORD), National Institutes of Health (NIH)

Description ➢ Clinical data on 6,000 rare diseases, research, and clinical trials for patients, providers, and researchers

Data type ➢ Text; tables

Access requirements ➢ Open

Supplemental resources ➢ ORD homepage **(http://rarediseases.info.nih.gov/ord/index.html)**
Investigator research resources **(http://rarediseases.info.nih.gov/ord/r_res.htm)**

User tips ➢ Check free access to National Library of Medicine (NLM) Medline database

Keywords ➢ rare diseases
orphan diseases

Rare disorders database

http://www.nord-rdb.com/~orphan/rdb/rd0057.htm

Sponsor ➢ National Organization for Rare Disorders, Inc. (NORD)

Description ➢ Database of orphan diseases; full text disease information for 140 health organizations

Data type ➢ Text

Access requirements ➢ Open; search by synonyms, disorder subdivisions, symptoms, or causes

Supplemental resources ➢ NORD homepage **(http://www.pcnet.com/~orphan/welcome.htm)**
Amyotrophic lateral sclerosis (ALS) **(http://www.nord-rdb.com/~orphan/rdb/rd0057.htm)**

User tips ➢ Check newsletter, *Orphan Disease Update*

Keywords ➢ orphan diseases
amyotrophic lateral sclerosis (ALS)

Sanitation inspections of international cruise ships, Green Sheet
http://www.cdc.gov/nceh/programs/sanit/vsp/scores/scores.htm

Sponsor ➢ National Center for Environmental Health (NCEH), Centers for Disease Control and Prevention (CDC)

Description ➢ Recent sanitation inspection scores and explanations for cruise ships

Data type ➢ Text

Access requirements ➢ Open

Supplemental resources ➢ Public health response to Pfiesteria **(http://www.cdc.gov/nceh/press/1997/970930pf.htm)**
Online abstracts, June, 1996–March 1997, *Journal of Travel Medicine* **(http://www.istm.org/jtm/index.html)**

User tips ➢ Cruise ship inspection data updated frequently

Keywords ➢ travel medicine
Pfiesteria

Search results for immunization and infectious diseases
http://www.healthfinder.gov/htmlge...MUNIZATION+AND+INFECTIOUS+DISEASES

Sponsor ➢ Healthfinder, Department of Health and Human Services (DHHS)

Description ➢ Hyperlinked results of search of Healthfinder site which produces Web and other resources for infectious diseases

Data type ➢ Variable

Access requirements ➢ Open

Supplemental resources ➢ Healthfinder homepage **(http://www.healthfinder.gov/)**

User tips ➢ Search for specific topics or diseases

Keywords ➢ epidemiology
medical information

Toxicology Internet resources

http://www.pitt.edu/~martint/welcome.htm#mothp

Sponsor ➢ Toxicology Treatment Program (TTP), University of Pittsburgh

Description ➢ Clinical and occupational toxicology links for practitioners, educators, and researchers in medical settings

Data type ➢ Variable

Access requirements ➢ Open

Supplemental resources ➢ Cysticercosis **(http://www.usc.edu/hsc/neurosurgery...ture_Series/Cysticercosis/cyst.html)**
Chart, title organ, disease **(http://korb1.sote.hu/KKK/LISTTYPE/D/DIA3E.HTM)**

User tips ➢ TTP site welcomes site or Web links suggestions

Keywords ➢ cirrhosis
cysticercosis

Weekly Epidemiological Record (WER)

http://www.who.ch/wer/wer_home.htm

Sponsor ➢ World Health Organization (WHO)

Description ➢ Weekly electronic edition of epidemiologic information on cases and outbreaks under the International Health Regulations

Data type ➢ Text

Access requirements ➢ Open; requires Acrobat Reader for viewing

Supplemental resources ➢ WER, past issues **(http://www.who.ch/wer/wer_home.htm)**
Pan American Health Organization (PAHO) country health profiles **(http://www.paho.org/english/country.htm)**

User tips ➢ Free WER bilingual English/French edition distributed every Friday

Keywords ➢ epidemiology
international health

Yellow Book Online: Health information for international travel, 1996–1997

wysiwyg://119/http://www.cdc.gov/travel/yellowbk/home.htm

Sponsor ➢	National Center for Infectious Diseases (NCID), Centers for Disease Control and Prevention (CDC)
Description ➢	Vaccinations, health risks, and other international travel tips according to country
Data type ➢	Reference; search enabled
Access requirements ➢	Open; requires Adobe Reader to download
Supplemental resources ➢	The Blue Sheet, health information for international travel **(wysiwyg://225/http://www.cdc.gov/travel/blusheet.htm)** Vaccine recommendations **(wysiwyg://88/http://www.cdc.gov/travel/travel.html)**
User tips ➢	Contact 1-800-CDC-SHOT for updated vaccine recommendations
Keywords ➢	immunization sanitation, cruise ships

Gastroenterology

Acute stress ulceration

http://gasbone.herston.uq.edu.au/te...hvc_stul/stressul.html#Pathogenesis

Sponsor ➢	Dr. Philip Cumpston
Description ➢	Definition, etiology, pathogenesis, prevention, and management of stress ulceration
Data type ➢	Text
Access requirements ➢	Open
Supplemental resources ➢	Postgraduate course materials; namely, lecture slides, online tutorial **(http://gasbone.herston.uq.edu.au/pg.html)**
User tips ➢	Table of contents indexed according to subject and expertise level
Keywords ➢	stress ulceration

Adenocarcinoma of the esophago-gastric junction

http://nt1.chir.med.tu-muenchen.de/slides/igcc/classificat/epi/sld019.htm

Sponsor ➢ 2nd International Gastric Cancer Congress

Description ➢ Issues presented during the Consensus Conference, Munich, April 27–30, 1997

Data type ➢ Slides of meeting lectures

Access requirements ➢ Open

Supplemental resources ➢ Congress homepage **(http://nt1.chir.med.tu-muenchen.de/GCC/index.htm)**

User tips ➢ A well executed interactive experience

Keywords ➢ cancer, gastric

Approach to patient with acute hepatitis

http://uhs.bsd.uchicago.edu/uhs/topics/hepatitis.html

Sponsor ➢ Topics in Primary Care, University Health Services, University of Chicago

Description ➢ Outline of hepatitis definition; etiology; clinical manifestations; complications

Data type ➢ Text

Access requirements ➢ Open

Supplemental resources ➢ Self-test on helicobacter pylori **(http://uhs.bsd.uchicago.edu/uhs/topics/helico.tf.html)**

User tips ➢ Good source for professionals

Keywords ➢ epidemiology
hepatitis

Diabetes Research International Network (DRI NET)

http://drinet.med.miami.edu/

Sponsor ➢ Academy for the Advancement of Diabetes Research and Treatment

Description ➢ Diabetes research, laboratory protocols, pancreas and islet transplant registries

Data type ➢ Text

Access requirements ➢ Open

Supplemental resources ➢ Mosby, University of Iowa *Family Practice Handbook*: Chapter 5: Diabetes mellitus **(http://vh.radiology.uiowa.edu/Provi...nRef/FPHandbook/Chapter05/10-5.html)**
Pancreatic Islet Cell Transplantation Text Book **(http://drinet.med.miami.edu/)**

User tips ➢ See homepage for diabetes support groups

Keywords ➢ transplants

Electrogastrography

http://www.ee.ualberta.ca/~mintchev/www.html

Sponsor ➢ Dr. Martin P. Mintchev, University of Calgary

Description ➢ Cyberzine on electrogastrography methodology and clinical applicability

Data type ➢ Text; introductory pictures

Access requirements ➢ Open

Supplemental resources ➢ Gastric electrical activity recorded "in vitro" **(http://www.enel.ucalgary.ca/People/Mintchev/gea.htm#EGG)**

User tips ➢ See homepage for overview of gastric electrical activity (GEA)

Keywords ➢ electrogastrography

Fundoplication

http://www.motility.org/fundo.htm

Sponsor > Children's Motility Disorder Foundation

Description > Procedures and contraindications for fundoplication

Data type > Text; diagrams

Access requirements > Open

Supplemental resources > Children's Motility Disorder Foundation homepage
(http://www.motility.org/index.htm)
Gastroesophageal reflux disease in children
(http://kidshealth.org/ai/service/general_ped_surgery.reflux.html)

User tips > See physician alert for Reglan on homepage

Keywords > fundoplication
pediatric digestive disorders

Gastroenterology training

http://www.gastrojournal.org/policy/v110n4p1266.html

Sponsor > American Gastroenterological Association (AGA)

Description > Core curriculum for training gastroenterologists of the future

Data type > Text

Access requirements > Open

Supplemental resources > AGA homepage
(http://www.gastro.org/)

User tips > Separate sections for physicians and the public

Keywords > gastroenterology training

GastroLinks
http://pharminfo.com/disease/gastro/gastrolinks.html#body

Sponsor ➢ PharmInfoNet's Digestive Disease Center

Description ➢ Gastroenterologic data according to organ system; disease and medical condition; drug information

Data type ➢ Text; diagrams

Access requirements ➢ Open

Supplemental resources ➢ Digestive Disease Center homepage **(http://pharminfo.com/disease/gastro.html)**
Discussions of research and clinical treatment guidelines (Gastro-EHLB) **(http://pharminfo.com/disease/gastro.html)**

User tips ➢ Check Center homepage for *Medical Sciences Bulletin*

Keywords ➢ gastroenterologic disorders

Hans Popper Society: Histopathological cases
http://hepar-sfgh.ucsf.edu/popper.htm

Sponsor ➢ American Association for the Study of Liver Diseases (AASLD)

Description ➢ Case diagnosis and treatment of liver conditions

Data type ➢ Text

Access requirements ➢ Open

Supplemental resources ➢ AASLD homepage **(http://hepar-sfgh.ucsf.edu/)**
Case: Intractable ascites after liver transplantation **(http://hepar-sfgh.ucsf.edu/popper/cases96/cases.htm)**

User tips ➢ See homepage for AASLD publications

Keywords ➢ liver histopathology

Helicobacter pylori
http://www.helico.com/

Sponsor ➢ International Foundation for Helicobacter and Intestinal Immunology

Description ➢ Latest information about Helicobacter pylori diagnosis, treatment, history, and clinical correlations

Data type ➢ Text; multimedia

Access requirements ➢ Open

Supplemental resources ➢ Diagnostic devices for H. Pylori
(http://www.helico.com/web/devices.html)
Helicobacter: The movie
(http://www.helico.com/web/movie1.html)

User tips ➢ Downloading movie requires fast modem

Keywords ➢ Helicobacter pylori

Incontinence and irritable bowel syndrome research
http://www.execpc.com/iffgd/research.html

Sponsor ➢ International Foundation for Functional Gastrointestinal Disorders (IFFGD)

Description ➢ Report on recent IFFGD research results

Data type ➢ Text

Access requirements ➢ Open

Supplemental resources ➢ Medical therapy for inflammatory bowel disease
(http://www.sma.org/smj/96jun2.htm)
Ostomy insurance and reimbursement for United States only
(http://www.convatec.com/osinsurc.htm#overview)

User tips ➢ IFFGD (toll free number: 1-888-964-2001)

Keywords ➢ bowel disease
ostomy insurance

Introduction to gastroesophageal reflux disease (GERD)

http://www.gerd.com/intro/home.htm

Sponsor ➢ GERD Information Resource Center, Astra Merck Inc.

Description ➢ Primer on general anatomy and pathophysiology of GERD

Data type ➢ Multimedia

Access requirements ➢ Site includes downloads for Shockwave plug-in and Netscape Navigator

Supplemental resources ➢ GERD homepage **(http://www.gerd.com/)**

User tips ➢ Information intended for residents of the United States and its territories only; contact number: 1-800-236-9933

Keywords ➢ gastroenterologic disorders

Laparoscopic surgery during pregnancy

http://www.sages.org/sg_pub23.html

Sponsor ➢ Society of American Gastrointestinal Endoscopic Surgeons (SAGES)

Description ➢ SAGES guidelines for laparoscopic surgery

Data type ➢ Text

Access requirements ➢ Open

Supplemental resources ➢ SAGES homepage **(http://www.sages.org/sages.html)**

User tips ➢ Check gastrointestinal links for additional information

Keywords ➢ pregnancy

Legislative action: Colorectal cancer screening

http://www.asge.org/doc/85

Sponsor ➢ American Society for Gastrointestinal Endoscopy (ASGE)

Description ➢ ASGE position on colorectal cancer screening

Data type ➢ Text

Access requirements ➢ Open

Supplemental resources ➢ ASGE homepage **(http://www.asge.org/)**
ASGE legislative actions **(http://www.asge.org/doc/82)**

User tips ➢ See bin for gastroenterology and hepatology fact sheet

Keywords ➢ gastrointestinal endoscopy

The Longitudinal Muscle in Esophageal Disease

http://www.inxpress.net/~oastiennon/

Sponsor ➢ O. Arthur Stiennon, M.D.

Description ➢ Reference on longitudinal muscle; topics include Boolean model of the esophagus; sphincter; Mallory-Weiss syndrome; and other topics

Data type ➢ Text

Access requirements ➢ Open

Supplemental resources ➢ Chapter: Gas/bloat and physiology of belching **(http://www.inxpress.net/~oastiennon/webdoc10.htm)**
Chapter: Function of hiccups **(http://www.inxpress.net/~oastiennon/webdoc21.htm)**

User tips ➢ Hard copy available with complete set of illustrations

Keywords ➢ esophageal disease

Minimally invasive surgery for heartburn
http://www.ccf.org/pc/misc/nfnissen.htm

Sponsor ➢	Minimally Invasive Surgery Center, Cleveland Clinic Foundation (CCF)
Description ➢	Report on heartburn surgery
Data type ➢	Text; some graphics
Access requirements ➢	Open
Supplemental resources ➢	CCF homepage **(http://www.ccf.org/pc/misc/mishome.htm)**
User tips ➢	Check homepage link to surgical procedures
Keywords ➢	heartburn surgery

National Digestive Diseases Information Clearinghouse (NDDIC)
http://www.niddk.nih.gov/Brochures/NDDIC.htm

Sponsor ➢	National Institute of Diabetes and Digestive and Kidney Diseases (NIDDK), National Institutes of Health (NIH)
Description ➢	Information and referral service regarding digestive and kidney diseases
Data type ➢	Database of text; journals; directories
Access requirements ➢	Open
Supplemental resources ➢	NIDDK homepage **(http://www.niddk.nih.gov/)** Digestive diseases dictionary **(http://www.niddk.nih.gov/DDDCTNRY/INDEX.HTM)**
User tips ➢	See databases for health professionals
Keywords ➢	digestive diseases dictionary diabetes

Overview of UK national groin hernia outcomes project

http://www.rcseng.ac.uk/res&aud/audit/hernia/

Sponsor ➢ Royal College of Surgeons of England

Description ➢ Overview, aims, and methodology of project

Data type ➢ Text

Access requirements ➢ Open

Supplemental resources ➢ Stapling technique for prosthetic hernia repair **(http://www.2020tech.com/hernia/stapling.html)**
Hernia repair methods, Lichtenstein Hernia Institute **(http://www.2020tech.com/hernia/index.html)**

User tips ➢ See Lichtenstein bins for additional hernia surgical data

Keywords ➢ hernia

Pressure ulcer research

http://www.npuap.org/prevmon.html

Sponsor ➢ National Pressure Ulcer Advisory Panel (NPUAP)

Description ➢ Prevention monograph: Ulcer etiology, assessment, and early intervention

Data type ➢ Monograph

Access requirements ➢ Open

Supplemental resources ➢ NPUAP homepage **(http://www.npuap.org/)**
Introduction to NPUAP **(http://www.npuap.org/historg.html)**

User tips ➢ See link for European Pressure Ulcer Advisory Panel (EPUAP)

Keywords ➢ digestive disorders

Prevention and treatment of complications of diabetes
http://www.cdc.gov/nccdphp/ddt/ddt/brn_tx2.htm

Sponsor ➢ National Center for Chronic Disease Prevention and Health Promotion (NCCDPHP), Centers for Disease Control and Prevention (CDC)

Description ➢ Guide for primary care practitioners

Data type ➢ Text

Access requirements ➢ Open

Supplemental resources ➢ Diabetes homepage **(http://www.cdc.gov/nccdphp/ddt/ddthome.htm)**

User tips ➢ Check homepage for diabetes gallery of clip art

Keywords ➢ diabetes

Research agenda on liver and related diseases
http://gi.ucsf.edu/alf/alf/alfpubpol.html

Sponsor ➢ American Liver Foundation (ALF)

Description ➢ Draft of ALF federal public policy agenda through December 31, 1998, rated according to priority level

Data type ➢ Text

Access requirements ➢ Open

Supplemental resources ➢ ALF homepage **(http://sadieo.ucsf.edu/alf/alffinal/homepagealf.html)**
Diet and hepatitis C **(http://gi.ucsf.edu/alf/info/diethcv.html)**

User tips ➢ Check homepage for ALF policy on needle exchange policy

Keywords ➢ liver research
needle exchange policy

Treatment of reflux esophagitis
http://pharminfo.com/meeting/ACG/acg_ehlb12.html

Sponsor ➢ American College of Gastroenterology (ACG)

Description ➢ Highlights from ACG 60th Annual Scientific Meeting

Data type ➢ Text

Access requirements ➢ Open

Supplemental resources ➢ Pharmaceutical Information Network (PharmInfoNet) gastroenterological resources **(http://pharminfo.com/meeting/ACG/acg_hp.html)**
Heartburn **(http://pharminfo.com/meeting/ACG/acg_ehlb1.html)**

User tips ➢ Check homepage for complete index of bulletins

Keywords ➢ heartburn
reflux esophagitis

General Medicine

Adolescent health, state of the nation
http://www.cdc.gov/nccdphp/dash/ahson/ahson/htm

Sponsor ➢	Division of Adolescent and School Health (DASH), National Center for Chronic Disease Prevention and Health Promotion (NCCDPHP), CDC
Description ➢	Monograph on pregnancy, sexually transmitted diseases, and risk behaviors among U.S. adolescents
Data type ➢	Monograph
Access requirements ➢	Open
Supplemental resources ➢	What is DASH? **(http://www.cdc.gov/nccdphp/dash/what.htm)** School health program funding opportunities **(http://www.cdc.gov/nccdphp/dash/funding.htm)**
User tips ➢	Monograph includes individual state profiles
Keywords ➢	adolescent health health funding, school

Adolescent suicide prevention
http://hiru.mcmaster.ca/ohcen/groups/hthu/95-12.htm

Sponsor ➢	Ontario Health Care Evaluation Network (OHCEN)
Description ➢	Curriculum-based suicide prevention program emphasizing teen suicide risk factors, implications for research and public health nursing practice
Data type ➢	Report
Access requirements ➢	Open
Supplemental resources ➢	Overview of adolescent suicide prevention programs **(http://hiru.mcmaster.ca/ohcen/groups/hthu/95-12sum.htm)** Radio transcript, youth suicide **(http://www.abc.net.au/rn/talks/8.30/helthrpt/hstories/hr070805.htm)**
User tips ➢	Note: Site no longer updated due to funding problems
Keywords ➢	adolescent suicide

African-American crisis in health care
http://www.unctv.org/localpro/local01/bifserie/bif00g.htm

Sponsor ➢	UNC-TV
Description ➢	Article, African-American health care
Data type ➢	Text
Access requirements ➢	Open
Supplemental resources ➢	Questionnaire assessing cultural issues in health care **(http://fbhc.org/Professionals/CulturalComp/assess.html)** Association of American Indian Physicians (AAIP), traditional medicine clerkship program **(http://www.aaip.com/tmclerk.html)**
User tips ➢	See terms and concepts for cultural issues assessment
Keywords ➢	cross-cultural medicine

AMA Physician Select (online doctor finder)

http://www.ama-assn.org/aps/amahg.htm

Sponsor ➢ American Medical Association (AMA)

Description ➢ AMA database on 650,000 U.S. licensed physicians

Data type ➢ Search enabled

Access requirements ➢ Open

Supplemental resources ➢ Reference library, migraine, asthma, HIV/AIDS **(http://www.ama-assn.org/aps/amahg.htm)**

User tips ➢ Search for physician by name, condition, or medical specialty

Keywords ➢ U.S. physician database

Ambulatory research with family physicians

http://www.tafp.com/starnet.htm

Sponsor ➢ State of Texas Ambulatory Research Network, Texas Academy of Family Physicians

Description ➢ Starnet, network to assist family physicians in designing and implementing practice-based research projects

Data type ➢ Text

Access requirements ➢ Open

Supplemental resources ➢ Rad tech compliance
(http://www.tafp.org/)
Texas Academy homepage
(http://www.tafp.org/)

User tips ➢ Research initiative restricted to Texas family physicians

Keywords ➢ family physicians
ambulatory research

Annals clinical extracts

http://www.acponline.org/index.htm

Sponsor ➢ American College of Physicians (ACP)

Description ➢ New ways to look at clinical information online

Data type ➢ Text

Access requirements ➢ Open; some sites restricted to members

Supplemental resources ➢ ACP homepage
(http://www.acponline.org/index.html)
Guidelines, laboratory evaluation of diagnosis of Lyme disease (December 15, 1997 issue)
(http://www.acponline.org/journals/annals/annaltoc.htm)

User tips ➢ Current on-line edition of *Annals of Internal Medicine* available

Keywords ➢ Lyme disease

Anti-aging data sources

http://worldhealth.net/

Sponsor ➢ World Health Network, American Academy of Anti-Aging Medicine

Description ➢ News, publications, and clinics describing longevity and anti-aging research

Data type ➢ Text; graphics

Access requirements ➢ Open

Supplemental resources ➢ Longevity Institute International
(http://www.liilongevity.com/test.cfm)

User tips ➢ Check homepage for anti-aging clinics

Keywords ➢ anti-aging
longevity

Certification of foreign medical graduates

http://www.ecfmg.org/

Sponsor ➢ Educational Commission for Foreign Medical Graduates (ECFMG)

Description ➢ Overview of certification program for foreign medical school graduates

Data type ➢ Text

Access requirements ➢ Open

Supplemental resources ➢ Clinical skills assessment **(http://www.ecfmg.org/csa.htm)**

User tips ➢ Graduates should obtain the most current information booklet

Keywords ➢ medical certification, foreign

EthnoMed: Ethnic Medicine Guide

http://www.hslib.washington.edu/clinical/ethnomed/

Sponsor ➢ Harborview Medical Center, University of Washington

Description ➢ Cultural profiles (Cambodian, Vietnamese, etc.) as related to health

Data type ➢ Text

Access requirements ➢ Open; search enabled

Supplemental resources ➢ Report, patient materials in languages using non-Roman alphabets **(http://www.hslib.washington.edu/clinical/ethnomed/pateduc.html#background)**
Cambodian cultural profile **(http://www.hslib.washington.edu/clinical/ethnomed/cambcp.html#food)**

User tips ➢ See sample of non-Roman text

Keywords ➢ cross-cultural medicine

European pancreas transplant activities
http://www.transplant.org/eur/WWW/Organs/Pancreas/rechts.html

Sponsor ➢ Eurotransplant Foundation, The Netherlands

Description ➢ Transplant references, medication, and organizations

Data type ➢ Text; photographs; images

Access requirements ➢ Open

Supplemental resources ➢ Eurotransplant transplant facts and figures **(http://www.transplant.org/eur/WWW/FactFigures/tabel.html)**
About Eurotransplant **(http://www.transweb.org/eur/WWW/Eurotransplant/rechts.html)**

User tips ➢ Check links for patient organizations

Keywords ➢ transplantation

Family health
http://www.tcom.ohiou.edu/family-health.html

Sponsor ➢ College of Osteopathic Medicine and the Telecommunications Center, Ohio University

Description ➢ Series of 2½ minute audio family health programs such as arthritis in children, cookware, hormone replacement therapy, and other topics

Data type ➢ Audio tapes

Access requirements ➢ Requires 14.4 modem; RealAudio player

Supplemental resources ➢ Index **(http://www.tcom.ohiou.edu/family-health.html)**

User tips ➢ Free family health recipe substitution guide available

Keywords ➢ family health
nutrition

Generalist Physician Initiative (GPI)

http://charlotte.hsc.missouri.edu/

Sponsor ➢ Robert Wood Johnson Foundation

Description ➢ Primary care education for the 21st century; lessons from national initiatives

Data type ➢ Reports

Access requirements ➢ Open

Supplemental resources ➢ Progress reports, 1996, 1997 **(http://charlotte.hsc.missouri.edu/progress/index.html)**

User tips ➢ See "call for papers"

Keywords ➢ primary care

Guidelines for Adolescent Preventive Services (GAPS)

http://www.ama-assn.org/adolhlth/recomend/monogrf1.htm#immunizations

Sponsor ➢ American Medical Association (AMA)

Description ➢ Guideline recommendations for physicians and other health professionals

Data type ➢ Text; graphics

Access requirements ➢ Open

Supplemental resources ➢ AMA health focus for teens **(http://www.ama-assn.org/insight/h_focus/adl_hlth/teen/teen.htm)**

User tips ➢ Check AMA homepage for additional medical links

Keywords ➢ adolescent health

Health care quality registers in Sweden
http://www.sos.se/mars/kva040/kva040.htm#why

Sponsor ➢ National Board of Health and Welfare, Sweden

Description ➢ Descriptions and categories of health care quality registers in Sweden, 1996–1997

Data type ➢ Text

Access requirements ➢ Open

Supplemental resources ➢ National Board homepage
(http://www.sos.se/sosmenye.htm)
Postgraduate training programs in international health
(http://www.medicusmundi.ch/courses.htm)

User tips ➢ See Board homepage for major projects

Keywords ➢ health care registers, Sweden
international health, postgraduate level

Healthy People 2000 fact sheet
http://nhic-nt.health.org/nmp/hp2kpage/hp2kfct1.htm

Sponsor ➢ Office of Public Health and Science (OPHS), U.S. Department of Health and Human Services (DHHS)

Description ➢ Healthy People 2000 goals and midcourse review of objectives

Data type ➢ Text

Access requirements ➢ Open

Supplemental resources ➢ Healthy People 2000 family planning resource list
(http://nhic-nt.health.org/nmp/hp2kpage/5family2.htm)
OPHS homepage
(http://phs.os.dhhs.gov/progorg/ophs/index3.htm)

User tips ➢ Check homepage menu of topics

Keywords ➢ public health

High blood cholesterol in adults
http://dragon.labmed.umn.edu/~relson/atp_home.html

Sponsor ➢ National Cholesterol Education Program (NCEP), National Heart, Lung, and Blood Institute (NHLBI), NIH

Description ➢ Second report on detection, evaluation, and treatment of high blood cholesterol in adults

Data type ➢ Report

Access requirements ➢ Open

Supplemental resources ➢ Executive summary **(http://dragon.labmed.umn.edu/~relson/atpsum.html)**
Contents page **(http://dragon.labmed.umn.edu/~relson/atptoc.html)**

User tips ➢ Complete report available

Keywords ➢ cholesterol

Hospice fact sheet
http://www.nho.org/facts.htm

Sponsor ➢ National Hospice Organization (NHO)

Description ➢ Hospice and patient counts, updated July 1, 1997

Data type ➢ Text

Access requirements ➢ Open

Supplemental resources ➢ NHO resolution on assisted suicide (adopted November 1996) **(http://www.nho.org/pasres2.htm)**
NHO statement opposing legalization of euthanasia and assisted suicide **(http://www.nho.org/pasposition.htm)**

User tips ➢ See NHO homepage for additional data

Keywords ➢ hospice

Information for providers

http://www.health.state.ny.us/nysdoh/provider/provider.htm

Sponsor ➢ New York State Department of Health

Description ➢ Files for biomedical ethics; clinical practice guidelines; financial/health care reform; hospital occupancy statistics

Data type ➢ Text; tables

Access requirements ➢ Open; for health care providers

Supplemental resources ➢ Public health priorities **(http://www.health.state.ny.us/nysdoh/phforum/summary.htm)**

User tips ➢ See bin for researchers

Keywords ➢ health policy

Information overload of physicians

http://ahcpr.gov/research/physprac.htm

Sponsor ➢ Agency for Health Care Policy and Research (AHCPR), U.S. Department of Health and Human Services (DHHS)

Description ➢ Summary of report: Information to guide physician practice; analyzes opportunities and problems posed by electronic information sources

Data type ➢ Text

Access requirements ➢ Open

Supplemental resources ➢ Clinical guidelines and reports for medical professionals **(http://www.ahcpr.gov/clinic/clintxt.htm)**
AHCPR homepage **(http://www.ahcpr.gov/data/)**

User tips ➢ Study available on disk; see site for instructions

Keywords ➢ medical computers
clinical guidelines

The interactive patient

http://medicus.marshall.edu/medicus.htm

Sponsor ➢ Marshall University School of Medicine

Description ➢ Teaching tool using interactive responses to patient complaint

Data type ➢ Interactive tool with answers submitted and evaluated

Access requirements ➢ Open to physicians, residents and medical students

Supplemental resources ➢ Interactive program **(http://medicus.marshall.edu/cgi-win/imagemap.exe/histmenu?50,48)**

User tips ➢ Users encouraged to submit diagnosis and treatment plan

Keywords ➢ medical education

Medic Alert purpose

http://www.medicalert.org/Pages/Pages/b_atrisk/b_risk01.html

Sponsor ➢ Medic Alert

Description ➢ Descriptions of 200 conditions requiring Medic Alert identification

Data type ➢ Text; graphics

Access requirements ➢ Open

Supplemental resources ➢ International medical links **(http://www.ama-assn.org/med_link/wintnatl.htm)**

User tips ➢ Hyperlinked search available for international medical links site

Keywords ➢ Medic Alert
international health

Medical palmtop PCs

http://med-amsa.bu.edu/AMSA/palmtop/writing.html#Article 1

Sponsor ➢ University of Arizona College of Medicine

Description ➢ Patient care using Hewlett-Packard palmtop PCs

Data type ➢ Report

Access requirements ➢ Open

Supplemental resources ➢ Newton Medical site and archive of software for patient management **(http://med-amsa.bu.edu/newton.medical/newton.medical.PM.html)**

User tips ➢ Hyperlinks provided for patient management software

Keywords ➢ medical computers, palmtop PCs
patient management software

Medical robotics

http://robotics.eecs.berkeley.edu/~mcenk/medical#vr

Sponsor ➢ Robotics and Intelligent Machines Laboratory, University of California at Berkeley

Description ➢ Report describing telesurgical workstations, virtual reality training simulator, and other robotics in minimally invasive surgery (MIS)

Data type ➢ Report

Access requirements ➢ Open

Supplemental resources ➢ Laboratory homepage **(http://robotics.eecs.berkeley.edu/)**

User tips ➢ Check homepage for list of additional topic papers

Keywords ➢ medical robotics
telemedicine

Minority Health Resource Center

http://www.omhrc.gov/welcome.htm#TOC

Sponsor ➢ Office of Minority Health (OMH), U.S. Department of Health and Human Services (DHHS)

Description ➢ News and programs from the Office of Minority Health

Data type ➢ Text

Access requirements ➢ Open

Supplemental resources ➢ Legislative report **(http://www.omhrc.gov/Legis/Current.HTM#7)**
Office of Minority Health homepage **(http://www.hhs.gov/progorg/ophs/omh/)**

User tips ➢ Check OMH headline page

Keywords ➢ minority health

Multimedia clinical examination

http://www.crc.nus.sg/CH/students/mce.html

Sponsor ➢ Eugene Loke and the National University of Singapore

Description ➢ Summarized reference notes of modules for psychological medicine, neonatology, pediatrics, and surgical approaches

Data type ➢ Multimedia

Access requirements ➢ For medical students

Supplemental resources ➢ Stones in urology **(http://ch.nus.sg/CH/students/mce/surgery/k-stones.html)**
Surgical module contents **(http://ch.nus.sg/CH/students/mce/surgery/surgery.html)**

User tips ➢ Check link for Cyberspace Hospital

Keywords ➢ clinical examination
medical education

National Pain Data Bank
http://www.AAPAINMANAGE.org/npdb/graphs.html

Sponsor ➢ American Academy of Pain Management (AAPM)

Description ➢ Approach for assessing patient responses to pain management treatment

Data type ➢ Data bank and instructions for utilization

Access requirements ➢ Open; primarily a professional resource

Supplemental resources ➢ AAPM homepage
(http://www.AAPAINMANAGE.org/)
Patient's bill of rights
(http://www.AAPAINMANAGE.org/)

User tips ➢ Data bank is presented as an experimental page

Keywords ➢ pain management

National Resident Matching Program (NRMP)
http://www.aamc.org/about/progemph/nrmp/start.htm

Sponsor ➢ Association of American Medical Colleges (AAMC)

Description ➢ Organizational data describing resident matching process

Data type ➢ Data

Access requirements ➢ Open

Supplemental resources ➢ AAMC homepage
(http://www.aamc.org/start.htm)
American Medical Student Association
(http://www.amsa.org/)

User tips ➢ See AMSA statement on affirmative action

Keywords ➢ affirmative action
medical education

Policies for graduate medical education review

http://www.acgme.org/acgme/polprod/MPCONTS.htm

Sponsor ➢ Accreditation Council for Graduate Medical Education (ACGME)

Description ➢ ACGME accreditation procedures for graduate medical programs

Data type ➢ Text

Access requirements ➢ Open

Supplemental resources ➢ ACGME homepage **(http://WWW.ACGME.ORG/)**
Types of graduate medical education programs **(http://www.acgme.org/acgme/polprod/types.htm)**

User tips ➢ See ACGME homepage for site index

Keywords ➢ medical education, graduate

Post-traumatic stress disorder and aircraft incidents

http://www.gretmar.com/webdoctor/aviation.html

Sponsor ➢ Aerospace Medical Association

Description ➢ Site features data related to aeromedical aspects of flight; topics include neurological fitness in pilots, night takeoffs, and other topics

Data type ➢ Data; images

Access requirements ➢ Open

Supplemental resources ➢ Federal Aviation Administration (FAA), U.S. Department of Transportation, aviation medicine report indexes **(http://amelia.db.erau.edu/Reference/faa_indexes.html)**
Aerospace Medical Association homepage **(http://www.asma.org/index.html)**

User tips ➢ FAA medicine reports can be accessed by year, author, or subject

Keywords ➢ aerospace medicine

Poverty reduction and the World Bank, 1996 and 1997

http://www.worldbank.org/html/extdr/pov_red/default.htm

Sponsor ➢	World Bank Group
Description ➢	Report reviews progress in implementation of the World Bank's poverty reduction strategy
Data type ➢	Report
Access requirements ➢	Open
Supplemental resources ➢	Executive summary **(http://www.worldbank.org/html/extdr/pov_red/execsum.htm)** World Bank and HIV/AIDS **(http://www.worldbank.org/html/Welcome.html)**
User tips ➢	See World Bank Annual Report 1997
Keywords ➢	poverty HIV/AIDS

Primary care baseline

http://www.med.ufl.edu/medinfo/baseline/index.html

Sponsor ➢	Richard Rathe, MD, Office of Medical Informatics, University of Florida
Description ➢	Medical notebook of primary care pearls on clinical algorithms and list of drugs
Data type ➢	Text; graphics; professional resource
Access requirements ➢	Open
Supplemental resources ➢	How to use this notebook **(http://www.med.ufl.edu/medinfo/baseline/extras/help.html)** Comparison of informatics curricula at various institutions **(http://www.med.ufl.edu/medinfo/sgea/infocurr.html)**
User tips ➢	See homepage for additional Internet medical education data
Keywords ➢	medical computers medical education

Rural health services

http://www.nal.usda.gov/ric/richs/

Sponsor ➢	Rural Information Center Health Services, Office of Rural Health Policy, Health Resources Services Administration (HRSA)
Description ➢	Information on rural health issues, including funding resources, telecommunications, and health care projects
Data type ➢	Text
Access requirements ➢	Open
Supplemental resources ➢	Telemedicine rural systems **(http://www.nal.usda.gov/ric/richs/chapter.htm)** Occupational definition of rural areas **(http://www.nal.usda.gov/ric/richs/goldsmit.htm)**
User tips ➢	Check research centers
Keywords ➢	rural health telemedicine

Transformation of the U.S. health care market

http://www.rwjf.org/health/dec95.htm

Sponsor ➢	Robert Wood Johnson Foundation
Description ➢	Health tracking: Lessons from 15 communities
Data type ➢	Report
Access requirements ➢	Open
Supplemental resources ➢	Applying for a grant **(http://www.rwjf.org/grant/jgrant.htm)** Health tracking index **(http://www.rwjf.org/health/jhealth.htm)**
User tips ➢	Check Robert Woods Johnson Foundation 1997 media resource guide on tobacco
Keywords ➢	managed care smoking

Transplantation resources on the Internet

http://www.transweb.org/resources_index.html

Sponsor ➢ TransWeb

Description ➢ Transplant centers with Web sites for organ-sharing networks, hospitals, compliance, and donations

Data type ➢ Text

Access requirements ➢ Open

Supplemental resources ➢ Transplant research developments **(http://www.transweb.org/news/research_index.html)**
Post-renal transplant compliance (cognition, emotions, and coping behaviors) **(http://www.transweb.org/news/siegal.html)**

User tips ➢ See link for organ and tissue donation, issues and answers

Keywords ➢ transplants
organ-tissue donations

Twin-to-twin transfusion

http://www.tttsfoundation.org/

Sponsor ➢ Twin-to-Twin Transfusion Syndrome (TTTS) Foundation

Description ➢ Data describing organizational support for TTTS placenta disease

Data type ➢ Text; some graphics

Access requirements ➢ Open

Supplemental resources ➢ Medical professional's guide to TTTS **(http://www.tttsfoundation.org/ProGuide.htm)**

User tips ➢ See incidence figures of twin-to-twin syndrome

Keywords ➢ twin-to-twin syndrome

Health Funding Policy

Acronym dictionary
http://www.wpc-edi.com/AcronymDictionary/Dictionary.html

Sponsor ➢	Washington Publishing Company
Description ➢	Dictionary of abbreviations utilized by electronic data and commerce
Data type ➢	Text
Access requirements ➢	Free download for Electronic Data Interchange (EDI)
Supplemental resources ➢	Health claim adjustment reason codes **(http://www.wpc-edi.com/Health/a.htm)** Implementation guides for Health Insurance Portability and Accountability Act (HIPAA) **(http://www.wpc-edi.com/hipaa/)**
User tips ➢	Required user ID and password are free
Keywords ➢	health insurance

Advocacy papers: Improving Medicare and Medicaid

http://www.aha.org/AdvPapers.html

Sponsor ➢ American Hospital Association (AHA)

Description ➢ Advocacy papers on Medicare managed care payments, skilled nursing facilities, outpatient services, and other issues

Data type ➢ Text

Access requirements ➢ Open

Supplemental resources ➢ AHA homepage **(http://www.aha.org/default.html)**

User tips ➢ Check AHA homepage for 1998 public policy advocacy agenda

Keywords ➢ hospitals
Medicare, Medicaid

AHCPR data and surveys

http://www.ahcpr.gov/data/

Sponsor ➢ Agency for Health Care Policy and Research (AHCPR)

Description ➢ Statistical data according to diagnosis, hospital inpatient, HIV-AIDS costs and utilization, and other information

Data type ➢ Tables and research notes

Access requirements ➢ Download with free Adobe Acrobat Reader software

Supplemental resources ➢ Healthcare Cost and Utilization Project (HCUP-3) **(http://www.access.gpo.gov/ahcpr/index.html)**
Clinical classifications for health policy research, version 2 software **(http://www.access.gpo.gov/ahcpr/hcuprn2.html#note2)**

User tips ➢ Check homepage for HIV-AIDS costs and utilization

Keywords ➢ HIV-AIDS costs
medical software

AMA releases on physician assisted suicide
http://www.ama-assn.org/ad-com/releases/1996/tr329.htm

Sponsor ➢	American Medical Association (AMA)
Description ➢	AMA releases on court decisions related to physician assisted suicide
Data type ➢	Text
Access requirements ➢	Open
Supplemental resources ➢	Maclean Center for Clinical Medical Ethics (CCME) end of life resources (euthanasia, assisted suicide ethics) **(http://ccme-mac4.bsd.uchicago.edu/CCMEDocs/Death)**
User tips ➢	See CCME sites for links to international death and dying resources
Keywords ➢	assisted suicide euthanasia

Assisted suicide in Canada
http://www.parl.gc.ca/english/senate/com-e/euth-e/rep-e/lad-tc-e.htm

Sponsor ➢	Special Senate Committee on Euthanasia and Assisted Suicide, Canada
Description ➢	Of Life and Death—Final Report, June 1995
Data type ➢	Report
Access requirements ➢	Open
Supplemental resources ➢	Special Senate homepage **(http://www.parl.gc.ca/english/senate/com-e/euth-e.htm)**
User tips ➢	Available in French and English
Keywords ➢	assisted suicide

Assisted suicide statement

http://www.aahpm.org/main.shtml

Sponsor ➢ American Academy of Hospice and Palliative Medicine

Description ➢ Guidelines by the Academy

Data type ➢ Text

Access requirements ➢ Open

Supplemental resources ➢ Certification in hospice and palliative medicine **(http://www.aahpm.org/main.shtml)**

User tips ➢ Check Academy funding opportunities

Keywords ➢ assisted suicide

Congressional Medicare testimony, 1997

http://www.PPRC.GOV/congtest.htm

Sponsor ➢ Medicare Payment Advisory Commission

Description ➢ Hyperlinked files of Congressional testimony by the Commission

Data type ➢ PDF files

Access requirements ➢ Open; direct access

Supplemental resources ➢ Commission responsibilities **(http://www.PPRC.GOV/respons2.htm)**
Physician Payment Review Commission **(http://www.PPRC.GOV/)**

User tips ➢ See list of Physician Payment Review Commission meetings

Keywords ➢ Medicare

Death and dying

http://www.nap.edu/readingroom/books/approaching/

Sponsor ➢ Division of Health Care Services, Institute of Medicine

Description ➢ Reference: *Approaching Death: Improving Care at the End of Life*

Data type ➢ Book

Access requirements ➢ Open

Supplemental resources ➢ Institute of Medicine homepage **(http://www.nas.edu/)**
Institute of Medicine, full report on emergency preparation for handling terrorist attacks **(http://www.nas.edu/)**

User tips ➢ See Institute homepage for report on blood banking and regulation, procedures, problems, and alternatives

Keywords ➢ emergency
death-dying

Federal research and education funding opportunities

http://www.rams-fie.com/opportunity.htm

Sponsor ➢ FEDIX

Description ➢ Search tool for funding announcements from eleven federal participating agencies, including Departments of Energy, Defense, Agriculture, and others

Data type ➢ Text

Access requirements ➢ Open

Supplemental resources ➢ FEDIX homepage **(http://web.fie.com/htdoc/fed/all/any/any/menu/any/index.htm)**
Grant related electronic newsletter **(http://www.rams-fie.com/opportunity.htm)**

User tips ➢ Register for e-mail announcements of funding opportunities

Keywords ➢ funding

Funding opportunities database
http://cos.gdb.org/repos/fund/

Sponsor ➢ Cleveland Clinic Foundation

Description ➢ Funding opportunities database for participating institutions and specific disciplines

Data type ➢ Database

Access requirements ➢ Open; search enabled site

Supplemental resources ➢ Expertise database
(http://www.ccf.org/ri/CCFCOS.html)
Databases of federally funded research in the United States
(http://www.ccf.org/ri/CCFCOS.html)

User tips ➢ Add your credentials to the expertise database

Keywords ➢ funding

Health care for the homeless
http://www.nashville.net/~hch/index.html

Sponsor ➢ National Health Care for the Homeless Council

Description ➢ Resources for improved health for the homeless

Data type ➢ Text

Access requirements ➢ Open

Supplemental resources ➢ Clinical guidelines for tuberculosis prevention among the homeless
(http://www.nashville.net/~hch/clinical.html)
National Coalition for the Homeless
(http://nch.ari.net/)

User tips ➢ Free mobile health care planning kit available

Keywords ➢ homelessness
tuberculosis control

Managed care
http://www.hrsa.dhhs.gov/hrsa/mngdcare/cmc.htm

Sponsor ➢ Center for Managed Care, Health Resources and Services Administration (HRSA), DHHS

Description ➢ HRSA managed care activities, publications, and data sources

Data type ➢ Text

Access requirements ➢ Open

Supplemental resources ➢ National Center for Health Workforce Information and Analysis, HRSA
(http://www.hrsa.dhhs.gov/bhpr/ORP/wiaaproj.htm)
Bureau of Health Professions (BHPr), HRSA homepage
(http://www.hrsa.dhhs.gov/bhpr/bhpr.html)

User tips ➢ Download report on HRSA and managed care

Keywords ➢ health workforce data
managed care

Medicaid consumer information
http://www.hcfa.gov/medicaid/mcaicnsm.htm

Sponsor ➢ Health Care Financing Administration (HCFA)

Description ➢ Site includes files on Medicaid information, Welfare Reform, fraud and abuse, state and federal 800 contact numbers

Data type ➢ Text

Access requirements ➢ Open

Supplemental resources ➢ Professional/technical information
(http://www.hcfa.gov/medicaid/mcaidpti.htm)

User tips ➢ Check link for Medicaid policies under the Balanced Budget Act of 1997

Keywords ➢ Medicaid

Medicaid managed care

http://www.chcs.org/mmcp.htm

Sponsor ➢ Center for Health Care Strategies (CHCS)

Description ➢ CHCS funding activities for Medicaid managed care strategies

Data type ➢ Text

Access requirements ➢ Open

Supplemental resources ➢ Medicaid managed care alphabet soup **(http://www.chcs.org/mmcsoup.htm)**

User tips ➢ See CHCS homepage for grant information

Keywords ➢ managed care
health funding

Medicare-Medicaid public use data files

http://www.hcfa.gov/stats/stats.htm

Sponsor ➢ Health Care Financing Administration (HCFA)

Description ➢ Statistics, tutorials, and resource files on Medicare-Medicaid

Data type ➢ Text; tutorials; databases

Access requirements ➢ Open; decompressed files require PKWare for unzipping

Supplemental resources ➢ Public use data files for providers, cost limits, renal dialysis facilities **(http://www.hcfa.gov/stats/pufiles.htm)**
HCFA Research Data Assistance Center (ResDac) for researchers **(http://www.hcfa.gov/ord/resdac0.htm)**

User tips ➢ See stats and data page for National Health Expenditures, 1960–1995

Keywords ➢ Medicare
Medicaid

Medicine and public health
http://www.nyam.org/pubhlth/medpubl.html

Sponsor ➢	New York Academy of Medicine
Description ➢	Paper emphasizing the relationship between medicine and public health; Academy is a premier source of current and historical medical data
Data type ➢	Text
Access requirements ➢	Open
Supplemental resources ➢	American Public Health Association (APHA) homepage **(http://www.apha.org/)** APHA legislative affairs and advocacy **(http://www.apha.org/)**
User tips ➢	See APHA homepage for public health resources
Keywords ➢	public health

National and international standards for healthcare codes
http://www.mcis.duke.edu/standards/HL7/termcode/codehome.htm

Sponsor ➢	Duke University Medical Center
Description ➢	Links to coding systems representing health care concepts; LOINC (laboratory and clinical terms); Snomed (multi-axial code for medical vocabulary); National Library of Medicine Unified Medical Language System (UMLS); and others
Data type ➢	Hyperlinks
Access requirements ➢	Open
Supplemental resources ➢	Healthcare informatics standards homepage **(http://www.mcis.duke.edu/standards/guide.htm)** *Dx International Classification of Diseases, 9th Revision, Clinical Modification* (ICD-9-CM) **(http://www.mcis.duke.edu/standards/HL7/termcode/icd9cm.htm)**
User tips ➢	Check homepage for links to medical informatics standards groups
Keywords ➢	health care coding systems

National Health Security Plan

http://sunsite.unc.edu:80/nhs/NHS-T-o-C.html

Sponsor ➢ Task Force, National Health Care Reform

Description ➢ Text and supporting documents of the National Health Security Plan

Data type ➢ Text

Access requirements ➢ Open

Supplemental resources ➢ Executive summary **(http://sunsite.unc.edu:80/nhs/executive/X-Summary-toc.html)**

User tips ➢ Check for links for full text of Health Security Act of 1993

Keywords ➢ health reform

National Institutes of Health (NIH) consensus and technology assessment reports

http://text.nlm.nih.gov/ftrs/pick?c...nih&cc=1&oldK=48264&t=884114739

Sponsor ➢ NIH Consensus Development Program, National Institutes of Health (NIH)

Description ➢ Collection of current and outdated consensus conference statements and technology assessment workshop reports

Data type ➢ Text

Access requirements ➢ Open

Supplemental resources ➢ Continuing medical education (CME) examinations for selected conferences **(http://text.nlm.nih.gov/ftrs/pick?c...nih&cc=1&oldK=48264&t=884114739)**
Search page for Technology Assessment Statements **(http://text.nlm.nih.gov/ftrs/pick?f...1&t=884114823&collect=nih&dbName=ta)**

User tips ➢ Search Technology Statements by diagnosis, symptom, or keyword

Keywords ➢ NIH Consensus Conference Reports

National Practitioner Data Bank (NPDB)

http://www.hrsa.dhhs.gov/bhpr/dqa/factshts/fsreport.htm

Sponsor ➢ Bureau of Health Professions, Health Resources and Services Administration, DHHS

Description ➢ Background and purpose of the National Practitioner Data Bank

Data type ➢ Text

Access requirements ➢ Open

Supplemental resources ➢ NPDB fact sheets
(http://www.hrsa.dhhs.gov/bhpr/dqa/factshts.htm)
Executive summary, annual report
(http://www.hrsa.dhhs.gov/bhpr/dqa/96es.htm)

User tips ➢ See NPDB homepage for Healthcare Integrity and Protection Data Bank; contact number: 1-800-767-6732

Keywords ➢ health quality assurance

New Supplemental Security Income (SSI) childhood disability legislation

http://www.ssa.gov/policy/child.htm

Sponsor ➢ Social Security Administration (SSA)

Description ➢ Review of SSA's implementation of childhood disability legislation

Data type ➢ Report

Access requirements ➢ Open

Supplemental resources ➢ SSA online
(http://www.ssa.gov/)
News release, December 19, 1997: SSA review of children with ceased disability benefits
(http://www.ssa.gov/press/childhood_press.html)

User tips ➢ Available in Spanish

Keywords ➢ disability
SSI benefits

Pfizer venture philanthropy

http://www.pfizer.com/pfizerinc/philanthropy/grant/grant.html

Sponsor ➢	Pfizer Corporate Philanthropy Program
Description ➢	Grants assistance for nonprofit organizations
Data type ➢	Text
Access requirements ➢	Open
Supplemental resources ➢	Guidelines **(http://www.pfizer.com/pfizerinc/philanthropy/grant/grant.html)**
User tips ➢	Check link for Foundation Center, New York City, for comprehensive grant and other funding resources
Keywords ➢	funding

Prevailing healthcare charges system (PHCS)

http://www.hiaa.org/healthcare/index.html

Sponsor ➢	Health Insurance Association of America (HIAA)
Description ➢	Description of PHCS data compilation, methodology, and services for professional providers, hospital facilities, and more
Data type ➢	Text
Access requirements ➢	Open; for healthcare providers
Supplemental resources ➢	HIAA homepage **(http://www.hiaa.org/)**
User tips ➢	See homepage for consumer insurance information
Keywords ➢	Prevailing healthcare charges system (PHCS) health insurance

Privatization and public health
http://www.phf.org/priv_execsumm.htm

Sponsor ➢ Public Health Foundation (PHF)

Description ➢ Study of initiatives and early lessons learned from privatization of public health services

Data type ➢ Report

Access requirements ➢ Open

Supplemental resources ➢ PHF homepage
(http://www.phf.org/index.htm)
Management training and distance learning programs and materials
(http://www.phf.org/distance_learning.htm)

User tips ➢ See PHF's Public Health Network for linking public health professionals

Keywords ➢ privatization
distance learning

U.S. medical insurance coverage, 1992–1993
http://www.census.gov/hhes/www/hlth9293.html

Sponsor ➢ U.S. Census Bureau

Description ➢ Statistical breakdown of U.S. medical insurance coverage by sex, race, education, residence, and other characteristics

Data type ➢ Statistical tables and text

Access requirements ➢ Open

Supplemental resources ➢ Highlights of child health insurance provisions, August 1, 1997
(http://www.npnd.org/Childlns.htm)
State initiatives for increasing health insurance access for children
(http://www.ASTHO.org/html/body_featured_state_initiatives.html)

User tips ➢ See *Current Population Reports*, P70-54, Census Bureau, for additional health insurance information

Keywords ➢ health insurance
child health insurance

HIV/AIDS

Abstracts, XI International Conference on AIDS
http://sis.nlm.nih.gov/aidsabs.htm

Sponsor ➢	Organizing Committee of the XI International Conference on AIDS and the National Library of Medicine (NLM)
Description ➢	Search and query tool for program abstracts
Data type ➢	Text
Access requirements ➢	Open
Supplemental resources ➢	Model Performance Evaluation Program (MPEP) **(http://www.cdc.gov/phppo/dis/peppt.htm)** Slide presentation: Quality assurance in HIV testing **(http://www.cdc.gov/phppo/dis/peppt.htm)**
User tips ➢	See HIV/AIDS resource page
Keywords ➢	AIDS abstracts

AIDS health fraud
http://www.applicom.com/tcrs/Fraud.htm

Sponsor ➢	Florida AIDS Health Fraud Task Force
Description ➢	Identification and prevention of AIDS health fraud
Data type ➢	Text
Access requirements ➢	Open
Supplemental resources ➢	Article: AIDS Fraud Task Force **(http://www2.immunet.org/immunet/atn.nsf/page/ZQX04001.html)** National Fraud Information Center (1-800-876-7060) **(http://www.fraud.org)**
User tips ➢	Check list of phone numbers for reliable AIDS treatment resources
Keywords ➢	AIDS fraud

AIDS patent database
http://patents.cnidr.org/welcome.html

Sponsor ➢	U.S. Patent and Trademark Office
Description ➢	AIDS bibliographic and patent databases issued by U.S., Japanese, and European patent offices
Data type ➢	Database
Access requirements ➢	Open
Supplemental resources ➢	AIDS patent browse page **(http://aids.uspto.gov/AIDS/access/browse.html)** AIDS patent search page **(http://aids.uspto.gov/AIDS/access/search.html)**
User tips ➢	All data are public domain documents; site is regularly updated
Keywords ➢	medical informatics

AIDS prevention strategies

http://www.epibiostat.ucsf.edu/capsweb/index.html

Sponsor ➢	Center for AIDS Prevention Studies (CAPS), University of California, San Francisco
Description ➢	AIDS prevention science, program, opportunities, and evaluation
Data type ➢	Reports, monographs, and bibliography
Access requirements ➢	Open
Supplemental resources ➢	Evaluating behavior change efforts **(http://chanane.ucsf.edu/capsweb/toolbox/EVAL02.html)** HIV, STD and unintended pregnancy prevention **(http://www.epibiostat.ucsf.edu/capsweb/STD-HIV.html)**
User tips ➢	See prevention programs, some include full curricula
Keywords ➢	AIDS prevention

The body: A multimedia AIDS and HIV information resource

http://www.thebody.com/cgi-bin/body.cgi

Sponsor ➢	Body Health Resources Corp. and Bristol-Myers, Roxane, Chiron, and Ortho Biotech
Description ➢	Multimedia materials on AIDS basics, treatment, quality of life, and conferences
Data type ➢	Multimedia; search enabled
Access requirements ➢	Open
Supplemental resources ➢	Links for medications, alternative medicine **(http://www.thebody.com/cgi-bin/body.cgi)**
User tips ➢	Register online for updates
Keywords ➢	AIDS treatment

Drug development and approval process in the '90s
http://www.critpath.org/research/process.htm

Sponsor ➢	Critical Path AIDS Project
Description ➢	Description of U.S. system of new drug approval mechanism
Data type ➢	Text; images; diagrams
Access requirements ➢	Open
Supplemental resources ➢	Critical Path AIDS Project homepage **(http://www.critpath.org/critpath.htm)** Three-dimensional diagram of human immunodeficiency virus **(http://www.critpath.org/maturhiv.gif)**
User tips ➢	Project founded by persons with AIDS (PWAs) to provide AIDS resource data
Keywords ➢	AIDS resource AIDS drugs

Framework for antiretroviral therapy
http://www.bmaids.demon.co.uk/pubs/antiret.htm

Sponsor ➢	National Association for Providers of AIDS Care and Treatment (PACT)
Description ➢	Approved PACT framework for antiretroviral therapy
Data type ➢	Text
Access requirements ➢	Open
Supplemental resources ➢	News and policy watch **(http://www.bmaids.demon.co.uk/news.htm)** British Medical Association (BMA) Foundation for AIDS **(http://www.bmaids.demon.co.uk/index.htm)**
User tips ➢	Specialized education tool for health workers
Keywords ➢	AIDS treatment antiretroviral therapy

Guidelines for antiretroviral agents for HIV in adults and adolescents

http:/207.226.163.175/hiv/nihreport/guide/acute.html

Sponsor ➢ Health Care Communications Group

Description ➢ Clinical care options for HIV treatment issues and guidelines

Data type ➢ Report

Access requirements ➢ Open

Supplemental resources ➢ *Antiviral Agents Bulletin* **(http://www.bioinfo.com/antiviral.html)**

User tips ➢ Bulletin; very large file (15 pages)

Keywords ➢ antiviral agents
antiretroviral therapy

HIV/AIDS and health care workers

http://aepo-xdv-www.epo.cdc.gov/wonder/prevguid/p0000344/p0000344.htm

Sponsor ➢ Centers for Disease Control and Prevention (CDC)

Description ➢ HIV/AIDS among health care workers

Data type ➢ Text

Access requirements ➢ Open

Supplemental resources ➢ National AIDS Fund homepage **(http://www.aidsfund.org/)**
Workshop summary: The HIV positive worker **(http://siksik.learnnet.nt.ca/HIV-Aids/hivPosWorker.html)**

User tips ➢ See National AIDS Fund homepage for additional programs

Keywords ➢ occupational health
legal medicine

HIV/AIDS drug assistance programs

http://www.hivpositive.com/f-Resour...-16-PharmDrugPgms/PharmCoPgrms.html

Sponsor ➢ HIV Positive Resources and Assistance

Description ➢ Directory of drugs, companies, and telephone numbers of pharmaceutical company indigent patient programs

Data type ➢ Directory

Access requirements ➢ Open

Supplemental resources ➢ National AIDS hotlines
(http://www.hivpositive.com/f-Resources/f-15A-Hotlines/15-HotNews.html)
HIV testing facts from the Gay Men's Health Committee (GMHC)
(http://www.hivpositive.com/f-TestingHIV/f-Testing/1-HIVtesting.html#test6)

User tips ➢ AIDS hotlines cite 800 numbers

Keywords ➢ AIDS hotline
drug assistance programs

HIV/AIDS treatment information

http://www.hivatis.org/

Sponsor ➢ HIV/AIDS Treatment Information Service (ATIS)

Description ➢ Data about federally approved treatment guidelines for HIV/AIDS

Data type ➢ Text

Access requirements ➢ Open

Supplemental resources ➢ Revised guidelines for use of antiretroviral agents in pediatric HIV infections
(http:/www.hivatis.org/)
CDC NCHSTP Daily News Update, 12/29/97
(http://www.cdcnac.org/summary.txt)

User tips ➢ ATIS bilingual (English and Spanish) staff available

Keywords ➢ AIDS antiretroviral agents
AIDS guidelines

HIV/AIDS treatment

http://www.ama-assn.org/special/hiv/treatmnt/treatmnt.htm

Sponsor ➢ HIV/AIDS Information Center, *Journal of the American Medical Association* (JAMA)

Description ➢ Clinical guidelines; clinical trials resources; treatment updates; drug information

Data type ➢ Text; reports; peer-reviewed resources

Access requirements ➢ Open

Supplemental resources ➢ HIV/AIDS Information Center homepage **(http://www.ama-assn.org/special/hiv/hivhome.htm)**
Ask an expert (for health professionals) **(http://www.ama-assn.org/special/hiv/treatmnt/ask.htm)**

User tips ➢ Expert fax number: 212-354-1169

Keywords ➢ AIDS treatment

HIV/STD prevention in rural America

http://www.indiana.edu/~aids/news/news7.html

Sponsor ➢ Rural Center for AIDS/STD Prevention (RCAP), Indiana University, and Purdue University

Description ➢ Report on rural HIV/AIDS prevention; successful prevention projects; study of rural jails

Data type ➢ Report

Access requirements ➢ Open

Supplemental resources ➢ Rural Center homepage **(http://www.indiana.edu/~aids/)**
AIDS in Botswana, Harvard AIDS Institute **(http://www.hsph.harvard.edu/Organiz...ai_ini/conferen/Botswana/index.html)**

User tips ➢ See list of RCAP projects on homepage

Keywords ➢ AIDS prevention
rural health

Inmates' HIV prevention needs
http://www.epibiostat.ucsf.edu/capsweb/inmatetext.html

Sponsor ➢ Marin AIDS Project (MAP), Center for AIDS Prevention Studies

Description ➢ Report on the impact of HIV and incarceration; obstacles to prevention; and other issues

Data type ➢ Report

Access requirements ➢ Open

Supplemental resources ➢ Marin AIDS Project **(http://www.epibiostat.ucsf.edu/capsweb/projects/mapindex.html)**
Immunet treatment info for AIDS/HIV caregivers **(http://www.immunet.org/immunet/home.nsf/page/homepage)**

User tips ➢ Check Immunet link for online AIDS bookstore

Keywords ➢ HIV in prisons
AIDS prevention

National AIDS Clearinghouse
http://www.cdcnac.org/nacdb.html

Sponsor ➢ Centers for Disease Control and Prevention (CDC)

Description ➢ Directory of 19,000 verified sources, services, and organizations for AIDS

Data type ➢ Text, graphics

Access requirements ➢ Open; search enabled

Supplemental resources ➢ Acquired Immunodeficiency Syndrome **(http://web.fie.com/htdoc/fed/nih/ali/any/text/mti/nihtni15.htm)**
HIV/AIDS Surveillance Report **(http://www.cdc.gov/nchstp/hiv_aids/stats/hasrlink.htm)**

User tips ➢ Select your topics before searching

Keywords ➢ AIDS resource
HIV-AIDS statistics

1997 National Conference on Women and HIV (NCWH)
http://www.iapac.org/clinmgt/ncwh/index.html

Sponsor ➢	International Association of Physicians and AIDS Care (IAPAC)
Description ➢	Abstracts archive featuring behavioral, epidemiology, and policy issues related to HIV in adolescents, adult women, and their families
Data type ➢	Abstracts archive
Access requirements ➢	Open
Supplemental resources ➢	1997 NCWH abstract index **(http://www.iapac.org/clinmgt/ncwh/ncwhtoc.html)** Index, AIDS News Service, Veterans Administration (VA) **(http://gopher.hivnet.org:70/1s/magazines/ans)**
User tips ➢	Review NCWH search and browse instructions
Keywords ➢	women's health

Nutrition in pediatric HIV infection
http://www.hivpositive.com/f-Nutrition/f-3-PediatricNeut/n-Zafonte.html

Sponsor ➢	HIV Positive
Description ➢	Glutathione, vitamin A, and other deficiencies related to HIV infection
Data type ➢	Text
Access requirements ➢	Open
Supplemental resources ➢	HIV and nutrition **(http://www.hivpositive.com/f-Nutrition/NutritionMenu.html)** Pediatric HIV/AIDS links **(http://mail.med.upenn.edu/~jstoller/pedaids.html)**
User tips ➢	Hyperlinked pediatric links include organizations, fact sheets, and articles
Keywords ➢	HIV and nutrition pediatrics

Pediatric AIDS Clinical Trials Group (PACTG)
http://pactg.s-3.com/pinfo.htm

Sponsor ➢	National Institute of Allergy and Infectious Diseases (NIAID) and National Institute for Child Health and Human Development
Description ➢	Overview and background of evaluation initiatives of pediatric AIDS initiatives
Data type ➢	Text
Access requirements ➢	Open
Supplemental resources ➢	Outline of train-the-trainer program for educating school nurses in HIV **(http://www.pedhivaids.org/training/program8.html)**
User tips ➢	See background of PACTG
Keywords ➢	pediatric AIDS

Skin diseases in patients with HIV infection
http://www.mediconsult.com/noframes...rgies/shareware/allergies/9736.html

Sponsor ➢	The Virtual Medical Center
Description ➢	Article summary; professional version available through PharmInfoNet
Data type ➢	Text
Access requirements ➢	Open
Supplemental resources ➢	Cutaneous manifestations of HIV disease **(http://pharminfo.com/disease/immun/aaaai/aai9736p.html)**
User tips ➢	Search site for other HIV topics
Keywords ➢	dermatology

State of the art: HIV vaccines
http://www.critpath.org/aric/dirt/10/index.htm

Sponsor ➢ *The Dirt (on AIDS)*, Direct Information on Research and Treatment

Description ➢ Quarterly newsletter for AIDS service

Data type ➢ Newsletter

Access requirements ➢ Open

Supplemental resources ➢ Main index of current and past issues of *The Dirt* **(http://www.critpath.org/aric/dirtidx.htm)**
FDA/Drug Watch: HIV protease inhibitors **(http://www.critpath.org/aric/dirt/10/fdawatch.htm)**

User tips ➢ See index for Carter's index of AIDS treatments

Keywords ➢ AIDS treatment
AIDS vaccine

Strategic United Nations plan for AIDS (1996–2000)
http://www.us.unaids.org/highband/projects/strat_plan.html#what

Sponsor ➢ Joint United Nations Programme on HIV/AIDS (UNAIDS)

Description ➢ Report on strategic plan (1996–2000) for addressing global AIDS

Data type ➢ Report

Access requirements ➢ Open

Supplemental resources ➢ AIDS Education Global Information System (AEGIS)
(http://www.aegis.com/)

User tips ➢ Check AEGIS for latest world news about AIDS

Keywords ➢ AIDS prevention

Textbook on HIV Disease, 2nd edition

http://hivinsite.ucsf.edu/akb/1994/index.html

Sponsor ➢ AIDS Knowledge Base, University of California; and the San Francisco General Hospital

Description ➢ Complete downloadable textbook on AIDS epidemiology; malignancies, legal issues, and other topics

Data type ➢ Textbook

Access requirements ➢ Open

Supplemental resources ➢ Chapt. 1.11, Table 1: Health-care workers with occupationally acquired HIV infection **(http://hivinsite.ucsf.edu/akb/1994/1-11/toctable1.html)**
Chapter index: The law and health care workers **(http://hivinsite.ucsf.edu/akb/1994/9-1/index.html#9-1-AaA)**

User tips ➢ Check homepage for tables of contents

Keywords ➢ AIDS reference
patient confidentiality

Legal Medicine

Declaration of Helsinki

http://www.ams.med.uni-goettingen.de/~rhilger/dek_htv.html

Sponsor ➢	Gottingen University
Description ➢	Basic principles for guiding physicians in clinical and nontherapeutic biomedical research involving human subjects
Data type ➢	Text
Access requirements ➢	Open
Supplemental resources ➢	ACHRE report, Chapter 1: Use of human subjects **(http://tis-nt.eh.doe.gov/ohre/roadmap/achre/chap1_4.html)** Department of Energy (DOE) openness: Human radiation experiments **(http://tis-nt.eh.doe.gov/ohre/index.html)**
User tips ➢	Gottingen University site in English and German
Keywords ➢	human research subjects medical ethics

Ethics and computerization of medicine
http://ccme-mac4.bsd.uchicago.edu/CCMEdocs/Info

Sponsor ➢ MacLean Center for Clinical Medical Ethics (CCME), University of Chicago

Description ➢ Files on informatics; expert systems in medicine; medical records confidentiality; electronic medical records

Data type ➢ Text

Access requirements ➢ Open

Supplemental resources ➢ Ethics Internet resources
(http://ccme-mac4.bsd.uchicago.edu/CCME.html)
News regarding health information security
(http://www.irongateinc.com/articles.html)

User tips ➢ Check link for medical records and the law

Keywords ➢ medical ethics
medical computers

Federal health care liability reform data
http://www.wp.com/hcla/page.htm

Sponsor ➢ Health Care Liability Alliance (HCLA)

Description ➢ Legislative and background information for resolving health injury disputes

Data type ➢ Text

Access requirements ➢ Open

Supplemental resources ➢ Health care product liability
(http://www.wp.com/hcla/hclaprod.htm)
Federal legislation on medical liability reform
(http://www.wp.com/hcla/hclaleg.htm)

User tips ➢ See homepage for background data regarding lawsuits and higher health care costs

Keywords ➢ medical liability
malpractice

Federal judicial health decisions
http://www.fjc.gov/

Sponsor ➢ Federal Judicial Center

Description ➢ Court decisions regarding MDL-Breast Implant litigation and other health-related decisions

Data type ➢ Searchable index of information

Access requirements ➢ Open

Supplemental resources ➢ U.S. Court of Appeals, Fourth Circuit—1996 decisions
(http://www.law.emory.edu/4circuit/index.1996.html)
Additional legal information servers
(http://www.fjc.gov/WWWlinks/govlinks.html)

User tips ➢ See server page for link to Findlaw database of Supreme Court decisions since 1937

Keywords ➢ legal decisions
breast implants

Health research and public health sites
http://weber.u.washington.edu/~hserv/hsic/resource/phlinks.html

Sponsor ➢ School of Public Health and Community Medicine, University of Washington

Description ➢ Sites with health services and public health information

Data type ➢ Database organized by subject

Access requirements ➢ Open

Supplemental resources ➢ Health care quality assurance
(http://weber.u.washington.edu/~hserv/hsic/resource/q-subj.html)
Report: Managed care quality
(http://www.ncqa.org/news/report.htm)

User tips ➢ Site updated regularly

Keywords ➢ managed care

Law and the physician

http://plague.law.umkc.edu/Xfiles/x_t.htm

Sponsor ➢ Public Health Law Project, University of Missouri at Kansas City

Description ➢ Online book: Rathbun and Richards, *Law and the Physician: A Practical Guide*

Data type ➢ Textbook with hyperlinked chapters

Access requirements ➢ Open

Supplemental resources ➢ Detailed table of contents **(http://plague.law.umkc.edu/Xfiles/xfc.htm)** Medical malpractice costs **(http://www.wp.com/hcla/tilling.htm)**

User tips ➢ Reference topics include physicians as related to patients, public health, family, and other issues

Keywords ➢ legal issues

Legal Medicine Open File 97

http://www.afip.mil/legalmed/openfile97/toc97.html

Sponsor ➢ Department of Legal Medicine, Armed Forces Institute of Pathology (AFIP)

Description ➢ Articles on clinical practice, quality assurance, risk management, and malpractice

Data type ➢ Text

Access requirements ➢ Open

Supplemental resources ➢ Department of Legal Medicine homepage **(http://www.afip.mil/homes/legalmed.html)**

User tips ➢ See instructions for obtaining continuing medical education (CME) credits in legal risk management

Keywords ➢ medical education

List of top health frauds

http://www.fda.gov/opacom/backgrounders/tophealt.html

Sponsor ➢	U.S. Food and Drug Administration (FDA)
Description ➢	Leading health frauds involving products, clinics, and cures
Data type ➢	Text
Access requirements ➢	Open
Supplemental resources ➢	Quackwatch **(http://www.quackwatch.com/index.html)** Health quackery, National Institute on Aging **(http://www.nih.gov/nia/health/pubpub/healthqy.htm)**
User tips ➢	Contact FDA, Consumer Affairs regarding mislabeled or misrepresented products
Keywords ➢	health fraud

Managed health care

http://www.chipp.cahwnet.gov/mctf/front.htm

Sponsor ➢	Managed Health Care Improvement Task Force
Description ➢	Task force report on managed care in California (CA)
Data type ➢	Report
Access requirements ➢	Open
Supplemental resources ➢	Homepage **(http://www.chipp.cahwnet.gov/mctf/front.htm)**
User tips ➢	See homepage for background papers
Keywords ➢	managed care

Medicine and law

http://www.physiciansnews.com/law/dvindex.html

Sponsor ➢ Physician's News Digest

Description ➢ Articles on physician-related legal issues

Data type ➢ Text

Access requirements ➢ Open

Supplemental resources ➢ Genetic testing law, September 11, 1997 **(http://www.physiciansnews.com/law/1197shay.html)**
Medicare chart documentation **(http://www.physiciansnews.com/law/1097reiss.html)**

User tips ➢ Digest updated regularly

Keywords ➢ genetics testing
Medicare documentation

Patient confidentiality

http://www.acep.org/POLICY/P0004155.HTM

Sponsor ➢ American College of Emergency Physicians (ACEP)

Description ➢ Statement on patient confidentiality

Data type ➢ Text

Access requirements ➢ Open

Supplemental resources ➢ Health information confidentiality, American College of Healthcare Executives (ACHE) **(http://www.ache.org/policy/policy12.html)**
Patient-therapist confidentiality protected, American Psychological Association (APA) **(http://www.apa.org/monitor/aug96/supreme.html)**

User tips ➢ See ACEP homepage for additional patient confidentiality data

Keywords ➢ patient confidentiality

Physician's guide to medical liability issues
http://www.afss.com/physguid.htm

Sponsor ➢ Fosmire Solka Stenton law firm

Description ➢ Physician's guide to medical liability litigation (applies only to State of Michigan)

Data type ➢ Text

Access requirements ➢ Open

Supplemental resources ➢ Negligence: Errors and carelessness in health care (for consumers)
(http://www.h-leelaw.com/page9.htm)
Research problems in malpractice
(http://plague.law.umkc.edu/Xfiles/x158.htm)

User tips ➢ Get the facts—check with an attorney

Keywords ➢ malpractice
medical liability

Rare case registry: Confidentiality submission issues
http://anes01.wustl.edu/RARE/Rare_guide.html

Sponsor ➢ Pediatric Critical Care Medicine (PedsCCM)

Description ➢ Patient confidentiality guidelines for submissions in rare case registry

Data type ➢ Text

Access requirements ➢ Open

Supplemental resources ➢ PedsCCM: Rare Case Registry
(http://anes01.wustl.edu/Rare_cases.html)
PIM (mortality prediction model for pediatric intensive care) software available for download
(http://anes01.wustl.edu/CLINICAL/PIM-ReadMe.html)

User tips ➢ Check homepage for PedsCCM file cabinet for pediatric critical care data

Keywords ➢ patient confidentiality
medical software

Medical Informatics

Biostatistics resources
http://www.sph.emory.edu/bios/bioslist.html

Sponsor ➢	Rollins School of Public Health, Emory University
Description ➢	Academic, federal, and public health statistical Web sites and databases
Data type ➢	Databases; reports; software
Access requirements ➢	Open; hyperlinked access
Supplemental resources ➢	Archival Data Online Repository, University of Wisconsin-Madison **(http://www.sph.emory.edu/bios/bioslist.html)** Hyperlinks to public health statistics online databases **(http://www.sph.emory.edu/bios/bioslist.html)**
User tips ➢	Comprehensive list of university statistical resources
Keywords ➢	biostatistics

CDC Wonder

http://wonder.cdc.gov/Wonder/background.html

Sponsor ➢	Centers for Disease Control and Prevention (CDC)
Description ➢	Free software for accessing public health information and communications system, provides query access to text-based and numeric databases on STD, cancer, mortality, and other topics
Data type ➢	Software; free download from site
Access requirements ➢	Open; see download instructions
Supplemental resources ➢	Guidelines for searches and queries **(http://wonder.cdc.gov/)** Wonder overview **(http://wonder.cdc.gov/Wonder/overview.html)**
User tips ➢	Read overview to differentiate canned resources from ad hoc queries
Keywords ➢	medical software

Combined Health Information Database (CHID)

http://chid.nih.gov/

Sponsor ➢	National Institutes of Health (NIH) and Centers for Disease Control and Prevention (CDC)
Description ➢	Megasite of health databases includes topics on AIDS, Alzheimer's disease; genetics; smoking; weight control
Data type ➢	Text; statistics; multimedia
Access requirements ➢	Open
Supplemental resources ➢	Database topics **(http://chid.nih.gov/subfile/subfile.html)** Deafness and communication disorders **(http://chid.nih.gov/subfile/contribs/dc.html)**
User tips ➢	Simple and detailed searches available
Keywords ➢	megasite

Congressional megasite
wysiwyg://56/http://lcweb.loc.gov/global/legislative/mega.html

Sponsor ➢ Library of Congress

Description ➢ Megasite of government and commercial resources for Congressional legislative information; sites include House Web, Senate Web, C-Span, FedNet, and many others

Data type ➢ Hyperlinked sites

Access requirements ➢ Open; subscription sites included

Supplemental resources ➢ Search of *Congressional Record*, 104th Congress **(http://rs9.lco.gov/home/r104query.html)**

User tips ➢ Check index of Congressional megasites

Keywords ➢ legislation sources

Doctor's Guide to the Internet
http://www.pslgroup.com/DOCGUIDE.HTM

Sponsor ➢ P/S/L/ Consulting Group, Inc.

Description ➢ Medical news, conferences, and announcements

Data type ➢ Variable

Access requirements ➢ Open; for professionals

Supplemental resources ➢ Achoo health care online directory **(http://www.achoo.com/directory/humanhealthanddisease/index.htm)**
Biotechnology Information Institute homepage **(http://www.bioinfo.com/outline.html)**

User tips ➢ Hyperlinked text for most of the databases

Keywords ➢ medical resources

Electronic Development and Environment Information System (ELDIS)

http://www.ids.ac.uk/eldis/eldis.html

Sponsor ➢ British Library for Development Studies

Description ➢ ELDIS databases on poverty in developing countries; rural appraisal bibliography

Data type ➢ Databases

Access requirements ➢ Open

Supplemental resources ➢ ELDIS search and browse tools **(http://www.ids.ac.uk/eldis/eldis.html)**
Index of nongovernmental organizations (NGOs) cited on World Health Organization (WHO) site **(http://www.who.ch/programmes/ina/ngo/1index.htm)**

User tips ➢ WHO site lists broad range of international health organizations

Keywords ➢ international data resources

Electronic information resources for health officers

http://www.cdc.gov/elecinfo.htm

Sponsor ➢ Centers for Disease Control and Prevention (CDC) and Agency for Toxic Substances and Disease Registry (ATSDR)

Description ➢ Review of CDC and ATSDR systems for querying, finding, and retrieving CDC files

Data type ➢ Text

Access requirements ➢ Open

Supplemental resources ➢ Computer retrieval of information on scientific projects (CRISP) **(http://www.ncrr.nih.gov/grants/crisp.htm)**
Tulane Medical Library's homepage **(http://www.tulane.edu/~matas/index.html)**

User tips ➢ See section on obtaining access to electronic resources

Keywords ➢ electronic resources

Evaluating Internet medical information

http://www.fda.gov/fdac/features/596_info.html#site

Sponsor ➢ U.S. Food and Drug Administration (FDA)

Description ➢ Tips for evaluating Internet medical information

Data type ➢ Text

Access requirements ➢ Open

Supplemental resources ➢ Guide to Internet discovery tools
(http://www.nnlm.nlm.gov/tools.html)
Images from History of Medicine (IHM), search enabled site
(http://wwwihm.nlm.nih.gov/)

User tips ➢ Check links for Internet health mailing lists

Keywords ➢ medical computers

Federal statistical databases

http://www.fedstats.gov/search.html

Sponsor ➢ Federal Interagency Council on Statistical Policy (Fedstats)

Description ➢ Statistics from seventy federal agencies including the Economic Research Service; Environmental Protection Agency (EPA); Bureau of Transportation

Data type ➢ Text; statistical tables

Access requirements ➢ Open

Supplemental resources ➢ *Statistical Abstract of the United States*, 1996
(http://www.census.gov/prod/2/gen/96statab/96statab.html)
White House social statistics briefing room
(http://www.whitehouse.gov/fsbr/health.html)

User tips ➢ All are hyperlinked sites

Keywords ➢ social science statistics
megasite

Federal Web Locator (FedWeb)

http://www.law.vill.edu/Fed-Agency/fedwebloc.html

Sponsor ➢ Villanova Center for Information Law and Policy

Description ➢ Megasite, one-stop data point for Federal government information on the Web

Data type ➢ Text; search enabled

Access requirements ➢ Open

Supplemental resources ➢ Department of Health and Human Services (DHHS) search bill reports since 1985 **(http://www.hhs.gov/search/bill_rep.html)**
Federal government Web servers **(http://www.law.vill.edu/fed-agency/fedwebloc.html)**

User tips ➢ Search engine exclusively for bills from the DHHS Office of the Secretary and other DHHS agencies

Keywords ➢ megasite
policy

Health data warehouse

http://www.cdc.gov/nchswww/nchshome.htm

Sponsor ➢ National Center for Health Statistics (NCHS), U.S. Department of Health and Human Services (DHHS)

Description ➢ Megasite of health statistics and data

Data type ➢ Variable

Access requirements ➢ Open

Supplemental resources ➢ National Vital Statistics System **(http://www.cdc.gov/nchswww/about/major/nvss/nvss.htm)**
Bureau of Labor Statistics (BLS) **(http://stats.bls.gov/blshome.htm)**

User tips ➢ NCHS is a search enabled site

Keywords ➢ statistics, labor
statistics, health

Health/medical topics and resources
http://www.noah.cuny.edu/qksearch.html

Sponsor ➢	New York Online Access to Health (NOAH)
Description ➢	Comprehensive health and medical resource of organizations, disorders; and information for professionals and consumers
Data type ➢	Searchable database
Access requirements ➢	Open
Supplemental resources ➢	Genital herpes **(http://www.noah.cuny.edu/pregnancy/...are the symptoms of genital herpes)** Eating disorders: Anorexia and bulimia nervosa **(http://noah.cuny.edu/wellconn/eatdisorders.html)**
User tips ➢	Check Noah's most read documents
Keywords ➢	eating disorders herpes

Healthfinder: Medical and health information
http://www.healthfinder.gov/

Sponsor ➢	U.S. Department of Health and Human Services (DHHS)
Description ➢	Megasite directory of over 800 links to federal and private health Web sites and organizations
Data type ➢	Text; graphics
Access requirements ➢	Open; search enabled; hyperlinked access
Supplemental resources ➢	Search results for domestic violence **(http://www.healthfinder.gov/htmlge...word.cmf?Keyword=DOMESTIC+VIOLENCE)** Toll-free numbers for health information **(http://nysenet.org/bcic/numbers/NHIC-tollfree.html)**
User tips ➢	Megasite of health resources
Keywords ➢	megasite

HON Media Gallery

http://www.hon.ch/Media/media.html

Sponsor ➢ Health On the Net Foundation (HON)

Description ➢ Searchable database of medical movies, images, x-rays, and other media

Data type ➢ Multimedia

Access requirements ➢ Requires movie player; see homepage instructions

Supplemental resources ➢ Clickable anatomical medical images and movies **(http://www.hon.ch/Media/anatomy.html)**
Viewing and downloading instructions **(http://www.hon.ch/Media/media.html)**

User tips ➢ Movies available in different formats

Keywords ➢ medical movies

Index of Internet medical resources

http://www.gretmar.com/webdoctor/window.html

Sponsor ➢ WebDoctor

Description ➢ Internet medical resource links to 10,000 documents and Web sites

Data type ➢ Documents and files designed by and for physicians

Access requirements ➢ Open

Supplemental resources ➢ Galaxy professional medical database of diseases and disorders **(http://lmc.einet.net:8000/galaxy/Medicine/Diseases-and-Disorders.html)**
General medical and health web sites, North Carolina Industrial Commission **(http://www.comp.state.nc.us/ncic/pages/medsites.htm)**

User tips ➢ Search enabled sites

Keywords ➢ megasite

Integrated public use microdata series (IPUMS)
http://www.hist.umn.edu/~ipums/

Sponsor ➢ Minnesota Historical Census Projects, University of Minnesota

Description ➢ Computerized database of individual level samples of the U.S. population censuses, 1850–1990

Data type ➢ Tabular

Access requirements ➢ Open; IPUMS files must be decompressed

Supplemental resources ➢ IPUMS samples
(http://www.hist.umn.edu/~ipums/sample.html)
Documentation and sample download instructions
(http://www.hist.umn.edu/~ipums/)

User tips ➢ Download DOS decompression software

Keywords ➢ microdata documentation
census data

Internet Grateful Med
http://igm.nlm.nih.gov:80/

Sponsor ➢ U.S. National Library of Medicine (NLM), National Institutes of Health (NIH)

Description ➢ Internet Grateful Med edition of Medline, HealthStar, Aidsdrugs, SDILine, and other Medlars databases; comprehensive selection of published medical data

Data type ➢ Open

Access requirements ➢ Open; search enabled; downloads for full text files and abstracts

Supplemental resources ➢ New user's survival guide
(http://igm.nlm.nih.gov:80/)

User tips ➢ User ID no longer required for Medline search

Keywords ➢ megasite
medical literature

Karolinska Institute Library and Information Center

http://www.mic.ki.se/Diseases/index.html

Sponsor ➢	Karolinska Institute Library
Description ➢	Database of diseases, disorders, and other medical resources on the Internet
Data type ➢	Hyperlinked text; multimedia; graphics
Access requirements ➢	Open; hyperlinked files
Supplemental resources ➢	Alphabetical hyperlinks of specific diseases and disorders **(http://www.mic.ki.se/Diseases/alphalist.html)** Irish medical directory, international medical links **(http://www.iol.ie/imd/interlnk.htm)**
User tips ➢	Karolinska offers hundreds of resources
Keywords ➢	megasite

Martindale's "The Reference Desk"

http://www-sci.lib.uci.edu/

Sponsor ➢	Jim Martindale
Description ➢	Megasite of social science, medical, and business references, tutorials, databases, dictionaries, and calculators
Data type ➢	Multimedia
Access requirements ➢	Open; some sites require registration
Supplemental resources ➢	Virtual Medical Center (otolaryngology, ophthalmology, otorhinolaryngology) **(http://www-sci.lib.uci.edu/~martindale/MedicalAudio.html#OOO)** Science tables and databases **(http://www-sci.lib.uci.edu/~martindale/Ref3.html#RTT2)**
User tips ➢	Searches available for thousands of files; frequent updates
Keywords ➢	megasite

MedAccess On-Line
http://www.medaccess.com/

Sponsor ➢ MedAccess Corporation

Description ➢ Databases, newsletter, health quizzes; healthcare locator; data bank; health news

Data type ➢ Text, statistics; search enabled

Access requirements ➢ Open

Supplemental resources ➢ Health statistics, United States, 1993 **(http://www.medaccess.com/health93/health_a.htm)**
Health Information Resources in the Federal Government, 6th edition **(http://www.medaccess.com/address/hircatoc.htm)**

User tips ➢ Check MedAccess homepage for personalized workbook and online record keeper

Keywords ➢ health resource

MedExplorer health/medical Internet search engine
http://www.medexplorer.com/

Sponsor ➢ MedExplorer

Description ➢ Searchable database of medical topics including laboratory; pharmaceutical; imaging; nursing/allied health

Data type ➢ Text; graphics

Access requirements ➢ Open

Supplemental resources ➢ Database of health organizations **(http://www.social.com/health/nhic/data/index.html)**
Health organizations beginning with "E" **(http://www.social.com/health/nhic/data/e.html)**

User tips ➢ Enter up to three search keywords

Keywords ➢ megasite

Medical case presentations and teaching files

http://www.geocities.com/HotSprings/2255/index.html

Sponsor ➢ Med Files, Geocities

Description ➢ Case presentations and teaching files from various institutions for health professionals covering anesthesia, HIV/AIDS, emergency, and other medical topics

Data type ➢ Hyperlinked index of files for anesthesia; hematology; metabolic endocrinology; gastrointestinal medicine; and others

Access requirements ➢ Open

Supplemental resources ➢ Gastrointestinal case studies and teaching files **(http://www.geocities.com/HotSprings/2255/geeeye.html)**
Orthopedics teaching files **(http://www.geocities.com/~fnp/ortho.html)**

User tips ➢ Numerous tutorial files available

Keywords ➢ tutorials
medical education

Medical Encyclopedia on the Net—Diseases

http://www.mosbych1.com/mhc/index/

Sponsor ➢ Mosby Consumer Health

Description ➢ Online reference for consumers; disease definitions, causes, prevention, symptoms, and diagnosis

Data type ➢ Hyperlinked chapter links; graphics

Access requirements ➢ Open

Supplemental resources ➢ Gastric ulcer **(http://www.mosbych1.com/mhc/scr/000213sc.htm)**
Diseases reference (for index of “G” diseases) **(http://www.mosbych1.com/mhc/index/diseidxg.htm)**

User tips ➢ Extensive list of disease information files

Keywords ➢ epidemiology
ulcer

Medical journals

http://www.webmedlit.com/

Sponsor ➢	Silver Platter Information, Inc. and Physicians' homepage
Description ➢	Database tracking 21 medical journals on AIDS, cancer, diabetes, and medical economics
Data type ➢	Database of professional journals
Access requirements ➢	Access by journal or topic, i.e., AIDS, women's health, diabetes
Supplemental resources ➢	Search **(http://www.webmedlit.com/)** Penn State Geisinger Library, online publications and medical columns index **(http://www.geisinger.edu/ghs/pubtips/pubtips.htm)**
User tips ➢	Sites generally include the most recent journal articles or abstraccts
Keywords ➢	medical journals

Medical World Search

http://www.mwsearch.com/help.html

Sponsor ➢	Medical World Search
Description ➢	Plain English database search and retrieval of medical Web sites
Data type ➢	Database
Access requirements ➢	Open; registration (free) preferred
Supplemental resources ➢	Search instructions page **(http://www.mwsearch.com/)** National Network of Libraries of Medicine (NN/LM) for health professionals **(http://www.nnlm.nlm.nih.gov/)**
User tips ➢	Database utilizes the National Library of Medicine's Unified Medical Language System (UMLS)
Keywords ➢	medical database medical computer language

Medistat
http://biomed.nus.sg/MSTAT/welcome.html

Sponsor ➢ National University of Singapore, Centre for Medical Informatics and Biostatistics, Dr. K. C. Lun

Description ➢ Online health and population statistics database

Data type ➢ Statistical database

Access requirements ➢ Open

Supplemental resources ➢ Singapore statistics, mortality, hospital admission rates
(http://biomed.nus.sg:80/MSTAT/spore/gen/genmain.html)
About Medistat
(http://biomed.nus.sg/MSTAT/mstatnfo.html)

User tips ➢ International hospital data included

Keywords ➢ megasite
international health statistics

MedWeb
http://www.gen.emory.edu/MEDWEB/medweb.html

Sponsor ➢ Emory University Health Sciences Center Library

Description ➢ Searchable database of medical organizations; conditions; tutorials; conferences (the whole works) categorized according to major medical disciplines

Data type ➢ All types

Access requirements ➢ Open; hyperlinked files

Supplemental resources ➢ MedWeb site for the day: Gynecology and women's health
(http://www.gen.emory.edu/MEDWEB/wha...y/gynecology_and_womens_health.html)
MedWeb rheumatology
(http://www.gen.emory.edu/medweb/medweb/rheumatology.html)

User tips ➢ Thousands of sites; retrieve according to topic, keyword, or organization

Keywords ➢ megasite
gynecology

Merck Manual of Medical Information—Home edition, 1997
http://www.merck.com/!!tcfQIINcStcfRL31_X/pubs/mmanual_home/

Sponsor ➢	Merck & Company, Inc.
Description ➢	Home edition of medical information
Data type ➢	Text; graphics
Access requirements ➢	Online chapter and topic searches available; downloadable
Supplemental resources ➢	Chapter: Endocarditis **(http://www.merck.com/!!tcfQI1NcStcfRL31_X/pubs/mmanual_home/chapt21.htm)**
User tips ➢	Hard copy available for purchase
Keywords ➢	home medical guide endocarditis

Morbidity and Mortality Weekly Report (MMWR)
http://www.cdc.gov/epo/mmwr/mmwr.html)

Sponsor ➢	Centers for Disease Control and Prevention (CDC)
Description ➢	Weekly record of state reported epidemiologic and mortality data
Data type ➢	Text; tables; searchable index
Access requirements ➢	Open; PDF files viewed with Acrobat Reader
Supplemental resources ➢	MMWR, November 7, 1997 **(http://www.cdc.gov/epo/mmwr/mmwr_wk.html)** CDC scientific data, surveillance, statistics, and laboratory information **(http://www.cdc.gov/scientific.htm#stats)**
User tips ➢	Searchable index of MMWR publications from 1993 through the present
Keywords ➢	statistics, morbidity and mortality epidemiology

Natality, morbidity, mortality statistics

http://www.lib.umich.edu/libhome/PubHealth.lib/bib/statistics.html

Sponsor ➢ Documents Center, University of Michigan

Description ➢ Contents include data on vital statistics, health economics, international statistics, statistical journals

Data type ➢ Text; statistics; multimedia

Access requirements ➢ Open; quick jump searches

Supplemental resources ➢ Statistical resources on the Web **(http://www.lib.umich.edu/libhome/Documents.center/stats.html)**
Selected sources on health statistics **(http://www.lib.umich.edu/libhome/PubHealth.lib/bib/statistics.html)**

User tips ➢ Frame and no-frame versions available

Keywords ➢ megasite
statistics

New England Journal of Medicine online

http://www.nejm.org/

Sponsor ➢ Massachusetts Medical Society

Description ➢ Weekly journal reporting worldwide medical research

Data type ➢ Journal

Access requirements ➢ Open; some full text files

Supplemental resources ➢ Collection of recent full text articles **(http://www.nejm.org/collections/1.htm)**
Images in clinical medicine (ICM) quiz **(http://www.nejm.org/scripts/icm/icm.cgi)**

User tips ➢ See homepage for archives search

Keywords ➢ medical journal

NIH Health Information Index, 1997

http://www.nih.gov/news/96index/pubincov.htm

Sponsor ➢ Office of Communications, National Institutes of Health (NIH)

Description ➢ Directory of diseases currently under investigation or targeted by NIH

Data type ➢ Alphabetized index with topic, funding agency, and telephone number

Access requirements ➢ Open

Supplemental resources ➢ Index of "P-T" topics **(http://www.nih.gov/news/96index/pubinp-t.htm)**
Licensing electronic resources, Medical Library Association Network of Health Information Professions **(http://mlahq.org/)**

User tips ➢ Area code for NIH telephone numbers is 301, unless otherwise indicated

Keywords ➢ health data index

Online medical journals and references

http://www-informatics.ucdmc.ucdavis.edu/informatics/MedRefs.html-ssi

Sponsor ➢ UCDHS Center for Medical Informatics and University of California at Davis Health System

Description ➢ Hyperlinks of Web-based Medline; journals; references; professional literature

Data type ➢ Hyperlinks to journals and references

Access requirements ➢ Open

Supplemental resources ➢ Medical Matrix **(http://www.medmatrix.org/index.asp)**

User tips ➢ See homepage for comprehensive list of online medical journals

Keywords ➢ breast cancer
medical journals

Recommendations for clinical software systems

http://amia2.amia.org/v04n06/442.htm

Sponsor ➢ American Medical Informatics Association (AMIA)

Description ➢ Abstract, recommendations for monitoring clinical software systems

Data type ➢ Text

Access requirements ➢ Open

Supplemental resources ➢ AMIA homepage
(http://amia2.amia.org/)
Electronic medical record–tracking specifications
(http://ncemi.org/docs/mercy-01.htm)

User tips ➢ Check AMIA job exchange bin

Keywords ➢ medical software
electronic records

Thomas Legislative Information on the Internet

http://thomas.loc.gov/

Sponsor ➢ Library of Congress

Description ➢ Searchable database of Congressional text of bills; House and Senate directories; bill summary and status; committee reports

Data type ➢ Text; search enabled

Access requirements ➢ Open

Supplemental resources ➢ About Thomas
(http://thomas.loc.gov/home/abt_thom.html)
C-Span online: Congress Today
(http://congress.nw.dc.us/c-span/)

User tips ➢ See Thomas homepage for historical and early Congressional documents

Keywords ➢ Congressional documents
legislation

U.S. National Library of Medicine (NLM)

http://www.nlm.nih.gov/

Sponsor ➢ U.S. National Library of Medicine (NLM)

Description ➢ Medical databases; extramural and intramural research programs; GenBank; images; library services; free Medline

Data type ➢ Open

Access requirements ➢ Open; search tools; download of full text files, abstracts

Supplemental resources ➢ Fact sheet: Unified Medical Language System (UMLS)
(http://www.nlm.nih.gov/pubs/factsheets/umls.html)
Toxicology and Environment Health Information Program
(http://www.nlm.nih.gov/)

User tips ➢ Comprehensive selection of published medical data

Keywords ➢ megasite
medical databases

United States Congress

http://www.access.gpo.gov/congress/index.html

Sponsor ➢ United States Congress

Description ➢ Congressional bills; directory; reports; bill history; publications

Data type ➢ Hyperlinked sites

Access requirements ➢ Open; search enabled

Supplemental resources ➢ History of Bills online (1983–1997)
(http://www.access.gpo.gov/su_docs/aces/aaces200.html)
The Congressional Institute
(http://www.conginst.org/conginst.nsf?OpenDatabase)

User tips ➢ See homepage for Congressional index

Keywords ➢ legislation sources
Congressional documents

World Health Organization Statistical Information System (WHOSIS)

http://www.who.ch/whosis/whosis.htm#databases

Sponsor ➢ World Health Organization (WHO)

Description ➢ Health related global statistical data and tools including the international classification of diseases

Data type ➢ Databases; statistical tables

Access requirements ➢ Open; search for WHO data by disease topic or keywords

Supplemental resources ➢ WHOSIS homepage, European health-for-all statistical database **(http://www.who.ch/whosis/whosis.htm#databases)**

User tips ➢ Check WHOSIS homepage for Health Futures 2025 study

Keywords ➢ international health statistics

W3-Electronic Medical Record System (W3-EMRS)

http://www.emrs.org/medweb/

Sponsor ➢ Boston Children's Hospital

Description ➢ Demonstration of a real medical database with simulated immunization information

Data type ➢ Demo

Access requirements ➢ Open

Supplemental resources ➢ Instructions **(http://www.emrs.org/medweb-bin/front-page)** Sample data page **(http://www.emrs.org/medweb-bin/record/cover-sheet?patient_id=4)**

User tips ➢ Multi-institutional demonstration database in progress

Keywords ➢ electronic records
medical software

Medical Specialties

ANESTHESIOLOGY

Blood, fluid, and electrolyte replacement lecture

http://www.med.virginia.edu/som-cl/anesth/education/blood.htm

Sponsor ➢ Department of Anesthesiology, University of Virginia

Description ➢ Lecture contents and study questions include topics on intravascular volume assessment and fluid replacement, electrolyte replacement, and others

Data type ➢ Text

Access requirements ➢ Open

Supplemental resources ➢ Anesthesia for liver transplantation (online publication) **(http://www.med.virginia.edu/som-cl/anesth/education/educatio.htm)**

User tips ➢ See homepage for lecture schedule

Keywords ➢ anesthesia
transplantation

Global Textbook of Anesthesiology

http://www.gasnet.eur.nl/gta/

Sponsor ➢ GASNet, Keith Ruskin, Yale University School of Medicine

Description ➢ Textbook covering acid-base physiology, airway management, anesthetic complications, malignant hyperthermia, obstetric anesthesia and other topics, along with phrase book

Data type ➢ Textbook for professionals

Access requirements ➢ Open

Supplemental resources ➢ Techniques of orbital regional anaesthesia **(http://www.iea.com/~dans/OAS/regional/Ophth_Regional.html)**

User tips ➢ Preview copyright instructions on homepage

Keywords ➢ anesthesiology
trauma anesthesiology

Practice parameters for physicians

http://gasnet.med.yale.edu/mirror/asa/Practice_Parameters/prac_TOC.html

Sponsor ➢ American Society of Anesthesiologists

Description ➢ Practice guidelines for blood component therapy, acute or chronic cancer pain, pulmonary artery catheterization, and other categories

Data type ➢ Text

Access requirements ➢ Open

Supplemental resources ➢ Guidelines for management of the difficult airway **(http://gasnet.med.yale.edu/mirror/a...rameters/Diff_Airway/difficult.html)**
Guidelines for sedation and analgesia by non-anesthesiologists **(http://gasnet.med.yale.edu/mirror/a...e_Parameters/Sedation/Sedation.html)**

User tips ➢ Hit bin for patient information

Keywords ➢ anesthesia guidelines

ENDOCRINOLOGY

Clinical guidelines for endocrine conditions

http://www.aace.com/guidelines/

Sponsor ➢	American Association of Clinical Endocrinologists (AACE) and American College of Endocrinology (ACE)
Description ➢	Guidelines for hypogonadism, thyroid carcinoma, diabetes, and other topics
Data type ➢	Text; graphics
Access requirements ➢	Open
Supplemental resources ➢	Thyroid self-neck check **(http://www.aace.com/guidelines/card.html)** AACE/ACE position statement on prevention, diagnosis, and treatment of obesity **(http://www.aace.com/guidelines/obesity.html)**
User tips ➢	Check thyroid nodule guidelines
Keywords ➢	thyroid endocrine guidelines

Endocrine surgery

http://endocrine-surgery.com/Welcome.html

Sponsor ➢	James Norman, M.D.
Description ➢	Guide to endocrine disorders of the thyroid, parathyroid, adrenal, and neuroendocrine tumors of the pancreas
Data type ➢	Text; some graphics
Access requirements ➢	Open
Supplemental resources ➢	Endocrine surgery index page **(http://endocrine-surgery.com/indexpg.html)** Thyroid goiter **(http://endocrine-surgery.com/goiter.html)**
User tips ➢	Files for physicians and patients
Keywords ➢	endocrine glands endocrine surgery

FORENSIC MEDICINE

Autopsy diagrams
http://www.afip.mil/oafme/diagrams.html

Sponsor ➢ Armed Forces Institute of Pathology (AFIP), Center for Advanced Pathology

Description ➢ Anatomical autopsy diagrams

Data type ➢ Images; text

Access requirements ➢ Open

Supplemental resources ➢ Office of the Armed Forces Medical Examiner
(http://www.afip.mil/homes/afmi.html)
Center for Advanced Pathology homepage
(http://www.afip.mil/homes/cap.html)

User tips ➢ AFIP provides consultation, education, and research

Keywords ➢ autopsy
pathology

Forensic odontology certification
http://www.abfo.org/qualific.htm

Sponsor ➢ American Board of Forensic Odontology, Inc. (ABFO)

Description ➢ Forensic odontology certification qualifications

Data type ➢ Text

Access requirements ➢ Open

Supplemental resources ➢ ABFO homepage
(http://www.abfo.org/)
Forensic odontology in the United Kingdom
(http://www.users.dircon.co.uk/~jasburns/index.html?34,10)

User tips ➢ Check ABFO homepage for membership application procedure

Keywords ➢ forensic odontology

Forensic protocols in human hair comparisons
http://olmec.lab.r1.fws.gov/proto/methods.htm

Sponsor ➢ Forensics Laboratory, U.S. National Fish and Wildlife Service

Description ➢ Equipment, supplies, and procedures for human hair analysis

Data type ➢ Text; some graphics

Access requirements ➢ Open

Supplemental resources ➢ Abstracts of professional papers
(http://olmec.lab.r1.fws.gov/abstract/ab-pprs.htm)
Animal forensic protocols
(http://olmec.lab.r1.fws.gov/labweb/labstart.htm)

User tips ➢ Forensics Lab investigates crimes involving wildlife

Keywords ➢ forensics, animals
forensic protocols

Forensic resources
http://www.hypernet.on.ca/quincy/formedic.htm

Sponsor ➢ The Forensic Scientist

Description ➢ Directory of international forensic medical professional organizations, directories, bibliographies, and databases

Data type ➢ Directory

Access requirements ➢ Open

Supplemental resources ➢ Forensic directories, bibliographies, databases
(http://www.hypernet.on.ca/quincy/dirbib.htm)
Forensic training, Forensic Science Society
(http://www.demon.co.uk/forensic/fortraining.html)

User tips ➢ Check homepage for forensic degree programs

Keywords ➢ forensic training

Landmark cases in forensic psychiatry
http://ua1vm.ua.edu/~jhooper/landmark.html

Sponsor ➢ Psychiatry and the Law, University of Alabama and the Alabama Department of Mental Health and Mental Retardation

Description ➢ Psychiatric issues of famous cases

Data type ➢ Text

Access requirements ➢ Open; all cases in one file

Supplemental resources ➢ National Forensic Hospital Data Network **(http://ua1vm.ua.edu/~jhooper/data.html)**
Forensic psychiatry resource page **(http://ua1vm.ua.edu/~jhooper/index.html)**

User tips ➢ Hospital data network includes rates of seclusion, restraint, medication errors, and other topics

Keywords ➢ insanity defense
forensic psychiatry

Medical examiner and coroner information sharing program
http://www.cdc.gov/nceh/pubcatns/1994/cdc/brosures/me-cbro.htm

Sponsor ➢ National Center for Environmental Health (NCEH), Centers for Disease Control and Prevention (CDC)

Description ➢ Collaborative program for death investigation practices

Data type ➢ Text

Access requirements ➢ Open

Supplemental resources ➢ Medical examiner briefs, AFIP **(http://www.afip.mil/homes/afmi.html)**

User tips ➢ Check CDC brochures

Keywords ➢ death investigation
forensics

Qualifications for forensic psychiatry
http://www.cc.emory.ed/AAPL/abpn.htm

Sponsor ➢ American Board of Psychiatry and Neurology, Inc. (ABPN)

Description ➢ Qualifications and fellowships in forensic psychiatry

Data type ➢ Text

Access requirements ➢ Open

Supplemental resources ➢ Feminism and forensic psychiatry **(http://www.priory.com/psych/feminism.htm)**
American Academy of Psychiatry and the Law (AAPL) homepage **(http://www.cc.emory.edu/AAPL/)**

User tips ➢ Check AAPL homepage for forensic psychiatry resources

Keywords ➢ forensic psychiatry

Writing cause-of-death statements
http://WWW.TheNAME.org:80/main.htm

Sponsor ➢ National Association of Medical Examiners (NAME)

Description ➢ Tutorial of basic principles; quick tips; CODWriter utility; and writing cause of death statements

Data type ➢ Interactive tutorial

Access requirements ➢ Open

Supplemental resources ➢ Pediatric toxicology (PedTox) registry information **(http://WWW.TheNAME.org:80/pedtox/pedtox.htm)**
NAME homepage **(http://WWW.TheNAME.org:80/info/info.htm)**

User tips ➢ Check link for death investigation careers

Keywords ➢ pediatric deaths
forensic careers

GENETICS

DNA vaccine

http://www.genweb.com/Dnavax/dnavax.html

Sponsor ➢ Robert Whalen

Description ➢ Article, resources about DNA

Data type ➢ Text; graphics

Access requirements ➢ Open

Supplemental resources ➢ DNA vaccine references
(http://www.genweb.com/Dnavax/dnavax.html)
Medical genetics, Glaxo Wellcome
(http://www.glaxowellcome.co.uk/home.html)

User tips ➢ Check bin for U.S. Patent and Trademark Office for full text articles of DNA vaccine–related patents

Keywords ➢ DNA

Human cloning ban advances in the U.S. House of Representatives

http://www.scienceXchange.com/aai/newsletter/November/cloning.htm

Sponsor ➢ American Association of Immunologists (AAI)

Description ➢ Synopsis of cloning ban advances in the U.S. House of Representatives, November 1997

Data type ➢ Text

Access requirements ➢ Open

Supplemental resources ➢ AAI homepage
(http://scienceXchange.com/aai/)
Glossary of immunology
(http://www-micro.msb.le.ac.uk/MBChB/ImmGloss.html)

User tips ➢ See AAI homepage for research fellowships at the postdoctoral or clinical fellow levels

Keywords ➢ human cloning
education funding

Human genome maps
http://www.oxmol.com/biolib/map/

Sponsor ➢	BioLib Project, Bioinformatics Library
Description ➢	Database search of human genome maps
Data type ➢	Demonstration database (Java applet)
Access requirements ➢	Open; slow running with some connections
Supplemental resources ➢	About BioLib project **(http://www.oxmol.com/biolib/)** GeneMap **(http://www.oxmol.com/biolib/map/)**
User tips ➢	Check UniGene human gene sequence collection
Keywords ➢	genetics chromosomes

PATHOLOGY

Human anatomy online
http://www.innerbody.com/indexbody.html

Sponsor ➢	Informative Graphics Corp.
Description ➢	Animated views of the human body with descriptive hyperlinks
Data type ➢	Multimedia
Access requirements ➢	Uses Java applets to show clickable images
Supplemental resources ➢	Animation index **(http://www.innerbody.com/htm/anim.html)** Mouth and throat (cut view) **(http://www.innerbody.com/anim/mouth.html)**
User tips ➢	Anatomy lessons included
Keywords ➢	anatomy

Pathology mini-tutorials
http://www-medlib.med.utah.edu/WebPath/TUTORIAL/TUTORIAL.html#3

Sponsor ➢ Internet Pathology Laboratory for Medical Education

Description ➢ Tutorials of gross and microscopic pathologic findings associated with human disease states of AIDS, diabetes, phlebotomy, and renal cystic disease

Data type ➢ Tutorials; 1,800 clickable images

Access requirements ➢ Open; also available on WebPath CD-ROM

Supplemental resources ➢ Laboratory homepage **(http://www-medlib.med.utah.edu/WebPath/webpath.html#menu)**
Tutorial, pathology of systemic lupus erythematosus **(http://www-medlib.med.utah.edu/WebPath/TUTORIAL/SLE/SLE.html)**

User tips ➢ See pathology tutorials

Keywords ➢ medical education

Visible embryo project
http://magenta.afip.mil/embryo/HomePage.html

Sponsor ➢ Human Developmental Anatomy Center, Armed Forces Institute of Pathology (AFIP)

Description ➢ Movies, models, and database of an embryo

Data type ➢ Multimedia

Access requirements ➢ Open; relevant viewers include GIF, JPEG, MPEG, TIFF

Supplemental resources ➢ Late stage 10 embryo of 3 weeks **(http://magenta.afip.mil/embryo/s10-movie.html)**
Mpeg movies **(http://magenta.afip.mil/embryo/movies.html)**

User tips ➢ See viewing instructions for Macintosh, Windows, and UNIX

Keywords ➢ embryo development

RADIOGRAPHY

Medical radiography homepage
http://www.aers.org

Sponsor ➢ Association of Educators in Radiological Sciences, Inc. (AERS)

Description ➢ Internet resources for radiologic science professionals

Data type ➢ Graphics; text

Access requirements ➢ Open

Supplemental resources ➢ Mandatory continuing education (CE) **(http://web.wn.net/~usr/ricter/web/Digest151.html)**
Radiation protection resources on the Internet **(http://www.radscice.com/dowd.html)**

User tips ➢ Radiation Internet resources subject to change with updates

Keywords ➢ continuing education
radiation protection resources

Medical radiography resources
http://web.wn.net/~usr/ricter/web/medradhome.html

Sponsor ➢ Massachusetts General Hospital

Description ➢ Medical imaging, radiologic anatomy, radiography software, and other Internet resources for radiologic science professionals

Data type ➢ Variable

Access requirements ➢ Open

Supplemental resources ➢ Rad Sci Online: Continuing education for radiologic science professionals **(http://www.radscice.com)**
Comparison of Internet medical search engine user interface capabilities **(http://web.wn.net/~usr/ricter/web/med.html)**

User tips ➢ See homepage for quick search for medical resources

Keywords ➢ radiography
medical education

Radiographic anatomy of the skeleton
http://www.scar.rad.washington.edu/RadAnatomy.html

Sponsor ➢ Michael L. Richardson, M.D.

Description ➢ Modules of spine and upper and lower extremities

Data type ➢ Graphics; text

Access requirements ➢ Open

Supplemental resources ➢ Radiographic anatomy of the wrist **(http://www.scar.rad.washington.edu/RadAnat/Wrist.html)**
Radiographic anatomy of the cervical spine **(http://www.scar.rad.washington.edu/RadAnat/CSpine.html)**

User tips ➢ Clickable anatomical views

Keywords ➢ radiographic anatomy
radiography

TELEMEDICINE

European telepathologist sites
http://europath.imag.fr/vpage/V.EPS.html

Sponsor ➢ Europath

Description ➢ List of European pathologists equipped to provide telepathology consultation

Data type ➢ Multimedia

Access requirements ➢ For pathologists

Supplemental resources ➢ List of sites **(http://europath.imag/fr/vpage/V.EPS.html)**
Telepathology Newsletter 1 **(http://ampat.amu.edu.pl/czasopis/ejp2-3/963-09.htm)**

User tips ➢ See Europath homepage for consultation instructions

Keywords ➢ telepathologists

Reimbursement of telemedicine consultations
http://206.156.10.7/scripts/esrimap.dll?name=Reporter&cmd=Report_1

Sponsor ➢ Federal Telemedicine Gateway, Joint Working Group on Telemedicine (JWGT) Inventory

Description ➢ Information about active, federally funded telemedicine projects providing direct patient care

Data type ➢ Text; graphics

Access requirements ➢ Open

Supplemental resources ➢ Key terms used in the JWGT telemedicine inventory
(http://www.tmgateway.org/gateway/key_defs.html)
Gateway homepage
(http://www.tmgateway.org/gateway/)

User tips ➢ Register to receive updates

Keywords ➢ telemedicine reimbursement
telemedicine glossary

Telemedicine and technology transfer sites
http://ourworld.compuserve.com/home.../global_telemedicine_apex/sites.htm

Sponsor ➢ Global Telemedicine Technologies II

Description ➢ Hyperlinks to telemedicine government, academic, and health facility transfer sites

Data type ➢ Text; graphics

Access requirements ➢ Open

Supplemental resources ➢ Telemedicine academic organizations and articles, Galaxy
(http://lmc.tradewave.com/galaxy/Med...lemedicine/Remote-Consultation.html)

User tips ➢ Check telemedicine publications

Keywords ➢ telemedicine resources

Telemedicine and the law
http://www.arentfox.com/telemedicine.html

Sponsor ➢ Arent Fox
Description ➢ Liability of telemedical transactions
Data type ➢ Text
Access requirements ➢ Open
Supplemental resources ➢ Executive action regarding telemedicine (federal notices) **(http://www.arentfox.com/telemed/fed.executive.html)**
Telemedicine legal issues **(http://www.netreach.net/~wmanning/telemedov.htm)**
User tips ➢ See Fox homepage for state telemedicine legislation
Keywords ➢ legal medicine

Telemedicine confidentiality statements
http://www.vtmednet.org/telemedicine/privacy.htm

Sponsor ➢ Fletcher Allen Health Care (FAHC)
Description ➢ Center policies to protect patients' privacy during teleconferences
Data type ➢ Text
Access requirements ➢ Open
Supplemental resources ➢ Overview, FAHC telemedicine program **(http://www.vtmednet.org/telemedicine/page1.htm)**
American Telemedicine Association (ATA) homepage **(http://www.atmeda.org/)**
User tips ➢ See ATA homepage for definition of telemedicine
Keywords ➢ telemedicine
patient confidentiality

Telemedicine in action
http://www.va.gov/telemed/teleactn.htm

Sponsor ➢ Department of Veterans Affairs (VA), Veterans Health Administration

Description ➢ VA funded program descriptions for teleradiology, telepathology, telecardiology, telemental health, and telemedicine

Data type ➢ Text

Access requirements ➢ Open

Supplemental resources ➢ VA telemedicine initiatives by state
(http://www.va.gov/mediauto/telemed/ar_t.htm)
Mexican-U.S. telemedicine program
(http://www.fc.net:80/~dlojacon/nafta.html#vc)

User tips ➢ See VA teledermatology for assessing skin conditions

Keywords ➢ teledermatology
telepathology

Telemedicine research
http://www.matmo.org/

Sponsor ➢ Telemedicine and Advanced Technology Research Center (TATRC), U.S. Department of Defense (DOD)

Description ➢ Telemedicine strategies for improving health systems, role of nursing in telemedicine, and other topics

Data type ➢ Text

Access requirements ➢ Open

Supplemental resources ➢ *TeleMed News*
(http://www.matmo.org/)
Telemedicine reports and reviews (DOD)
(http://www.matmo.org/)

User tips ➢ Audio available for Pacific site

Keywords ➢ telemedicine
nursing

Telepathology tips from Armed Forces Institute of Pathology (AFIP)
http://www.afip.mil/telepath/tips/tip1.html

Sponsor ➢ U.S. Department of Defense (DOD)

Description ➢ Site describes telepathology program for consultation, systems, rotation and practicum, and tips

Data type ➢ Text

Access requirements ➢ Open

Supplemental resources ➢ Telepathology system components **(http://www.vtmednet.org.:80/telemedicine/path.htm)**
Telepathology at AFIP **(http://www.afip.mil/homes/telepath.html)**

User tips ➢ Check instructions for sending consultation cases to AFIP through telepathology

Keywords ➢ telepathology
teleradiology

UROLOGY

End-stage renal disease
http://www.niddk.nih.gov/EndStageRenalDisease/EndStageRenalDisease.html

Sponsor ➢ National Institute of Diabetes and Digestive and Kidney Diseases (NIDDK), NIH

Description ➢ Booklet on end-stage renal disease

Data type ➢ Text

Access requirements ➢ Open

Supplemental resources ➢ NIDDK homepage for megasite on diabetes, digestive, endocrine, and other diseases **(http://www.niddk.nih.gov/NIDDK_HomePage.html)**

User tips ➢ See databases of clinical studies for health professionals

Keywords ➢ renal disease
urologic statistics

Laboratory regulation in urological offices

http://auanet.org/pub_pat/policies/...Laboratory regulation in urological

Sponsor ➢ American Urological Association (AUA)

Description ➢ Policy issues for improving urology laboratories

Data type ➢ Text

Access requirements ➢ Open

Supplemental resources ➢ AUA homepage
(http://auanet.org/pub_pat/policies/)
Kidney and urologic statistics, U.S.
(http://www.niddk.nih.gov/KU_Stats/kustats.htm)

User tips ➢ National Kidney Foundation contact number: 1-800-622-9010

Keywords ➢ urology laboratories
urology

Marketing continence

http://www.continenceworldwide.com/articles/3.html

Sponsor ➢ Continence Worldwide, Continence Foundation

Description ➢ Continence marketing strategies

Data type ➢ Text

Access requirements ➢ Open

Supplemental resources ➢ Managing urinary incontinence
(http://www.wellweb.com/acct/manage.html)
Videoscopic balloon bladder neck suspension; bladder control treatment options
(http://www.mdfinder.com/bns4.htm)

User tips ➢ Hit bin for additional information on videoscopic balloon

Keywords ➢ incontinence treatment

Urologic trauma

(http://indy.radiology.uiowa.edu/Pro...nRef/FPHandbook/Chapter01/15-1.html

Sponsor ➢ Mosby, *The Family Practice Handbook*, University of Iowa

Description ➢ Discussions of kidney, urethral, bladder and other urologic trauma

Data type ➢ Text

Access requirements ➢ Open

Supplemental resources ➢ Incontinence and PMD
(http://www.incontinet.com/professional.htm)
Impotence
(http://incontinet.com/articles/art_sex/impotenc.htm)

User tips ➢ See data on fecal incontinence and constipation

Keywords ➢ impotence
incontinence

Mental Health

Adolescent and child psychiatry

http://www.aacap.org/web/aacap/

Sponsor ➢	American Academy of Child and Adolescent Psychiatry (AACAP)
Description ➢	AACAP homepage featuring psychiatric services for families and children
Data type ➢	Text; graphics
Access requirements ➢	Open
Supplemental resources ➢	Report card on child and adolescent mental disorders research **(http://www.psych.med.umich.edu/web/aacap/rptcard.htm)** Facts for families, information sheets on topics such as stepfamily issues, depressed child, and other issues **(http://www.aacap.org/web/aacap/factsFam/)**
User tips ➢	Available in Spanish, English, and French
Keywords ➢	adolescent psychiatry

Anorexia/bulimia
http://members.aol.com/amanbu/index.html

Sponsor ➢	The American Anorexia/Bulimia Association, Inc. (AABA)
Description ➢	Support group for friends and families of anorexia/bulimia sufferers
Data type ➢	Text
Access requirements ➢	Open
Supplemental resources ➢	What should I do? **(http://members.aol.com/amanbu/fandf.html)**
User tips ➢	See AABA links for friends and families of sufferers
Keywords ➢	mental disorders nutrition

Calendar of events for mental health professionals
http://www.umdnj.edu/psyevnts/meet.FEB00.html#Date

Sponsor ➢	Myron Pulier
Description ➢	Worldwide list of mental health related meetings through Year 2004 arranged according to date and subject
Data type ➢	Search enabled
Access requirements ➢	Open
Supplemental resources ➢	Sample of mental health organization finder **(http://www.umdnj.edu/psyevnts/orgsH.html)** Pulier's psychiatry and behavioral resources for mental health professionals **(http://www.users.interport.net/~mpulier/)**
User tips ➢	Resources for 1,900 mental health organizations
Keywords ➢	mental health resources

Common misconceptions about suicide
http://www.save.org/misconc.html

Sponsor ➢ Suicide Awareness Voices of Education (SAVE)

Description ➢ Explanations of the truths and myths about suicide; consumer site

Data type ➢ Text; audiotapes

Access requirements ➢ Open

Supplemental resources ➢ Support for depressed hospitalized friends
(http://www.save.org/hospital.html)
SA\VE homepage
(http://www.save.org/)

User tips ➢ Check homepage for list of suicide education materials

Keywords ➢ suicide
depression

Computerized measurement of health and thermal pain perception
http://www.psychologie.uni-bonn.de/kap/for/bio/com.htm

Sponsor ➢ Department of Clinical and Applied Psychology, University of Bonn, Germany

Description ➢ Presentations from the Computers in Psychology Conference '96, York University

Data type ➢ Text; configurations

Access requirements ➢ Open

Supplemental resources ➢ WWW resources for clinical and abnormal psychology
(http://www.psychologie.uni-bonn.de/kap/li_home.htm)
National Academy of Neuropsychology homepage
(http://www.nan.drexel.edu/)

User tips ➢ Sponsors welcome suggestions for additional links

Keywords ➢ computers in psychology
pain perception

Consumer's guide to treatment of anxiety disorders

http://www.adaa.org/4_info/4a_cgt/4a_02.htm

Sponsor ➢ Anxiety Disorders Association of America (ADAA)

Description ➢ Treatment options for anxiety disorders

Data type ➢ Text

Access requirements ➢ Open

Supplemental resources ➢ Anxiety Disorders Association homepage **(http://www.adaa.org/)**
Chart outlining treatment modalities, goals, benefits, drawbacks for anxiety disorders **(http://www.adaa.org/4_info/4a_cgt/4a_02.htm)**

User tips ➢ See homepage for site search instructions

Keywords ➢ mental disorders

Crisis intervention

http://www.uic.edu/orgs/convening/Proceed21.htm

Sponsor ➢ 21st Annual Convening of Crisis Intervention Personnel, April 1997

Description ➢ Summaries of crisis intervention conference presentations

Data type ➢ Text

Access requirements ➢ Open

Supplemental resources ➢ Starting a crisis unit **(http://www.uic.edu/orgs/convening/Starting.htm)**
Adolescent suicide: Assessment and prevention **(http://www.uic.edu/orgs/convening/AdolesSuicide.htm)**

User tips ➢ Check links for crisis counseling with gay, lesbian, and bisexual clients

Keywords ➢ adolescent suicide
mental health therapy

Crisis intervention resource manual

http://www.bartow.k12.ga.us/psych/crisis/crisis.htm

Sponsor ➢ Office of Psychological Services, Bartow County School System

Description ➢ Step-by-step manual for crisis intervention in schools

Data type ➢ Text

Access requirements ➢ Open

Supplemental resources ➢ Description of suicide intervention plan **(http://www.bartow.k12.ga.us/psych/crisis/sueplan.htm)**

User tips ➢ Manual updated regularly

Keywords ➢ crisis intervention
suicide

Disorders and treatments index

http://www.cmhc.com/selfhelp.htm

Sponsor ➢ Mental Health Net, Community Mental Health Centers Systems

Description ➢ Alphabetized list of mental disorders

Data type ➢ Text for consumers

Access requirements ➢ Direct access to topics

Supplemental resources ➢ Resources for obsessive compulsive disorders (OCD) **(http://www.ocdresource.com/resources.html)**
Helping a loved one with OCD **(http://www.ocdresource.com/helpingocd.html)**

User tips ➢ Check homepage for downloads of *Self-Help Sourcebook Online* and *Psychological Self-Help*

Keywords ➢ mental health therapy
obsessive compulsive disorder (OCD)

Dissociative disorders
http://www.voiceofwomen.com/VOW2_11950/centerarticle.html

Sponsor ➢ The Center: Post-Traumatic and Dissociative Disorders Program

Description ➢ Articles and resources on the spectrum of diagnosis and treatment of dissociative disorders

Data type ➢ Text

Access requirements ➢ Open

Supplemental resources ➢ The Center homepage **(http://www.voiceofwomen.com/VOW2_11950/center.html)**
Educational resources on abuse, trauma, and dissociative disorders **(http://www.voiceofwomen.com/VOW2_11950/centerres.html#anchor715634)**

User tips ➢ References specified for professionals and survivors

Keywords ➢ dissociative disorders

Early diagnosis and management of psychosis
http://home.vicnet.net.au/~eppic/intervene.html#anchor436997

Sponsor ➢ Early Psychosis Prevention and Intervention Centre (EPPIC)

Description ➢ Report of early psychosis diagnosis and management

Data type ➢ Text

Access requirements ➢ Open

Supplemental resources ➢ EPPIC homepage **(http://home.vicnet.net.au/~eppic/frame2.html)**
Report: Systematic treatment of persistent positive symptoms **(http://www.vicnet.net.au/vicnet/community/sub.htm)**

User tips ➢ See early intervention framework

Keywords ➢ mental disorders

Electroconvulsive therapy (ECT)

http://www.mentalhealth.com/book/p45-ect1.html

Sponsor ➢ National Institutes of Health (NIH)

Description ➢ ECT Consensus Development Conference Statement, June 1985

Data type ➢ Report

Access requirements ➢ Open

Supplemental resources ➢ Pediatric ECT
(http://www.mhsource.com/exclusive/pedect.html)
American Psychiatric Association (APA) report on electroconvulsive therapy
(http://www.psych.org/clin_res/ect.html)

User tips ➢ See directions for future research

Keywords ➢ pediatrics
mental health therapy

European-American descriptions of disorders

http://www.mentalhealth.com/main.html

Sponsor ➢ Internet Mental Health, Philip W. Long, M.D.

Description ➢ American and European diagnostic criteria of mental health disorders

Data type ➢ Text

Access requirements ➢ Open

Supplemental resources ➢ Index of disorders according to category
(http://www.mentalhealth.com/p20.html)
American description, separation anxiety disorder
(http://www.mentalhealth.com/dis1/p21-ch03.html)

User tips ➢ See homepage links to online diagnosis, and medication

Keywords ➢ phobias
mental disorders

Gestalt therapy
http://www.behavior.net/mhn/bolfor...th=8&detail=description&lastread=5

Sponsor ➢	Behavior OnLine
Description ➢	Articles; online forum on gestalt therapy; for professionals
Data type ➢	Text
Access requirements ➢	Open
Supplemental resources ➢	Mental health and applied behavior online meeting place homepage **(http://www.behavior.net/)** Adlerian professional training for psychotherapists, Alfred Adler Institute **(http://www.behavior.net/orgs/adler/classica.html)**
User tips ➢	Check Behavior homepage for additional ongoing discussions
Keywords ➢	gestalt therapy

Index of reports on disorders
http://www.mhsource.com/disorders/

Sponsor ➢	Mental Health Infosource (MHI)
Description ➢	Index of reports on disorders, including attention deficit hyperactivity disorder, eating disorders, Tourette's syndrome, and sexual disorders
Data type ➢	Text
Access requirements ➢	Open
Supplemental resources ➢	Panic disorder treatment **(http://www.mhsource.com/edu/psytimes/p970358.html)**
User tips ➢	See MHI Professional Directory to search for mental health professionals
Keywords ➢	mental disorders

Insanity defense
http://www.psych.org/public_info/INSANI~1.HTM

Sponsor ➢ American Psychiatric Association (APA)

Description ➢ Article responding to insanity defense questions

Data type ➢ Text

Access requirements ➢ Open

Supplemental resources ➢ APA statement regarding HIV infection and psychiatric hospitalization of children and adolescents **(http://www.psych.org/libr_publ/aids_state3.html)**
HCFA guidelines for Medicare private contracts **(http://www.psych.org/pub_pol_adv/rushnotes_1297.html)**

User tips ➢ Check APA homepage for schizophrenia awareness video

Keywords ➢ psychiatric hospitalization
legal medicine

Interactive testing in psychiatry (ITP)
http://www.med.nyu.edu/Psych/ITP/gpm2.html

Sponsor ➢ New York University Department of Psychiatry

Description ➢ Testing modules and CME credit for psychiatrists

Data type ➢ Interactive text

Access requirements ➢ Open

Supplemental resources ➢ Online screening for anxiety **(http://www.med.nyu.edu/Psych/screens/anx.html)**
Psychiatry information for the public **(http://www.med.nyu.edu/Psych/public.html)**

User tips ➢ Public site includes online screenings for depression, sexual disorders, and personality disorders

Keywords ➢ mental disorders

Managed care and mental health program funding

http://mimh.edu/TM/T3780

Sponsor ➢ Missouri Institute of Mental Health (MIMH)

Description ➢ Resources for managed care issues

Data type ➢ Text

Access requirements ➢ Open

Supplemental resources ➢ MIMH homepage
(http://www.missouri.edu/~mimhmj)
Planning worksheet for children's mental health programs
(http://mimh.edu/TM/E22192T3780)

User tips ➢ See decision checklist for designing capitation projects for the severely mentally ill

Keywords ➢ managed care
mental health funding

Mental disorders

http://www.nimh.nih.gov/hotsci/hotsci.htm

Sponsor ➢ National Institute of Mental Health (NIMH)

Description ➢ Latest research results on obsessive compulsion disorder, schizophrenia, and depression

Data type ➢ Text

Access requirements ➢ Open

Supplemental resources ➢ Anxiety disorders
(http://www.nimh.nih.gov/publicat/anxiety.htm#anx2)
Mental illness in America: The NIMH agenda
(http://www.nimh.nih.gov/research/amer.htm)

User tips ➢ Toll free numbers for free publications: 1-888-8-ANXIETY and depression: 1-800-421-4211

Keywords ➢ mental disorders
anxiety

Mental health bill of rights
http://helping.apa.org/rights.html

Sponsor ➢ American Psychological Association (APA)

Description ➢ Text of patient mental health bill of rights

Data type ➢ Text

Access requirements ➢ Open

Supplemental resources ➢ PsychNet APA homepage
(http://www.apa.org/psychnet/)
APA PsycInfo (fee service)
(http://www.apa.org/psycinfo/)

User tips ➢ Download booklet on psychology careers for the 21st century

Keywords ➢ patient rights
psychology careers

Mental health research volunteer opportunities
http://www.nimh.nih.gov/~cng/volnteer.htm

Sponsor ➢ Clinical Neurogenetics Branch, National Institute of Mental Health (NIMH)

Description ➢ Research studies on schizophrenia, sexual orientation, neuroleptic side effects; seeking volunteers for compensation

Data type ➢ Text

Access requirements ➢ Open

Supplemental resources ➢ Pre-teen volunteers sought for mood study
(http://intramural.nimh.nih.gov/recruit/recruit.htm)
Homepage for searchable publications and abstracts
(http://www.nimh.nih.gov/~cng/cng-pg1c.htm)

User tips ➢ Teen volunteer study; contact NIMH: 301-496-1301

Keywords ➢ moods

Mental health services databases

http://www.mentalhealth.org/mhorgsdb/index.htm

Sponsor ➢ Center of Mental Health Services (CMHS), Knowledge Exchange Network (KEN)

Description ➢ Databases for mental health organizations, CMHS grantees, consumer/survivors, and publications

Data type ➢ Databases

Access requirements ➢ Open

Supplemental resources ➢ Glossary of terms in children's and adolescents' mental health
(http://www.mentalhealth.org/child/glossary.htm)
Violence in the schools: *Teacher Talk*
(http://educ.indiana.edu/cas/tt/v2i3/v2i3toc.html)

User tips ➢ *Teacher Talk*, publication for secondary teachers

Keywords ➢ mental health services
adolescent violence

Mental health statistics

http://www.mentalhealth.org/mhstats/index.htm

Sponsor ➢ Center for Mental Health Services (CMHS)

Description ➢ Statistical data of mental services utilization; mental hospital rates

Data type ➢ Text; statistical notes

Access requirements ➢ Open

Supplemental resources ➢ Mental health emergency services
(http://www.mentalhealth.org/emerserv/index.htm)
Psychological aspects of terrorism
(http://www.mentalhealth.org/emerserv/TERRORIS.HTM)

User tips ➢ See link to CMHS programs on homelessness

Keywords ➢ emergency medicine
mental health statistics

Multimedia library courses
http://www.mhsource.com/edu/hmstudy/all2.html#disorders

Sponsor ➢ Mental Health Infosource (MHI)

Description ➢ Home study courses on children and adolescents; psychiatric board preparation materials; psychopharmacology

Data type ➢ Audio- and videotapes

Access requirements ➢ Open

Supplemental resources ➢ *Psychiatric Times* **(http://www.mhsource.com/psychiatrictimes.html)**
Archives of General Psychiatry **(http://www.ama-assn.org/public/journals/psyc/psychome.htm)**

User tips ➢ Journals updated regularly

Keywords ➢ mental health training
mental health journals

Overview of depressive illness and symptoms
http://www.ndmda.org/depover.htm

Sponsor ➢ National Depressive and Manic-Depressive Association (NDMDA)

Description ➢ Introduction to affective disorders; depression symptoms

Data type ➢ Text; videotapes

Access requirements ➢ Open

Supplemental resources ➢ Overview of bipolar disorders **(http://www.ndmda.org/biover.htm)**
Diagnosis and treatment of depression in late life **(http://text.nlm.nih.gov/nih/cdc/www/86txt.html)**

User tips ➢ Download video on manic depression; DMDA contact number: 1-800-826-3632

Keywords ➢ depression
bipolar disorder

Personality disorders
http://www.ns.sympatico.ca/Contents/Health/LISTS/B4-C03-06_all1.html

Sponsor ➢ Sympatico
Description ➢ Reviewed sites describing mental health personality disorders
Data type ➢ Text
Access requirements ➢ Open
Supplemental resources ➢ Helping children cope with stress, Hoechst Marion Roussel
(http://www.thriveonline.com/@@JZjcA...brary/pedillsymp/pedillsymp583.html)
Internet resources for mental health professionals
(http://www.aatbs.com/internet.htm)
User tips ➢ Check Hoechst's health library
Keywords ➢ mental health resources

Psychiatry and the Web
http://www.psych.med.umich.edu/web/psytimes/psychwww.htm

Sponsor ➢ *Psychiatric Times*
Description ➢ Psychiatry navigates the Web; a review of psychiatric topics on the Web
Data type ➢ Text
Access requirements ➢ Open
Supplemental resources ➢ Psychiatric Society for Informatics (PSI) homepage
(http://www.psych.med.umich.edu/web/psi)
User tips ➢ Check PSI newsletter
Keywords ➢ informatics

Schizophrenia

http://www.cityscape.co.uk/users/ad88/schizo.htm

Sponsor ➢ Dr. B. Green, psychiatrist, UK, *Psychiatry On-Line*

Description ➢ Review of schizophrenia

Data type ➢ Text

Access requirements ➢ Open

Supplemental resources ➢ Ziegler mania rating scale **(http://www.mhsource.com/disorders/zieglerrating.html)**

User tips ➢ See schizophrenia glossary

Keywords ➢ mental disorders

Violence risk assessment study

http://ness.sys.virginia.edu/macarthur/violence.html

Sponsor ➢ MacArthur Research Network on Mental Health and the Law

Description ➢ Executive summary of study assessing violence potential of the mentally disturbed

Data type ➢ Text

Access requirements ➢ Open

Supplemental resources ➢ MacArthur Research Network homepage **(http://ness.sys.virginia.edu/macarthur/)**
Institute of Law, Psychiatry and Public Policy **(http://ness.sys.Virginia.EDU/ilppp/research.html)**

User tips ➢ See MacArthur homepage for bin on treatment competence

Keywords ➢ forensic medicine

Musculoskeletal Health

Acute low back problems in adults

http://text.nlm.nih.gov/ftrs/tocview

Sponsor ➢	National Institute of Arthritis and Musculoskeletal Diseases (NIAMS), NIH
Description ➢	Quick reference guide for medical history, examination, pain behavior, and other management considerations for low back problems in adults
Data type ➢	Text; interactive table of contents
Access requirements ➢	Open
Supplemental resources ➢	NIAMS homepage **(http://www.nih.gov/niams/)** NIH Consensus Statement: Total hip replacement, September 1994 **(http://www.nih.gov/niams/scientific/)**
User tips ➢	See space travel effects on musculoskeletal system
Keywords ➢	back pain space travel effects

Aquatic therapy
http://www.biomech.com/archive/1997/bdr97/aquatxt.html

Sponsor ➢ BioMechanics Desk Reference, 1997

Description ➢ Aquatic exercise in ACL reconstruction and rehabilitation

Data type ➢ Article

Access requirements ➢ Open

Supplemental resources ➢ BioMechanics homepage
(http://www.biomech.com/archive/1997/bdr97/index.html)
Knee braces: The injured knee
(http://www.biomech.com/archive/1997/bdr97/kneebracetxt.html)

User tips ➢ Check index for links to data on ankle braces and walkers

Keywords ➢ aquatic therapy
knee injury

Arthritis and lupus clinical trials
http://preferences.stanford.edu/arthritis/recruit.htm

Sponsor ➢ Stanford Arthritis and Rheumatology Research

Description ➢ Trials for systemic lupus erythematosus, particularly in the San Francisco Bay area

Data type ➢ Text

Access requirements ➢ Open

Supplemental resources ➢ Systemic lupus erythematosus (SLE) study of symptoms
(http://preferences.stanford.edu/arthritis/re00005.htm)
Hormonal drug trial for women with active SLE
(http://preferences.stanford.edu/arthritis/re00004.htm)

User tips ➢ Check site page for clinical trial contacts

Keywords ➢ clinical trials
rheumatology

Arthritis sites for consumers
http://www.nerdworld.com/cgi-bin/vdata.cgi?783

Sponsor ➢	Nerd World Media
Description ➢	Miscellaneous arthritis news, treatments, and self-help
Data type ➢	Text
Access requirements ➢	Open
Supplemental resources ➢	Diseases and conditions, Nerd World Media **(http:207.159.105.133/cgi-bin/vdata.cgi?cat=1460&mode=d)**
User tips ➢	Useful data on several sites
Keywords ➢	arthritis

Clinical guidelines for prevention of postmenopausal osteoporosis
http://www.aace.com/guidelines/osteoporosis.html

Sponsor ➢	American Association of Clinical Endocrinologists (AACE) and American College of Endocrinology (ACE)
Description ➢	Prevalence and clinical aspects of postmenopausal osteoporosis
Data type ➢	Report; images
Access requirements ➢	Open
Supplemental resources ➢	Osteoporosis definition **(http://www.aace.com/guidelines/osteoporosis.html)**
User tips ➢	Check section on clinical features and complications
Keywords ➢	osteoporosis prevention

Computers and arthritis
http://weber.u.washington.edu/~dboo...subjects/arthritis/xzzzzzzd3_1.html

Sponsor ➢ Bone and Joint Center, University of Washington (UW)

Description ➢ Article, "Can my computer be arthritis-friendly?"

Data type ➢ Text

Access requirements ➢ Open

Supplemental resources ➢ Arthritis index of conditions, diagnosis, and treatment
(http://weber.u.washington.edu/~dboo...bjects/arthritis/Arthritis.idx.html)
UW bone and joint sources
(http://weber.u.washington.edu/~dboo...subjects/arthritis/zzzzzzzz1_1.html)

User tips ➢ Check file on how joints work

Keywords ➢ arthritis
bone-joint data sources

***Cutting Edge Reports* on osteoporosis**
http://www.nof.org/cutedg3.html

Sponsor ➢ National Osteoporosis Foundation (NOF)

Description ➢ New research findings on osteoporosis prevention drugs

Data type ➢ Text

Access requirements ➢ Open

Supplemental resources ➢ National Osteoporosis Foundation homepage
(http://www.nof.org/)
Assessing impact of osteoporosis
(http://www.merck.com/!!tdgfB3RnJtd...osteoporosis/mebd0035.html#summary)

User tips ➢ See NOF homepage for link to professional data link

Keywords ➢ osteoporosis

Gait lab case presentations

http://gait.aidi.udel.edu/res695/ho...d_ortho/gait_lab/cases/casehome.htm

Sponsor ➢ Gait Laboratory, Alfred I. duPont Institute

Description ➢ Case presentations

Data type ➢ Text

Access requirements ➢ Open

Supplemental resources ➢ Gait case presentation, asymetric diplegia **(http://gait.aidi.udel.edu/res695/ho...e/pd_ortho/gait_lab/cases/case1.htm)**
Gait Analysis Laboratories homepage **(http://gait.aidi.udel.edu/res695/homepage/pd_ortho/gait_lab/page1.htm)**

User tips ➢ See homepage for link to cerebral palsy

Keywords ➢ gait disorders

Hand and finger pain

http://www-med.stanford.edu/school/DGIM/Teaching/Modules/handfinger.html

Sponsor ➢ Mark Musen, M.D., Stanford Division of General Internal Medicine

Description ➢ Teaching module for hand and finger pain and carpal tunnel syndrome

Data type ➢ Teaching module

Access requirements ➢ Open

Supplemental resources ➢ Links for podiatry management **(http://www.footdoc.com/footman/)**

User tips ➢ Check sample cases under teaching module

Keywords ➢ medical education
podiatry

Interactive test for knee injury
http://www.med.und.nodak.edu:80/depts/fpc/knee/knee.htm

Sponsor ➢ American Orthopaedic Society for Sports Medicine (AOSSM)

Description ➢ Interactive test with responses forwarded to site authors

Data type ➢ Text

Access requirements ➢ Open

Supplemental resources ➢ AOSSM homepage
(http://www.sportsmed.org/)
Ask the sports doctor
(http://www.sportsmed.org/d/d.htm)

User tips ➢ See football helmet removal guidelines

Keywords ➢ sports injuries

Lumbar laminectomy
http://familyinternet.com/mhc/scr/002973sc.htm

Sponsor ➢ Family Internet

Description ➢ Definition, description, indications, risks, and costs of lumbar disorder

Data type ➢ Text

Access requirements ➢ Open

Supplemental resources ➢ Homepage for Family Internet (megasite)
(http://www.familyinternet.com/mhc/menu.htm)
Hypophosphatasia
(http://www.osteo.org/hypoph.htm)

User tips ➢ Daily updates for Family Internet

Keywords ➢ bone disorders
lumbar disorders

Lupus
http://www.hamline.edu/lupus/

Sponsor ➢ Hamline University

Description ➢ Lupus overview, symptoms, and other associated conditions

Data type ➢ Text

Access requirements ➢ Open

Supplemental resources ➢ Lupus in men
(http://www.hamline.edu/lupus/articles/Lupus_in_Men.html)
Pregnancy and lupus
(http://www.hamline.edu/lupus/articles/Pregnancy_in_Lupus.html)

User tips ➢ Watch for conferencing center for the Lupus Internet Project

Keywords ➢ lupus, men
pregnancy

Muscular dystrophy research updates
http://www.mdausa.org/research/updates.html

Sponsor ➢ Muscular Dystrophy Association (MDA)

Description ➢ Bulletins summarizing latest findings in neuromuscular disease research

Data type ➢ Text

Access requirements ➢ Open

Supplemental resources ➢ MDA homepage
(http://www.mdausa.org/index.html)
Neuromuscular diseases in the MDA program
(http://www.mdausa.org/disease/index.html)

User tips ➢ See eligibility guidelines for MDA Research Grants Programs

Keywords ➢ muscular dystrophy
health funding

Orthopedic outcomes assessment
http://www.aaos.org/wordhtml/outcomes.htm

Sponsor ➢	American Academy of Orthopaedic Surgeons (AAOS)
Description ➢	Outcomes assessment for orthopaedic surgeons and other providers
Data type ➢	Text
Access requirements ➢	Open
Supplemental resources ➢	AAOS homepage **(http://www.aaos.org/wordhtml/home2.htm)** Accomplishments of orthopaedic research **(http://www.aaos.org/wordhtml/research/orthores.htm)**
User tips ➢	See AAOS homepage for legislative news
Keywords ➢	orthopedic research

Osteopathic medicine
http://www.aacom.org/what.htm

Sponsor ➢	American Association of Colleges of Osteopathic Medicine (AACOM)
Description ➢	Site describes osteopathic medicine, physicians, and manipulative treatment
Data type ➢	Text
Access requirements ➢	Open
Supplemental resources ➢	Index of osteopathic medicine, education, and treatment **(http://www.aacom.org/)** History of osteopathic medicine **(http://www.aacom.org/ats.htm)**
User tips ➢	See list of osteopathic medical colleges
Keywords ➢	osteopathic medicine

Osteoporosis and men

http://www.osteo.org/osteoinmen.html

Sponsor ➢	Osteoporosis and Related Bone Disease~National Resource Center (ORBD~NRC)
Description ➢	Article describing osteoporosis prevalence in men
Data type ➢	Text
Access requirements ➢	Open
Supplemental resources ➢	ORBD~NRC homepage **(http://www.osteo.org/)** Professional resources **(http://www.osteo.org/boneprof.html)**
User tips ➢	See links on Paget's disease; osteogenesis imperfecta
Keywords ➢	osteoporosis, men Paget's disease

Pediatric rheumatology

http://www.arthritis.org/ajao/athreya/athreya_part_1.shtml

Sponsor ➢	American Juvenile Arthritis Organization, Arthritis Foundation
Description ➢	Status of pediatric rheumatology
Data type ➢	Text
Access requirements ➢	Open
Supplemental resources ➢	Arthritis Foundation homepage **(http://www.arthritis.org/)** Diagnosis of juvenile rheumatoid arthritis **(http://www.rheumatology.org/guidelin/jra.htm)**
User tips ➢	Arthritis answers (1-800-283-7800)
Keywords ➢	pediatric rheumatoid arthritis

Rheumatology megasite
http://www.gen.emory.edu/medweb/medweb.rheumatology.html

Sponsor ➢ MedWeb
Description ➢ Megasite of rheumatology hyperlinked sites to organizations, research, and publications
Data type ➢ Hyperlinked directory
Access requirements ➢ Open
Supplemental resources ➢ Inconsistent findings and pain behavior (NIAMS) **(http://text.nlm.nih.gov/tempfiles/is/tempBrPg50397?t=883253571)**
User tips ➢ Check MedWeb for hundreds of medical sites
Keywords ➢ pain behavior
rheumatology

Rheumatology resources
http://www.rheumatology.org/patient/factsheet.html

Sponsor ➢ American College of Rheumatology (ACR)
Description ➢ Rheumatology disorders, and treatment for tendinitis, arthritis, osteoporosis, and osteoarthritis
Data type ➢ Text
Access requirements ➢ Open
Supplemental resources ➢ Gout diagnosis and treatment
(http://www.rheumatology.org/patient/gout.htm)
Grants for rheumatology research
(http://www.rheumatology.org/layorg.html)
User tips ➢ Participants sought for rheumatoid and osteoarthritis studies
Keywords ➢ arthritis
rheumatology

Wheeless' Textbook of Orthopaedics

http://www.medmedia.com/med.htm

Sponsor ➢	Anspach and Instrument Makar, Inc.
Description ➢	Orthopaedics reference topics include fracture menu, joints, muscles, medications, and lab tests
Data type ➢	Textbook; direct access to chapters
Access requirements ➢	Open; search enabled
Supplemental resources ➢	Chapter: Renal osteodystrophy **(http://www.medmedia.com/oa3/49.htm)** Infection risk from dental procedures after total knee arthroplasty **(http://www.aaos.org/wordhtml/press/dental.htm)**
User tips ➢	European and Australian online editions available
Keywords ➢	orthopedics reference dental health

Neurology

ANGEL Neurosurgical Information Resource

http://www.usc.edu/hsc/neurosurgery/Neurosurgeons/angindx.html

Sponsor ➢	Department of Neurosurgery, University of Southern California (USC)
Description ➢	Neurology lectures, grand rounds; international data for consumers, residents, and neuropractitioners
Data type ➢	Text; some graphics
Access requirements ➢	Open
Supplemental resources ➢	Abstracts and full text of articles from the *Archives of Neurology* **(http://www.ama-assn.org/public/journals/neur/toc.htm)** MedWeb megasite of neurology resources **(http://www.gen.emory.edu/medweb/medweb.neurology.html)**
User tips ➢	Check USC site for head trauma operations
Keywords ➢	head trauma medical education

Brain tumor noteworthy treatments

http://www.virtualtrials.com/noteworth.html

Sponsor ➢ Musella Foundation for Brain Tumor Research and Information and Johns Hopkins Stereotactic Radiosurgery

Description ➢ Noteworthy treatments include functional image guided surgery; gliadel wafers; stereotactic radiosurgery

Data type ➢ Text

Access requirements ➢ Open

Supplemental resources ➢ Interactive database search of 200 treatment trials **(http://www.virtualtrials.com/)**
Chemotherapy in brain tumors **(http://www.virtualtrials.com/levin1.html)**

User tips ➢ Keyword search available for clinical trials site clinical trials

Keywords ➢ brain tumor

Brain tumor online resources

http://www.tbts.org/onlinere.htm

Sponsor ➢ Brain Tumor Society

Description ➢ List servers, discussion groups, and WWW resources for brain tumor information and research

Data type ➢ Directory

Access requirements ➢ Open

Supplemental resources ➢ Children's Brain Tumor Foundation **(http://www.bethisraelny.org/inn/tumor/cbtf/cbtf_int.html)**
Cansearch: Guide to Cancer Resources, National Coalition for Cancer Survivorship **(http://www.access.digex.net/~mkragen/cansearch.html)**

User tips ➢ Contact number: 1-800-770-TBTS (8287)

Keywords ➢ brain tumor
cancer

Childhood Cancer Ombudsman Program
http://www.mnsinc.com/cbtf/ombuds.html

Sponsor ➢ Childhood Brain Tumor Foundation

Description ➢ Assistance for families of cancer victims in resolving health insurance and other problems associated with cancer treatment

Data type ➢ Text

Access requirements ➢ Open

Supplemental resources ➢ Foundation homepage **(http://www.mnsinc.com/cbtf/)**

User tips ➢ Check homepage for related articles

Keywords ➢ pediatric brain tumor
pediatric cancer

Chronic fatigue and immune dysfunction syndrome (CFIDS)
http://www.cfids.org/cfids.html

Sponsor ➢ CFIDS Association of America

Description ➢ CFIDS symptoms, diagnosis, treatment, risks, and online resources

Data type ➢ Text

Access requirements ➢ Open

Supplemental resources ➢ CFIDS Association homepage **(http://www.cfids.org/)**
Social Security Administration adjudication of claims involving chronic fatigue syndrome **(http://www.cfids.org/info/ssa.html)**

User tips ➢ Check CFIDS homepage for pediatric CFS

Keywords ➢ chronic fatigue
Social Security Administration (SSA)

Chronic fatigue syndrome (CFS)

http://weber.u.washington.edu/~dedra/aacfs1.html

Sponsor ➢ American Association for Chronic Fatigue Syndrome (AACFS)

Description ➢ CFS bibliographic database; research projects; teleconferences; publications

Data type ➢ Text

Access requirements ➢ Open

Supplemental resources ➢ AACFS speaker's bureau **(http://weber.u.washington.edu/~dedra/m-spkbur.html)**
CFS information for physicians, NIAID **(http://www.niaid.nih.gov/publications/cfs/contents.htm)**

User tips ➢ See list of speaker topics and other arrangement details

Keywords ➢ chronic fatigue syndrome

Chronic fatigue syndrome (CFS) treatments and studies

http://www.cdc.gov/ncidod/diseases/cfs/cfshome.htm

Sponsor ➢ National Center for Infectious Diseases, Centers for Disease Control and Prevention (CDC)

Description ➢ CFS definition; treatment; studies; and support groups

Data type ➢ Text

Access requirements ➢ Open

Supplemental resources ➢ Index, CFS treatments **(http://www.cdc.gov/ncidod/diseases/cfs/treatme0.htm)**
Antidepressant treatments for CFS **(http://www.cdc.gov/ncidod/diseases/cfs/treatme6.htm)**

User tips ➢ Check homepage for ongoing and future CFS studies

Keywords ➢ chronic fatigue syndrome

Costs and causes of traumatic brain injury (TBI)

http://www.biausa.org/costsand.htm

Sponsor ➢ Brain Injury Association, Inc.

Description ➢ Definition, scope, and costs related to brain injury

Data type ➢ Text; graphics

Access requirements ➢ Open

Supplemental resources ➢ Brain Injury Association homepage **(http://www.biausa.org/)**
Anatomy of a brain injury **(http://www.biausa.org/trauma.htm)**

User tips ➢ Check University of Washington link for brain injury services

Keywords ➢ brain injury
brain injury, rehabilitation

Dictionary of pain terms

http://weber.u.washington.edu/~crc/IASP/dict.html#RTFToC11

Sponsor ➢ International Association for the Study of Pain (IASP)

Description ➢ Pocket dictionary of pain terminology

Data type ➢ Dictionary

Access requirements ➢ Open

Supplemental resources ➢ IASP homepage **(http://weber.u.washington.edu/~crc/IASP/IASP3/IASPright.html)**

User tips ➢ Check homepage for unofficial resources for pain researchers and clinicians

Keywords ➢ pain

Headache causes

http://www.achenet.org/whatcause.htm

Sponsor ➢	American Council for Headache Education (ACHE)
Description ➢	Understanding causes and types of headaches
Data type ➢	Question and answer format on headache types and causes
Access requirements ➢	Open; some sites restricted to members
Supplemental resources ➢	Migraine diagnosis **(http://www.migrainehelp.com/diagnosis/index.html)** ACHE Web Forum headache menu **(http://neuro-www.mgh.harvard.edu/forum/HeadacheMenu.html)**
User tips ➢	See ACHE homepage for headache prevention link
Keywords ➢	pain, headache migraine

Human brain project

http://www-hbp.scripps.edu/Home.html

Sponsor ➢	National Institute of Mental Health (NIMH)
Description ➢	World Wide Web (WWW) servers for human brain project
Data type ➢	Text
Access requirements ➢	Open
Supplemental resources ➢	List of human brain project Web servers **(http://www-hbp.scripps.edu/HBP_html/HBPsites.html)**
User tips ➢	Check list of other WWW sites
Keywords ➢	brain

Huntington's disease latest news

http://www.angelfire.com/al/leonc/

Sponsor ➢	Carolyn Crowson and Noel Crowson
Description ➢	Summaries of 130 daily newspaper citations of Huntington's disease news
Data type ➢	News articles
Access requirements ➢	Open
Supplemental resources ➢	Huntington's disease summaries **(http://search.newsworks.com/aquery.html?qt=Huntington's+Disease&qp=&rf=2)**
User tips ➢	Consumer oriented site
Keywords ➢	Huntington's disease

Multiple sclerosis

http://www.nmss.org/home.html

Sponsor ➢	National Multiple Sclerosis (MS) Society
Description ➢	Multiple sclerosis resources
Data type ➢	Text; graphics
Access requirements ➢	Open
Supplemental resources ➢	Map of MS clinic locations **(http://www.nmss.org/resources/clinics.html)**
User tips ➢	National MS Society number: 1-800-Fight-MS (1-800-344-4867)
Keywords ➢	multiple sclerosis

Neurofibromatosis
http://www.nf.org/

Sponsor ➢	National Neurofibromatosis Foundation, Inc.
Description ➢	Neurofibromatosis (NF) diagnostic information for physicians and healthcare professionals
Data type ➢	Text
Access requirements ➢	Open
Supplemental resources ➢	Foundation homepage **(http://www.nf.org/)** Neurofibromatosis for patients and families **(http://www.nf.org/)**
User tips ➢	See homepage for distinction between NF1 and NF2
Keywords ➢	neurofibromatosis

Neurological clinical trials
http://www.innd.org/trials.htm

Sponsor ➢	Institute of Neurotoxicology and Neurological Disorders (INND)
Description ➢	Links for neurological clinical trials, new medications
Data type ➢	Text
Access requirements ➢	Open
Supplemental resources ➢	Neurological disorders (amyotrophic lateral sclerosis [ALS], Parkinson disease, etc.) **(http://www.innd.org/diseases.htm)**
User tips ➢	Check site for Lou Gehrig's disease (ALS) clinical trials consortium
Keywords ➢	neurologic disorders Lou Gehrig's disease (ALS)

Neuroscience for kids
http://weber.u.washington.edu/~chudler/neurok.html

Sponsor ➢	Eric H. Chudler, Ph.D.
Description ➢	Neuroscience games and activities for students and teachers
Data type ➢	Text; graphics
Access requirements ➢	Open
Supplemental resources ➢	Brain games **(http://weber.u.washington.edu/~chudler/chgames.html)**
User tips ➢	Try search engine for neuroscience page
Keywords ➢	neuroscience for children

Online neurosurgery resident's handbook
http://sunsite.unc.edu/Neuro/handbook/handbook.html

Sponsor ➢	Angiographic Anatomy, Syracuse Neurosurgery (SUNY-HSC)
Description ➢	Neurosurgery grading scale; drugs; MRI appearance of hemorrhage; spinal root compression syndromes
Data type ➢	Text; graphics
Access requirements ➢	Open
Supplemental resources ➢	Clinical guidelines for brain death declaration **(http://sunsite.unc.edu/Neuro/handbook/proc.html#bd)** University of North Carolina, Division of Neurosurgery homepage **(http://sunsite.unc.edu/Neuro/uncns/home.html)**
User tips ➢	Take guided tour of neurosurgery on the Web
Keywords ➢	neurosurgery

Patient information guide for neurology

http://www.aan.com/public/pig.html

Sponsor ➢ American Academy of Neurology (AAN)

Description ➢ Guide for identifying patient-oriented neurologic disorders materials and services

Data type ➢ Hyperlinked contents

Access requirements ➢ Open

Supplemental resources ➢ AAN homepage **(http://www.aan.com/home.html)**
Amyotrophic lateral sclerosis (ALS) brochure **(http://www.aan.com/public/bals.html)**

User tips ➢ Hit homepage for link to neurological conditions

Keywords ➢ neurologic disorders
Lou Gehrig's disease

Sleep medicine online

http://www.users.cloud9.net/~thorpy/sleepdoc.html

Sponsor ➢ SleepDocs Online, Sleep Multimedia, Inc.

Description ➢ E-mail help by board-certified sleep specialists of the American Board of Sleep Medicine

Data type ➢ Interactive service

Access requirements ➢ Sleep disorder questions and responses via e-mail, fax, or mail (fee service)

Supplemental resources ➢ Sleep problem symptoms, diagnoses, and treatment **(http://www.users.cloud9.net/~thorpy/sleepdoc.html)**

User tips ➢ See homepage for e-mail instructions; fee service

Keywords ➢ sleep disorders

Spike Train Analysis Graphical Environment (Stranger) package

http://biogfx.neuro.wfu.edu/stranger/analysis.html

Sponsor ➢ Bowman Gray School of Medicine, Wake Forest University

Description ➢ Database for graphical histograms and other analyses of neurons

Data type ➢ Downloadable demo software

Access requirements ➢ Open

Supplemental resources ➢ Free Stranger demo download and installation instructions
(http://biogfx.neuro.wfu.edu/stranger/download.html)
Neuroinformatics homepage
(http://biogx.neuro.wfu.edu/)

User tips ➢ See download requirements

Keywords ➢ neurologic diagnosis
medical software

Spine disorders

http://mcns10.med.nyu.edu/cases/spine.html

Sponsor ➢ New York University (NYU), Department of Neurosurgery

Description ➢ Discussions of anterior and posterior thoracic decompression, cervical synovial cyst, herniated thoracic disk, and other disorders

Data type ➢ Text; images

Access requirements ➢ Open

Supplemental resources ➢ Myxopapillary ependymoma of the cauda equina
(http://mcns10.med.nyu.edu/cases/epend/PG/PG.html)
Neurology Web Forums, Massachusetts General Hospital
(http://neuro-www.mgh.harvard.edu/forum/)

User tips ➢ Full size images available

Keywords ➢ spine disorders

Stroke emergency evaluation and treatment

http://www.stroke.org/First_Few_Hours.html

Sponsor ➢ National Stroke Association (NSA)

Description ➢ Emergency treatment of stroke during the first few hours

Data type ➢ Report

Access requirements ➢ Open

Supplemental resources ➢ NSA homepage
(http://www.stroke.org/)
NSA Stroke Center Network
(http://www.stroke.org/Network.html)

User tips ➢ See NSA newsletter, *Be Stroke Smart*

Keywords ➢ stroke
emergency

Stroke treatment in children

http://www.ninds.nih.gov/HEALINFO/D...ke%20proceedings/chd-resp.htm#Treat

Sponsor ➢ National Institute of Neurological Disorders and Stroke (NINDS)

Description ➢ Report on etiology; prehospital emergency care; rehabilitation for stroke in children

Data type ➢ Text

Access requirements ➢ Open

Supplemental resources ➢ NINDS homepage
(http://www.ninds.nih.gov/)
Arachnoiditis treatment and research
(http://www.ninds.nih.gov/healinfo/disorder/arachnoi/arachnoi.htm)

User tips ➢ Check NINDS homepage for job opportunities

Keywords ➢ pediatric stroke
neurologic disorders

Traumatic brain injury (TBI) in the United States

http://www.cdc.gov/ncipc/dacrrdp/tbi.htm

Sponsor ➢ National Center for Injury Prevention and Control, Centers for Disease Control and Prevention

Description ➢ Studies of TBI-related hospitalizations and deaths in the U.S.

Data type ➢ Text; tables

Access requirements ➢ Open

Supplemental resources ➢ Brain injury and brain death resources **(http://www.changesurfer.com/BD/Brain.html#4)**
Directory of information organizations for spinal cord injuries, strokes, and paralysis **(http://neurosurgery.mgh.harvard.edu/paral-r.htm)**

User tips ➢ See brain death resource site for anencephaly resources

Keywords ➢ traumatic brain injury
spinal cord

Whole brain atlas

http://www.med.harvard.edu/AANLIB/home.html

Sponsor ➢ Keith A. Johnson, M.D. and J. Alex Becker, Harvard Medical School

Description ➢ Neuroimaging primer atlas with lecture notes on normal brain, cerebrovascular, and neoplastic diseases

Data type ➢ Multimedia

Access requirements ➢ Open; for professionals

Supplemental resources ➢ Images, large cerebral infact **(http://www.med.harvard.edu/AANLIB/cases/case13/ct3/017.html)**
Malignant brain tumors and neuro-oncology resources, Massachusetts General Hospital **(http//neurosurgery.mgh.harvard.edu/nonc-hp.htm)**

User tips ➢ Clickable images

Keywords ➢ radiology
neuro-oncology

Women with epilepsy

http://www.efa.org/what/wei/wei.html

Sponsor ➢	Epilepsy Foundation of America (EFA)
Description ➢	Prevalence and conditions related to women with epilepsy
Data type ➢	Report
Access requirements ➢	Open
Supplemental resources ➢	EFA homepage **(http://www.efa.org/)**
User tips ➢	Check EFA news desk
Keywords ➢	women's health epilepsy

Nursing and Home Health Care

American Association of Colleges of Nursing
http://www.aacn.nche.edu/

Sponsor ➢	American Association of Colleges of Nursing (AACN)
Description ➢	Homepage for American Association of Colleges of Nursing
Data type ➢	Text
Access requirements ➢	Open
Supplemental resources ➢	National Student Nurses' Association (NSNA) **(http://www.nsna.org/index.html)** NSNA scholarships, funding database **(http://www.omhrc.gov/fund-db/F0573.htm)**
User tips ➢	Check AACN homepage for position statements
Keywords ➢	student nurses

American Association of Critical-Care Nurses (AACN)
http://www.aacn.org/

Sponsor ➢ American Association of Critical-Care Nurses (AACN)

Description ➢ Homepage for American Association of Critical Care nurses

Data type ➢ Text

Access requirements ➢ Open

Supplemental resources ➢ AACN public policy resources
(http://www.aacn.org/aacn/aacnhome....1047088256510007f0658?OpenDocument)
American Association of Spinal Cord Injury Nurses (AASCIN)
(http://www.epva.org/AASCIN.html)

User tips ➢ See AACN homepage for certification data

Keywords ➢ spinal cord injury nurses
critical care nurses

Continence program in long-term care settings
http://www.ahcpr.gov/clinic/uidon.htm

Sponsor ➢ Agency for Health Care Policy and Research (AHCPR), DHHS

Description ➢ Continence program in long-term care settings; alert for nursing home directors

Data type ➢ Text

Access requirements ➢ Open

Supplemental resources ➢ American Organization of Nurse Executives
(http://www.aone.org/index.htm)
Clinical information: Medical Treatment Effectiveness Program (MEDTEP)
(http://www.ahcpr.gov/clinic/clintxt.htm)

User tips ➢ AHCPR, an excellent resource; keep URL handy

Keywords ➢ continence program

Graduate education in nursing informatics
http://www.gl.umbc.edu/~abbott/NIprogram.htm

Sponsor ➢ Nursing Informatics Working Group, American Medical Informatics Association (AMIA)

Description ➢ Graduate programs and fellowships in nursing informatics

Data type ➢ Text

Access requirements ➢ Open

Supplemental resources ➢ Computers in nursing
(http://www.cini.com/cin/cin.htm)
Overview of nursing informatics
(http://www.ajn.org/treasures/NCNR/report/ov.html)

User tips ➢ See nursing informatics training programs

Keywords ➢ nursing informatics
medical education

Health care workers with bloodborne disease, HIV
http://www.aorn.org/nsgtoday/hiv.htm

Sponsor ➢ Association of Operating Room Nurses, Inc. (AORN)

Description ➢ AORN's revised statement on workers with bloodborne diseases

Data type ➢ Text

Access requirements ➢ Open

Supplemental resources ➢ AORN homepage
(http://www.aorn.org/nsgtoday/index.htm)
Links to surgery related sites (for patients)
(http://www.aorn.org/nsgtoday/index.htm)

User tips ➢ Check homepage for perioperative resource network directory of nurse experts

Keywords ➢ perioperative nursing
operating room nurses

Home care aide
http://www.nahc.org/HCA/home.html

Sponsor ➢ Home Care Aide Association of America (HCAAA), an affiliate of National Association for Home Care (NAHC)

Description ➢ Advocacy organization for paraprofessional home care aides

Data type ➢ Text

Access requirements ➢ Open

Supplemental resources ➢ White paper, delivery of long-term care **(http://www.nahc.org/HCA/whtppr.html)**
NAHC affiliates **(http://www.nahc.org/NAHC/Membership/affiliates.html)**

User tips ➢ White paper describes role of home care aides in long-term care

Keywords ➢ home care aides
long term care

Home care online
http://www.nahc.org/

Sponsor ➢ National Association for Home Care (NAHC)

Description ➢ Home health care news, legislation, and consumer information

Data type ➢ Text

Access requirements ➢ Open

Supplemental resources ➢ News release, Medicare Home Health Interim Payment System (IPS) **http://www.nahc.org/NAHC/NewsInfo/98nr/lewrptips.html)**
1998 NAHC legislative issues **(http://www.nahc.org/NAHC/NewsInfo/KeyIssues/98keys.html)**

User tips ➢ See NAHC homepage for certified home/hospice care executive certification

Keywords ➢ Medicare Interim Payment System (IPS)
home care executive

Home health care classification: Nursing diagnoses and interventions

http://www.dml.georgetown.edu/research/hhcc/

Sponsor ➢ Georgetown University School of Nursing

Description ➢ Classification of patients to determine resources required to provide home health services for Medicare population

Data type ➢ Report

Access requirements ➢ Open

Supplemental resources ➢ Home health care nursing interventions definition and coding scheme **(http://www.dml.georgetown.edu/research/hhcc/HHCNI.html)**
Report table of contents **(http://www.dml.georgetown.edu/research/hhcc/)**

User tips ➢ File can be downloaded in Word Perfect for PC

Keywords ➢ home health care

Hospital to home care for nurses

http://www.okqchomehealth.com/indepth/hospital.htm

Sponsor ➢ Home Health Care In Depth, Olsten Health Services

Description ➢ Nursing and home health care

Data type ➢ Text

Access requirements ➢ Open

Supplemental resources ➢ Home health care in depth index **(http://www.okqchomehealth.com/indepth/)**
National Association for Practical Nurse Education and Service (NAPNES) **(http://www.social.com/health/nhic/data/hr0170.html)**

User tips ➢ Check bin on disease state management

Keywords ➢ home health care

Influencing Congress: Ten commandments
http://www.nurse.org/acnp/leg/10com.shtml

Sponsor ➢ American College of Nurse Practitioners (ACNP)
Description ➢ Rules on how to influence Congress
Data type ➢ Text
Access requirements ➢ Open
Supplemental resources ➢ Changes in nurse practitioner reimbursement under the 1997 Balanced Budget Act
(http://www.nurse.org/acnp/facts/medicare.shtml)
Nurse practitioner statistics, Health Resources and Services Administration (HRSA)
(http://www.hrsa.dhhs.gov/bhpr/DN/npnmdata.htm)
User tips ➢ See ANCC nurse practitioner certification programs
Keywords ➢ nurse practitioner certification
political survival

Language for an interstate model of nursing regulation
http://www.ncsbn.org/files/newsreleases/nr971216.html

Sponsor ➢ American Nurses Association (ANA)
Description ➢ Boards of Nursing approval of proposal for interstate model of nursing regulation, December 16, 1997
Data type ➢ Text
Access requirements ➢ Open
Supplemental resources ➢ ANA homepage
(http://www.ana.org/index.htm)
ANA position statements on bloodborne and airborne diseases, ethics, health care
(http://www.ana.org/readroom/position/index.htm)
User tips ➢ Check ANA proceedings for data regarding a racist free nursing workplace
Keywords ➢ nursing occupational actions
economic equity

Legislative position statement on job protection
http://www.aana.com/notices/notice10.html

Sponsor ➢ American Association of Nurse Anesthetists (AANA)

Description ➢ Statement by AANA urging Congress to defeat Anesthesiologist Job Protection Act

Data type ➢ Text

Access requirements ➢ Open

Supplemental resources ➢ AANA homepage
(http://www.aana.com/)
Directory of volunteer anesthesia service
(http://www.aana.com/volunteer/frames/volmain.htm)

User tips ➢ See AANA link for the International Federation of Nurse Anesthetists

Keywords ➢ nurse anesthetists
medical volunteers

MedExplorer Internet nursing resources
http://www.medexplorer.com/m-nurse.htm

Sponsor ➢ MedExplorer

Description ➢ Internet search engine of nursing organizations

Data type ➢ Variable

Access requirements ➢ Open

Supplemental resources ➢ Healthweb Nursing of global nursing organizations
(http://www.lib.umich.edu/hw/nursingorgan.html)
National Black Nurses Association (NBNA)
(http://www.bronzeville.com/nbna/about.html)

User tips ➢ Most MedExplorer sites are hyperlinked files

Keywords ➢ nursing resources

Nursing and midwifery
http://www.who.ch/programmes/nur/wha455en.htm

Sponsor ➢	World Health Organization (WHO) Nursing Board
Description ➢	WHO resolution for strengthening nursing and midwifery
Data type ➢	Text
Access requirements ➢	Open
Supplemental resources ➢	Midwifery education **(http://www.acnm.org/prof/)** Report, nursing beyond the year 2000 (in progress) **(http://www.who.ch/programmes/nur/english.htm)**
User tips ➢	Check WHO site for bulletin board system (BBS)
Keywords ➢	midwifery anesthesia

Nursing education and practice, U.S.
http://www.bibl-u-szeged.hu/bibl/afit/nursingw.html

Sponsor ➢	Division of Nursing, Health Resources and Services Administration (HRSA), Department of Health and Human Services (DHHS)
Description ➢	Nursing workforce reports
Data type ➢	Report
Access requirements ➢	Open
Supplemental resources ➢	Minority registered nurses, HRSA **(http://www.hrsa.dhhs.gov/bhpr/DN/minorty.htm)** Nursing workforce data, HRSA **(http://www.hrsa.dhhs.gov/bhpr/dn/dn.htm)**
User tips ➢	See nursing homepage for procedure to obtain sample survey of registered nurses, March 1996
Keywords ➢	nursing workforce

Nursing ethical conflict in the workplace

http://www.bc.edu/bc_org/avp/son/ethics/research.html

Sponsor ➢ Nursing Ethics Network (NEN)

Description ➢ Report examines nurse executives' response to ethical conflict and choice in the workplace

Data type ➢ Report

Access requirements ➢ Open

Supplemental resources ➢ NEN homepage **(http://www.bc.edu/bc_org/avp/son/ethics/nen.html)**
HealthSeek employment site **(http://www.healthseek.com/forums/career/index.shtml#Database)**

User tips ➢ See NEN site for online inquiries

Keywords ➢ nursing ethics
nursing employment

Nursing informatics, enhancing patient care

http://www.nih.gov/ninr/vol4/index.html

Sponsor ➢ National Institute of Nursing Research (NINR), NIH

Description ➢ National nursing research agenda in informatics, including defining patient care data, training, and priorities

Data type ➢ Report

Access requirements ➢ Open

Supplemental resources ➢ Table of contents **(http://www.nih.gov/ninr/vol4/Contents.html)**
Worldwide Nurse, Internet nursing index **(http://www.wwnurse.com/)**

User tips ➢ Check nursing student resources in Worldwide Nurse

Keywords ➢ nursing informatics
informatics fellowships

Nursing malpractice
http://www.npg.com/npg/whocan.htm#0

Sponsor ➢ Nurses Protection Group (NPG) and Allied Health Providers

Description ➢ Tips regarding nursing malpractice

Data type ➢ Text; graphics

Access requirements ➢ Open

Supplemental resources ➢ Possible litigation conditions for nursing home residents
(http://www.rt66.com/~bdpersh/serlit.htm)
The myth of vicarious liability involving midwifery
(http://acnm.org/prof/vicaliab.htm)

User tips ➢ Full text of vicarious liability available

Keywords ➢ nursing malpractice
nursing homes

Nursing personnel in schools
http://www.aap.org/policy/01584.html

Sponsor ➢ American Academy of Pediatrics (AAP)

Description ➢ Policy statement: Qualifications and utilization of nursing personnel in schools

Data type ➢ Report

Access requirements ➢ Open

Supplemental resources ➢ Legislative actions, American Association of Occupational Health Nurses, Inc. (AAOHN)
(http://www.aaohn.org/govaff.htm#tuberculosis)
Hispanic Nurses Association
(http://www.hispanicnurses.org/)

User tips ➢ Check AAOHN employment information service

Keywords ➢ occupational health nurses
school nurses

Nursing role in the new marketplace
http://www.nursingcenter.com/career/guide97/articles/g7baer.html)

Sponsor ➢ 1997 *American Journal of Nursing (AJN) Career Guide*

Description ➢ Market perspective of nursing careers

Data type ➢ Article

Access requirements ➢ Open

Supplemental resources ➢ Directory of U.S. nursing boards, Whole Nurse **(http://www.wholenurse.com/nursing_boards.html)**
National Council of State Boards of Nursing **(http://www.ncsbn.org/)**

User tips ➢ Check AJN homepage for article on nursing graduate education

Keywords ➢ nursing careers
nursing boards

Pharmacotherapeutics for advanced practice nurses in rural Georgia
http://www2.gasou.edu/nursing/pharm#Program Driectors and Faculty

Sponsor ➢ Georgia Board of Nursing

Description ➢ Program curriculum and materials for pharmacotherapeutic diabetes, respiratory problems, women's health, and other topics

Data type ➢ Curriculum materials

Access requirements ➢ Open; download in Acrobat Reader

Supplemental resources ➢ Curriculum outline for diabetes treatment **(http://www2.gasou.edu/nursing/pharm/diabetes.html)**
Virtual Nursing Center, Martindale's Health Science Guide **(http://www-sci.lib/uci.edu/HSG/Nursing.html)**

User tips ➢ Curriculum emphasizes skill upgrading rather than basic skills

Keywords ➢ pharmacotherapeutics
rural health

Prescriptive privileges for nurse practitioners

http://www.nln.org/pr050104.htm

Sponsor ➢ National League for Nursing (NLN)

Description ➢ A curriculum model for acute care nurse practitioners

Data type ➢ Article

Access requirements ➢ Open

Supplemental resources ➢ Life-terminating choices, NLN
(http://www.nln.org/webnln/info-suicide.htm)
National Organization for Associate Degree Nursing (NOADN)
(http://www.podi.com/adnursing)

User tips ➢ NLN site of online abstracts in progress

Keywords ➢ nurse practitioners
assisted suicide

Private duty nursing services

http://www.cancer.org/rig/rigduty.html

Sponsor ➢ American Cancer Society (ACS)

Description ➢ How to select private duty nursing services

Data type ➢ Text

Access requirements ➢ Open

Supplemental resources ➢ Helping people cope: private duty nursing services
(http://www.oncolink.upenn.edu/psychosocial/cope/55.html)
Notice for oncology nursing certification (ONC)
(http://www.oncc.org/pages/about_certification/about_cert.htm)

User tips ➢ Bachelor's degree minimum requirement for ONC beginning January 1, 2000

Keywords ➢ private duty nursing
oncology nursing certification

State licensure guide

http://nursingcenter.com/career/guide/Licensure.cfm

Sponsor ➢ Lippincott Nursing Center

Description ➢ Licensure information includes addresses, fees, time limits, and other details, according to state

Data type ➢ Directory

Access requirements ➢ Open

Supplemental resources ➢ Lippincott's Nursing Center
(http://www.nursingcenter.com/)
Career Center
(http://www.nursingcenter.com/career/page 1.cfm)

User tips ➢ See nursing center homepage for continuing education information

Keywords ➢ medical education
nursing licensure

Telephone or triage nursing

http://www.katsden.com/telenurse/triage.html

Sponsor ➢ Telenursing Resources

Description ➢ Overview of telephone or triage nursing

Data type ➢ Text

Access requirements ➢ Open

Supplemental resources ➢ Employment in triage nursing
(http://www.katsden.com/telenurse/employ.html)
Occupational statistics for nursing supervisors and registered nurses, Canada
(http://www.hrdc-drhc.gc.ca/hrdc/cor...s/english/volume1/315/315.html#2000)

User tips ➢ See list of conferences on telephone triage and telenursing

Keywords ➢ triage nursing

Using anesthesia bags
http://www.hooked.net/~gtrimble/using_anesthesia_bags.html

Sponsor ➢ Emergency Nursing World

Description ➢ Instructions for using anesthesia bags

Data type ➢ Text

Access requirements ➢ Open

Supplemental resources ➢ Sedated procedures outline **(http://www.hooked.net/~gtrimble/sedation_guidelines.html)**
Emergency Nursing World homepage **(http://www.hooked.net/~ttrimble/enw/index.html)**

User tips ➢ Check homepage for discharge instructions

Keywords ➢ emergency nurses
anesthesia

Visiting Nurse Associations of America (VNAA)
http://www.vnaa.org/body_default.html

Sponsor ➢ Visiting Nurse Associations of America (VNAA)

Description ➢ Discussion of role and purpose of VNAA

Data type ➢ Text

Access requirements ➢ Open

Supplemental resources ➢ Selecting a home health care provider **(http://www.vnaa.org/html/body_picking_a_provider.html)**
Online resources for geriatric nurses, National Gerontological Nursing Association **(http://www.geriatricvideo.com/resource.htm)**

User tips ➢ Check links for specialty nursing organizations

Keywords ➢ nursing
home health care

Nutrition

Annual reports on family expenditures

http://www.usda.gov/fcs/cnpp.htm

Sponsor ➢	Center for Nutrition Policy and Promotion, U.S. Department of Agriculture (USDA)
Description ➢	Annual reports of expenditures on children by families, 1995 and 1996
Data type ➢	Text; some graphics
Access requirements ➢	Open
Supplemental resources ➢	Cost of food at home, May 1996-September 1997 **(http://www.usda.gov/fcs/cnpp.htm)**
User tips ➢	See homepage for report on dietary guidelines for Americans, 1995
Keywords ➢	nutrition

Aquaculture
http://www.ancs.purdue.edu/aquanic/home.htm

Sponsor ➢ Aquaculture Network Information Center (AquaNIC)

Description ➢ Publications, computer training, and resources for aquaculture species

Data type ➢ Text; multimedia

Access requirements ➢ Open; levels for beginners and discussion groups

Supplemental resources ➢ Species manuals for aquaculture education, National Council for Agricultural Education **(http://www.ansc.purdue.edu/aquanic/publicat/govagen/ncae/council.htm)**

User tips ➢ See reproduction, diseases, and farming of carp, crawfish, and catfish

Keywords ➢ seafood

The Bad Bug Book
http://vm.cfsan.fda.gov/~mow/intro.html

Sponsor ➢ Center for Food Safety and Applied Nutrition, U.S. Food and Drug Administration (FDA)

Description ➢ Handbook of facts on foodborne, pathogenic microorganisms and natural toxins

Data type ➢ Text with hypertext links

Access requirements ➢ Open

Supplemental resources ➢ *Salmonella* spp.
(http://vm.cfsan.fda.gov/%7Emow/chap1.html)
FDA press releases; Congressional testimony and *Federal Register* documents, 1997
(http://vm.cfsan.fda.gov/~lrd/press.html)

User tips ➢ Food information and seafood hotline (1-800-FDA-4010)

Keywords ➢ food safety
foodborne microorganisms

Catfish production teaching plan

http://www.catfishinstitute.com/home.html

Sponsor ➢ Catfish Institute

Description ➢ Teaching plans for catfish farming and marketing

Data type ➢ Instruction plan

Access requirements ➢ Open

Supplemental resources ➢ Catfish recipes with photos
(http://www.catfishinstitute.com/recipe/r5.html)
Food and Drug Administration (FDA) raw oysters alert, July 1995
(http://vm.cfsan.fda.gov/~lrd/oyster.html)

User tips ➢ Recipes photos can be enlarged

Keywords ➢ seafood

Closing the gap on food safety standards

http://ificinfo.health.org/insight/ih-cgof.htm

Sponsor ➢ International Food Information Council (IFIC)

Description ➢ International food safety standards involving the General Agreement of Tariffs and Trade (GATT), and other regulations

Data type ➢ Text; search enabled; glossary

Access requirements ➢ Open

Supplemental resources ➢ IFIC homepage
(http://ificinfo.health org/)
Presidential announcement of U.S. policy on imported and domestic foods, October 2, 1997
(http://vm.cfsan.fda.gov/~dms/fsfact2.html)

User tips ➢ See homepage links for reporters and educators

Keywords ➢ imported food safety

Crop production data

http://www.usda.gov/nass/aggraphs/graphics.htm

Sponsor ➢ National Agricultural Statistics Service (NASS), U.S. Department of Agriculture (USDA)

Description ➢ Graphics, historic data of crop production, livestock, economics, and research

Data type ➢ Graphics; tables

Access requirements ➢ Open

Supplemental resources ➢ Lentil production—Idaho and Washington **(http://www.usda.gov/nass/aggraphs/lentils.htm)**
Statistics, graphic data for dry beans, peas, and lentils production **(http://www.usda.gov/nass/aggraphs/drybeans.htm)**

User tips ➢ See homepage for agriculture census

Keywords ➢ agriculture production

Egg nutrition

http://www.aeb.org/

Sponsor ➢ American Egg Board

Description ➢ Egg industry information

Data type ➢ Text; some graphics

Access requirements ➢ Open

Supplemental resources ➢ Studies of plasma and dietary cholesterol **(http://www.enc-online.org/dietc.htm)**
Egg links **(http://www.roseacre.com/links.htm)**

User tips ➢ Check egg links for poultry science virtual library

Keywords ➢ eggs

Food and drug law history

http://www.fda.gov/opacom/backgrounders/miles.html

Sponsor ➢ U.S. Food and Drug Administration (FDA)

Description ➢ Milestones in U.S. food and drug law history, from 1785 to present

Data type ➢ Text

Access requirements ➢ Open

Supplemental resources ➢ FDA homepage **(http://www.fda.gov/)**

User tips ➢ Search FDA homepage for additional legislative actions

Keywords ➢ food legislation

Foodborne illness education

http://www.nal.usda.gov/fnic/foodborne/foodborn.htm

Sponsor ➢ Foodborne Illness Education Information Center, U.S. Department of Agriculture and Food and Drug Administration (FDA)

Description ➢ Index of foodborne illness resources and training database

Data type ➢ Text for consumers and professionals

Access requirements ➢ Open; some information available on floppy disk

Supplemental resources ➢ Food and Nutrition Information Center (FNIC) homepage
(http://www.nal.usda.gov/fnic/)
Salmonella monitoring in humans and cattle (10/94), USDA
(gopher://hal.aphis.usda.gov:70/0./Al.d/AHl.d/AHMRAE.d/salmmon.f)

User tips ➢ Check FNIC index of food and nutrition Internet resources

Keywords ➢ food safety
food illness

Hazard Analysis Critical Control Points (HACCP) training

http://www.nal.usda.gov/fnic/foodborne/haccp/index.shtml

Sponsor ➢	Food and Nutrition Information Center, USDA/FDA
Description ➢	HACCP training and resources for industry and food service professionals
Data type ➢	Database; search enabled
Access requirements ➢	Open
Supplemental resources ➢	HACCP training programs and resources database **(http://www.nal.usda.gov/fnic/foodborne/haccp/test/train.html)** News, HACCP inspection regulations for seafood industry **(http://www.mdsg.umd.edu/seagrantmediacenter/news/haccp.html)**
User tips ➢	Additional HACCP listings welcomed; e-mail to **croberts@nal.usda.gov**
Keywords ➢	food safety HACCP

Insects for food

http://www.ent.iastate.edu/Misc/InsectsAsFood.html

Sponsor ➢	Iowa State University
Description ➢	Recipes for banana worm bread, rootworm beetle dip, chirpie chip cookies, and others
Data type ➢	Photographs and text
Access requirements ➢	Open
Supplemental resources ➢	Insect cleaning and preparation, University of Kentucky **(http://www.uky.edu/Agriculture/Entomology/ythfacts/bugfood2.htm)** Insect snacks around the world **(http://www.uky.edu/Agriculture/Entomology/ythfacts/ythfacts/yf813.htm)**
User tips ➢	See data on baiting and preparing dragonflies in Bali
Keywords ➢	insect food entomology

Iodine deficiency disorders (IDD) database
http://www.idrc.ca/mi/idddocs/iddindex.htm

Sponsor ➢ International Council for Control of Iodine Deficiency Disorders

Description ➢ Technical database: index of IDD assessment, treatment, consequences, and legislation

Data type ➢ Index; search enabled by country, subject, or keywords

Access requirements ➢ Open

Supplemental resources ➢ *IDD Newsletter* **(http://www.idrc.ca/mi/dddocs/idd593.htm#Role)**
Micronutrient malnutrition and control program status, Global Micronutrient Network **(http://www.idrc.ca/mi/pre_con.htm)**

User tips ➢ See reports from world regions

Keywords ➢ iodine deficiency
micronutrients

Nutrition library catalog
http://www.geocities.com/HotSprings/2455/tableofcont.html

Sponsor ➢ Geocities.com

Description ➢ Consumer catalog of nutrition data files for cholesterol, food cravings, guide to fats, and food color

Data type ➢ Hyperlinked text

Access requirements ➢ Open

Supplemental resources ➢ Family recipes of Black American chefs, National Cancer Institute (NCI) **(http://www.geocities.com/HotSprings/2455/dnhealth.html)**

User tips ➢ Check summary on Black American diet

Keywords ➢ low fat diet

Poverty and nutrition in welfare societies

http://www.edv.agrar.tu-muenchen.de...es/9510-Poverty-Nutrition/agev1.htm

Sponsor ➢ 2nd European Interdisciplinary Meeting, Germany, 1995

Description ➢ Abstracts of meeting contributors

Data type ➢ Direct access; data for professionals

Access requirements ➢ Open

Supplemental resources ➢ Abstract: From food poverty to social exclusion **(http://www.edv.agrar.tu-muenchen.de...s/9510-Poverty-Nutrition/abs_01.htm)**

User tips ➢ See abstracts on hunger, careers of poverty in modern society

Keywords ➢ malnutrition and poverty

Protein Data Bank (PDB)

http://www.pdb.bnl.gov/

Sponsor ➢ Brookhaven National Laboratory

Description ➢ Archive of three-dimensional structures of biological macromolecules

Data type ➢ Data for researchers, educators, and students

Access requirements ➢ Open; direct access

Supplemental resources ➢ Protein software-related information **(http://www.pdb.bnl.gov/software.html)**

User tips ➢ Check software available through PDB

Keywords ➢ protein data bank

USDA Food Composition Databases

http://www.nal.usda.gov/fnic/foodcomp/

Sponsor ➢ Nutrient Data Laboratory, Agricultural Research Service (ARS), USDA

Description ➢ Database of food composition products data sets, nutrient data, and nutrition

Data type ➢ Database

Access requirements ➢ Open; data sets can be downloaded

Supplemental resources ➢ Instructions for submitting data to USDA Food Composition Databases
(http://www.nal.usda.gov/fnic/foodcomp/)
Interactive food guide pyramid
(http://www.nal.usda.gov/fnic/Fpyr/pyramid.html)

User tips ➢ Pyramid is a large file in PDF format

Keywords ➢ nutrient data sets
food guide pyramid

Vegetarian diets

http://www.fortran.com/%7Ernepomuc/heal/ada.htm#authors

Sponsor ➢ American Dietetic Association (ADA)

Description ➢ ADA position on vegetarian diets

Data type ➢ Text for consumers and professionals

Access requirements ➢ Open

Supplemental resources ➢ ADA homepage
(http://www.eatright.org/)
National Center for Nutrition and Dietetics
(http://www.eatright.org/ncnd.html)

User tips ➢ Consumer nutrition hotline (1-800-366-1655)

Keywords ➢ vegetarian diet
nutrition

Weight-control Information Network (WIN)

http://www.niddk.nih.gov/NutritionDocs.html

Sponsor ➢ National Institute of Diabetes and Digestive and Kidney Diseases (NIDDK)

Description ➢ Information on nutrition, obesity, eating disorders, statistics, and treatment medications

Data type ➢ Text; tables; graphics

Access requirements ➢ Open

Supplemental resources ➢ Gallstones **(http://www.niddk.nih.gov/Gallstones/Gallstones.html)**
Gastric surgery for severe obesity **(http://www.niddk.nih.gov/Gastric/Gastsurg.html)**

User tips ➢ Weight-control Information Network (WIN) (1-800-WIN-8098)

Keywords ➢ obesity
gastric surgery

Women, Infants, and Children (WIC) Nutrition Program

http://www.usda.gov/fcs/wic/wicfac~2.htm

Sponsor ➢ Food and Consumer Service, U.S. Department of Agriculture (USDA)

Description ➢ WIC program description and eligibility

Data type ➢ Text

Access requirements ➢ Open

Supplemental resources ➢ Food and Consumer Service homepage **(http://www.usda.gov/fcs/fcs.htm)**
WIC national breastfeeding promotion campaign **(http://www.usda.gov/fcs/brfdcpgn.htm)**

User tips ➢ Check homepage link for gleaning/food recovery

Keywords ➢ pediatric nutrition
WIC program

World food emergency weekly reports
http://www.vita.org/disaster/wfp/

Sponsor ➢	United Nations World Food Programme (WFP)
Description ➢	Weekly emergency reports
Data type ➢	Text
Access requirements ➢	Open
Supplemental resources ➢	WFP homepage **(http://www.wfp.org/Wfphome.html)** Report 49, 5 December 1997 **(http://www.vita.org/disaster/wfp/0022.html)**
User tips ➢	Check weekly operation report of major WFP relief activities
Keywords ➢	global food data disaster relief

Occupational Health

Accident causes and prevention
http://www.cdc.gov/niosh/nasd/video/av00400.html

Sponsor ➢	National Ag Safety Video Database (NASD)
Description ➢	Database of video abstracts and contacts on farming accidents, hazards, impact, and safety
Data type ➢	Video database
Access requirements ➢	Open
Supplemental resources ➢	NASD database **(http://www.cdc.gov/niosh/nasd/nasdhome.html)**
User tips ➢	Videos available for borrowing, rental, or purchase
Keywords ➢	agricultural safety preventive health

Census of occupational injuries, fatalities, and illnesses
http://stats.bls.gov/oshhome.htm

Sponsor ➢ Bureau of Labor Statistics (BLS)

Description ➢ Statistical database documentation of fatal, nonfatal, injuries, illnesses, and annual health care expenditures

Data type ➢ Text; statistics

Access requirements ➢ Open

Supplemental resources ➢ Census of fatal occupational injuries **(http://stats.bls.gov/oshfat1.htm)**
News releases and tables: Census of fatal occupational injuries **(http://stats.bls.gov/oshcftab.htm)**

User tips ➢ See homepage for list of electronic documents available for download

Keywords ➢ occupational fatalities
injury statistics

Cumulative trauma disorder (CTD)
http://ctdnews.com/

Sponsor ➢ Center for Workplace Health

Description ➢ Statistics, ergonomics, and research regarding CTD-related injuries

Data type ➢ Newsletter for health and safety professionals

Access requirements ➢ Open

Supplemental resources ➢ Cumulative trauma disorders (CTD) toll on workers' compensation **(http://ctdnews.com/comp.html)**
Backbelt research **(http://ctdnews.com/belt.html)**

User tips ➢ Check file for reports on ergonomic products

Keywords ➢ cumulative trauma disorder (CTD)
ergonomics

Dust sampling results (metal and nonmetal mines)

http://www.msha.gov/STATS/SAMPLING/MAINPGE.htm

Sponsor ➢ Mine Safety and Health Administration (MSHA), U.S. Department of Labor

Description ➢ Prevention of dust-related illnesses; MSHA compliance data

Data type ➢ Text

Access requirements ➢ Open

Supplemental resources ➢ Labor related data **(http://www.dol.gov/dol/asp/public/dollabdata/labdata.htm)**
Mine accidents, injury, and illness statistics **(http://www.msha.gov/STATS/STATSCR1.htm)**

User tips ➢ Check data from the U.S. Economics and Statistics Administration

Keywords ➢ mining safety
dust related illnesses

Ergonomics

http://ergo.human.cornell.edu/

Sponsor ➢ CUErgo: Cornell Ergonomics Web

Description ➢ Ergonomics research projects in keyboard, cumulative trauma disorders, and back injuries

Data type ➢ Text; slideshows

Access requirements ➢ Open

Supplemental resources ➢ Evaluation of keyboard research projects **(http://ergo.human.cornell.edu/AHProjects/kbdprojects.html)**
Preventing carpal tunnel syndrome, from the Cornell/Honeywell Study **(http://www.tc.cornell.edu/Research/MetaSoft/Articles/CIE/IRI/Hedge/hedge.html)**

User tips ➢ See postural risk factors for back injury—Cornell dairy study

Keywords ➢ carpel tunnel syndrome
ergonomics

Ergonomics—statistics

http://www.osha-slc.gov/ergo/Statistics.html

Sponsor ➢ U.S. Department of Labor, Occupational Safety and Health Administration (OSHA)

Description ➢ Disorders associated with repeated trauma according to industry

Data type ➢ Text; charts; graphics

Access requirements ➢ Open

Supplemental resources ➢ Ergonomics homepage
(http://www.osha-slc.gov/ergo/)
Line chart: Number of occupational illnesses
(http://www.osha-slc.gov/ergo/chart1.html)

User tips ➢ See OSHA homepage for training activities

Keywords ➢ repetitive stress injuries (RSIs)
ergonomics

Experiences of Texas workers denied spinal surgery

http://www.roc.capnet.state.tx.us/spinal.htm

Sponsor ➢ Research and Oversight Council on Workers' Compensation, Texas

Description ➢ Report on experiences of injured workers denied spinal surgery, June 1997

Data type ➢ Report

Access requirements ➢ Open

Supplemental resources ➢ Worker injury costs, National Safety Council
(http://www.nsc.org/lrs/statinfo/afp51.htm)
National Safety Council (NSC)
(http://www.nsc.org/)

User tips ➢ See NSC accident facts menu

Keywords ➢ worker compensation
neurology

Index of occupational safety and health files
http://osh.net/

Sponsor ➢	Occupational Safety and Health Net (OSHNET)
Description ➢	Files on ergonomics, radiation safety, safety management, violence, and professional certifications for industrial hygiene, construction, and other occupation
Data type ➢	Case studies, reports, guidebooks
Access requirements ➢	Open
Supplemental resources ➢	Safety software and analysis **(http://osh.net/soft.htm)** Occupational Safety and Health Web (OSHWEB) for chemical safety; electrical; risk management **(http://turva.me.tut.fi/~oshweb/)**
User tips ➢	Check safety job links
Keywords ➢	electrical safety chemical safety

1997 Decisions of the Occupational Safety and Health Review Commission (OSHRC)
http://www.oshrc.gov/comm97.html

Sponsor ➢	Occupational Safety and Health Review Commission (OSHRC)
Description ➢	Decisions resulting from Occupational Safety and Health Administration (OSHA) inspections of workplaces
Data type ➢	Dockets of case number, issuance date, and case name
Access requirements ➢	Cases viewed by Adobe Acrobat Reader
Supplemental resources ➢	OSHRC homepage **(http://www.oshrc.gov/index.html)**
User tips ➢	Full text legal files available
Keywords ➢	legal medicine

Nursing home occupational injuries

http://www.osha-slc.gov/SLTC/NursingHome/index.html

Sponsor ➢ Occupational Safety and Health Administration (OSHA), U.S. Department of Labor

Description ➢ Nursing home safety evaluation, control, compliance, training, and directives

Data type ➢ Text; search enabled

Access requirements ➢ Open

Supplemental resources ➢ OSHA homepage **(http://www.osha-slc.gov/)**
Case summaries, preventing injury in nursing homes **(http://www.osha-slc.gov/NewInit/NurseHome/cases.html)**

User tips ➢ See diagram of nursing home with potential hazards

Keywords ➢ nursing home safety

Occupational health issues

http://www.aiha.org:80/govt.html

Sponsor ➢ American Industrial Hygiene Association (AIHA)

Description ➢ Position and white papers on reporting occupational illnesses, certification for respiratory protection devices, and lead protection for industrial hygienists

Data type ➢ Text

Access requirements ➢ Open

Supplemental resources ➢ American College of Occupational and Environmental Medicine (ACOEM) homepage **(http://www.acoem.org:80/)**
Abstracts and articles from ACOEM's *Journal of Occupational and Environmental Medicine* **(http://www.acoem.org:80/pubs/joem/1197abs.htm)**

User tips ➢ ACOEM journal maintains abstracts of recent articles

Keywords ➢ occupational health
industrial hygienists

Occupational safety and health databases

http://turva.me.tut.fi/cis/occupational_safety_databases2.htm

Sponsor ➢ International Occupational Safety and Health Information Centre (CIS), International Labour Office (ILO)

Description ➢ Occupational safety and health database name, type, language, software information

Data type ➢ Directory

Access requirements ➢ Open

Supplemental resources ➢ CIS homepage
(http://turva.me.tut.fi/cis/epubgen.html)
Occupational health online resources
(http://www.einet.net/galaxy/Medici...edicine/Occupational-Medicine.html)

User tips ➢ Database in Spanish (in progress)

Keywords ➢ occupational safety resource

OSHA statistics and data

http://www.osha.gov/oshstats/index.html

Sponsor ➢ Occupational Safety and Health Administration (OSHA), Department of Labor (DOL)

Description ➢ OSHA inspections according to industry

Data type ➢ Text

Access requirements ➢ Search by establishment

Supplemental resources ➢ Compliance assistance
(http://www.osha.gov/compliance/)
Small entity compliance guide for OSHA's abatement verification regulation
(http://www.osha.gov/compliance/)

User tips ➢ See industry profile for OSHA standard

Keywords ➢ OSHA compliance
environmental health

Plain facts about farmer health

http://www.nsc.org/necas/aghealth.htm

Sponsor ➢ National Education Center for Agricultural Safety, National Safety Council

Description ➢ Occupational conditions affecting farmer health

Data type ➢ Text

Access requirements ➢ Open

Supplemental resources ➢ Center homepage
(http://www.nsc.org/necas.htm)
How farm accidents happen
(http://www.geisinger.edu/ghs/pubtips/F/FarmAccidents.htm)

User tips ➢ See homepage link to the agricultural industry

Keywords ➢ farm safety

State profiles of occupational safety and health

http://ftp.cdc.gov/niosh/ia.html

Sponsor ➢ National Institute for Occupational Safety and Health (NIOSH), CDC

Description ➢ Data regarding prevalence, costs, and prevention of occupational fatalities, injuries, and disease

Data type ➢ Text

Access requirements ➢ Open; or by phone (1-800-356-4674)

Supplemental resources ➢ NIOSH programs and standards for eye protection, respiratory, and hearing
(http://www.niehs.nih.gov/odhsb/ih/ihhome.htm)
Warning, hazards of flood cleanup work
(http://www.cdc.gov/niosh/flood.html)

User tips ➢ CDC emergency response number: 770-488-7100

Keywords ➢ laboratory safety
occupational health statistics

Trigger finger disorder
http://www.sechrest.com/mmg/ctd/trigger.html

Sponsor ➢	Medical Multimedia Group
Description ➢	Description of trigger finger anatomy, causes, and symptoms
Data type ➢	Text
Access requirements ➢	Open
Supplemental resources ➢	Neck, shoulder, and elbow disorders **(http://www.sechrest.com/mmg/ctd/stuff.html)** Video terminals no risk to pregnancy **(http://www.infoseek.com/Content?arn...earch&sv=N5&col=NX&kt=A&ak=news1486)**
User tips ➢	Consult physician for specific treatment recommendations
Keywords ➢	cumulative trauma disorder pregnancy

Workers compensation law materials
http://www.law.cornell.edu/topics/workers_compensation.html#menu

Sponsor ➢	Legal Information Institute, Cornell Law School
Description ➢	Overview and sources for workers compensation law materials
Data type ➢	Text
Access requirements ➢	Open
Supplemental resources ➢	Legal Information Institute homepage **(http://www.law.cornell.edu/index.html)**
User tips ➢	Check Institute homepage for downloads
Keywords ➢	worker compensation

Ophthalmology

Collaborative ocular melanoma study (COMS)

http://webeye.ophth.uiowa.edu/coms/

Sponsor ➢	National Eye Institute (NEI), National Cancer Institute (NCI), National Institutes of Health (NIH)
Description ➢	Description of multicenter randomized trial to determine most effective treatment for choroidal melanoma
Data type ➢	Study
Access requirements ➢	Open
Supplemental resources ➢	COMS glossary **(http://webeye.ophth.uiowa.edu/coms/booklet/book5.htm)** Myopia Control Network Service (MCNS) **(http://www.mcns.com/pateint.htm)**
User tips ➢	Check homepage for additional information and resources
Keywords ➢	ocular melanoma myopia

Computer vision

http://www.cs.cmu/edu/~cil/vision.html

Sponsor ➢ Computer Vision

Description ➢ Test images include mammography image databases (over 100 images); Los Alamos fingerprint images, Graz University of Technology stereo pairs, TIFF format

Data type ➢ Text; demos; databases

Access requirements ➢ Open

Supplemental resources ➢ Index, computer vision test images **(http://www.cs.cmu/edu/~cil/v-images.html)**

User tips ➢ Search computer vision homepage for additional links

Keywords ➢ computer vision tests
medical software

Current eye research

http://www.wilmer.jhu.edu/research.htm

Sponsor ➢ Wilmer Eye Institute

Description ➢ Research center for hereditary eye diseases; cornea and anterior segment; preventive ophthalmology; glaucoma

Data type ➢ Text

Access requirements ➢ Open

Supplemental resources ➢ Wilmer Eye Institute homepage **(http://www.wilmer.jhu.edu/)**
Earlier diagnosis of glaucoma using nerve fiber layer exam **(http://www.wilmer.jhu.edu/research.htm)**

User tips ➢ Check Center research file for hereditary eye data diseases

Keywords ➢ eye research

Eye Net

http://www.eyenet.org/member/visit_aao/fax_on_demand.html#seminars

Sponsor ➢ American Academy of Ophthalmology (AAO)

Description ➢ Academy documents include clinical education materials for students, physicians, and allied health staff

Data type ➢ Text

Access requirements ➢ Open

Supplemental resources ➢ American Society of Cataract and Refractive Surgery and American Society of Ophthalmic Administrators
(http://www.ascrs.org/)
International list of refractive surgeons and surgery centers (ASCRS)
(http://or.stanford.edu/~mob/RK/surgeon.html)

User tips ➢ Academy documents available by fax

Keywords ➢ ophthalmologic resources
medical education

Free eyeglasses for kids

http://www.tdl.com/~kids/FreeEyeglasses.html

Sponsor ➢ American Optometric Association (AOA)

Description ➢ Eligibility requirements for free eyeglasses for kids

Data type ➢ Text

Access requirements ➢ Open

Supplemental resources ➢ Kids Foundation Research Institute
(http://www.tdl.com/~kids)
Vision school program, grades 4-8
(http://www.nei.nih.gov/vision/vision.htm)

User tips ➢ Visual exam and spectacles are free

Keywords ➢ free eyeglasses
pediatrics

National eye-health related organizations

http://www.nei.nih.gov/publications/sel-org.htm

Sponsor ➢ National Eye Institute (NEI), National Institutes of Health (NIH)

Description ➢ Directory of name, address, phone, Web site, and e-mail numbers of eye organizations

Data type ➢ Directory

Access requirements ➢ Open

Supplemental resources ➢ Clinical studies and recruitment contacts for herpetic eye study, myopia
(http://www.nei.nih.gov/recruit.htm)
Information for health care professionals
(http://www.nei.nih.gov/professionals.htm)

User tips ➢ Toll free numbers available for most clinical trial studies

Keywords ➢ eye resources
clinical trials

Ophthalmic photography

http://webeye.ophth.uiowa.edu/ops/index.htm

Sponsor ➢ Ophthalmic Photographers' Society, Inc.

Description ➢ Description of ophthalmic photography

Data type ➢ Text; images

Access requirements ➢ Open

Supplemental resources ➢ What is ophthalmic photography?
(http://webeye.ophth.uiowa.edu/ops/op-photo/op-photo.htm)

User tips ➢ Check homepage for certification and educational programs

Keywords ➢ ophthalmic photography

Ophthalmology multimedia theater
http://www.eyeworld.org/October/theater.html

Sponsor ➢	ASCRS Ophthalmic Services Corp.
Description ➢	Clips on cataract, eye diseases, contact lenses, surgery, technology, and other topics
Data type ➢	Multimedia AVI movies
Access requirements ➢	Download AVI movie viewer
Supplemental resources ➢	Movies: Dot motion perimetry, trabeculoplasty **(http://www.eyeworld.org/October/theaterpic_glaucoma.html)**
User tips ➢	All clips available for slower connections
Keywords ➢	ophthalmology

Optometry career guidance
http://www.aoanet.org/career-guidance.html

Sponsor ➢	American Optometric Association (AOA)
Description ➢	Optometry schools and careers
Data type ➢	Text; audio
Access requirements ➢	Open
Supplemental resources ➢	AOA homepage **(http://www.aoanet.org/index-mainspace.html)** You want to be an optometrist **(http://www.aoanet.org/career-guidance.html)**
User tips ➢	AOA represents optometry doctors, students, and paraoptometric assistants
Keywords ➢	optometry allied health

Orbital and eye lesions
http://patho.wat.ch:80/ophthalmo/

Sponsor ➢ Patho.Wat.ch

Description ➢ Online relational database providing diagnosis for orbital and eye lesions

Data type ➢ Text; images

Access requirements ➢ Open; database searchable by preconfigured queries or image name fields

Supplemental resources ➢ Ophthalmic, pathology links **(http://patho.wat.ch/info/links.cfm)**
Topic search criteria **(http://patho.wat.ch/Ophthalmo/SearchSimple.cmf?Lang=E)**

User tips ➢ Check homepage for instructions on submitting comments

Keywords ➢ ophthalmology
pathology

Pediatric ophthalmology and strabismus
http://med-aapos.bu.edu/default.html

Sponsor ➢ American Association for Pediatric Ophthalmology and Strabismus (AAPOS)

Description ➢ Professional and general information on pediatric ophthalmology

Data type ➢ Text; multimedia

Access requirements ➢ Open

Supplemental resources ➢ Corneal and red reflex images **(http://med-aapos.bu.edu/AAPOS/MTI.html)**
Link for audio and video archives for professionals **(http://med-aapos.bu.edu/default.html)**

User tips ➢ See pedi-ophth consumer resource file

Keywords ➢ pediatric ophthalmology
strabismus

Photoreceptors

http://insight.med.utah.edu/Webvision/photo1.html

Sponsor ➢ Web Vision

Description ➢ Movies and text describing light microscopy, outer segments, visual transduction; types of cones

Data type ➢ Multimedia

Access requirements ➢ Open

Supplemental resources ➢ Index for WebVision homepage **(http://www.insight.med.utah.edu/Webvision/index.html)**
Patient handouts on contact lenses, corneal topography, and other topics **(http://www.slackinc.com/eye/osn/osnsupp.htm)**

User tips ➢ See index for link to retina facts and figures

Keywords ➢ retina
photoreceptor

Spatially guided navigation and infant vision

http://john.berkeley.edu/Features/demos.html

Sponsor ➢ Bankslab, Guided Navigation and Infant Vision Laboratory, University of California at Berkeley

Description ➢ Demos of real versus simulated eye rotation; stereo flow; Aubert-Fleischel reversal; and other topics

Data type ➢ Demos

Access requirements ➢ Downloadable demos

Supplemental resources ➢ Demo of the failure of Hering's law **(http://john.berkeley.edu/Figures_%26_Demos/monocularocclusion.html)**
Homepage **(http://john.berkeley.edu/)**

User tips ➢ Additional demos scheduled for future release

Keywords ➢ vision research
medical software

Vision research WWW servers

http://www.socsci.uci.edu:80/cogsci/vision.html

Sponsor ➢	University of California, Irvine Research
Description ➢	Alphabetized links of international schools and universities involved with human and primate vision research
Data type ➢	Hyperlinked directory
Access requirements ➢	Open; for professionals
Supplemental resources ➢	University of Genova, Italy: Physical structure of perception **(http://www.socsci.uci.edu:80/cogsci/vision.html)**
User tips ➢	International schools well represented in directory
Keywords ➢	vision research

Otolaryngology

Acoustic emissions from dysfunctional temporomandibular joints (TMJs)
http://www.geocities.com/CapeCanaveral/8462/index.html

Sponsor ➢	Geocities
Description ➢	Description of TMJ dysfunction and causes
Data type ➢	Text
Access requirements ➢	Open
Supplemental resources ➢	American Academy of Audiology **(http://www.audiology.com/)**
User tips ➢	Check TMJ links
Keywords ➢	temporomandibular joint (TMJ)

Clinical and special services for the deaf and hard of hearing

http://www.gallaudet.edu/~nicd/health.html

Sponsor ➢ National Information Center on Deafness (NICD), Gallaudet University

Description ➢ Resources for health care, devices, oral interpreters, text telephones, and other services for deafness and hearing loss

Data type ➢ Text

Access requirements ➢ Open

Supplemental resources ➢ NICD homepage **(http://www.gallaudet.edu:80/~nicd/)**

User tips ➢ Resources categorized according to state

Keywords ➢ deaf services

Deaf-blind children

http://www.tr.wou.edu/dblink/data/index.htm

Sponsor ➢ National Information Clearinghouse on Children Who Are Deaf-Blind (DB-Link), U.S. Department of Education

Description ➢ Deaf-blind catalog and resource databases for parents and providers

Data type ➢ Text; graphics; database

Access requirements ➢ Open; search enabled

Supplemental resources ➢ DB-Link homepage **(http://www.tr.wou.edu/dblink/)**
Bibliography from DB-Link **(http://www.tr.wou.edu/dblink/over-bib.htm)**

User tips ➢ See homepage link for additional online resources; contact number: 1-800-438-9376

Keywords ➢ deaf-blind children

Deafness and Communication Disorders Information Clearinghouse

http://www.aerie.com/nihdb/nidcd/dctest.html

Sponsor ➢ National Institute on Deafness and Other Communication Disorders (NIDCD), NIH

Description ➢ Database of titles, abstracts, and education materials

Data type ➢ Clearinghouse database

Access requirements ➢ Open; search enabled

Supplemental resources ➢ NIDCD homepage **(http://www.nih.gov/nidcd/)**

User tips ➢ See instructions for simple and detailed searches

Keywords ➢ communication disorders
deafness

Ear, Nose, and Throat Information Center

http://www.netdoor.com/entinfo/index.html

Sponsor ➢ American Academy of Otolaryngology–Head and Neck Surgery, Inc. (AAO-HNS)

Description ➢ Nose and sinus; ear and hearing related information

Data type ➢ Text; graphics for consumers

Access requirements ➢ Open

Supplemental resources ➢ Earache and otitis media **(http://www.netdoor.com/entinfo/omaao.html)**
What is an otolaryngologist-head-neck surgeon? **(http://www.netdoor.com/entinfo/otolaaao.html)**

User tips ➢ Check computer generated, stereoscopic movie on paranasal sinus embryology, anatomy, and surgery

Keywords ➢ sinus
ear-hearing disorders

Materials for acquired deaf-blindness
http://www.dbcent.dk/uk/materials.htm#faktatop

Sponsor ➢	Information Center for Acquired Deafblindness
Description ➢	Videos, booklets, and other materials on the deaf-blind
Data type ➢	Text
Access requirements ➢	Open
Supplemental resources ➢	Center homepage **(http://www.dbcent.dk/uk/menu_eng.htm)**
User tips ➢	Materials available in English and Danish
Keywords ➢	deaf-blind

Meeting the needs of the deaf-blind
http://www.vois.org.uk/vois-bin/chapter/sense?2

Sponsor ➢	Sense, the National Deafblind and Rubella Association
Description ➢	Parents' self-help group for deaf-blind persons
Data type ➢	Text; photos
Access requirements ➢	Open
Supplemental resources ➢	Sense homepage **(http://www.vois.org.uk/sense/)**
User tips ➢	Review links for additional information regarding services
Keywords ➢	deaf-blind

Net connections for communication disorders and sciences
http://www.mankato.msus.edu/dept/comdis/kuster2/welcome.html

Sponsor ➢	Judith M. Kuster, Mankato State University
Description ➢	Index of child and adult language disorders; voice; articulation; prevention of communication disorders
Data type ➢	Text
Access requirements ➢	Open
Supplemental resources ➢	Speech and language disorders **(http://www.mankato.msus.edu/dept/comdis/kuster2/splang.html)**
User tips ➢	Site for professionals and students
Keywords ➢	communication disorders

Technology 2000: Clinical applications for speech-language pathology
http://www.asha.org/professionals/tech_resources/tech2000/5.htm

Sponsor ➢	American Speech-Language-Hearing Association (ASHA)
Description ➢	Futuristic considerations for speech-language-hearing
Data type ➢	Text
Access requirements ➢	Open
Supplemental resources ➢	ASHA homepage **(http://www.asha.org/)**
User tips ➢	Check homepage for model bill for universal newborn/infant hearing screening
Keywords ➢	hearing disorders speech pathology

Vestibular rehabilitation

http://www.mayo.edu/vest-rehab/

Sponsor ➢	Mayo Medical Center
Description ➢	Services for vestibular rehabilitation
Data type ➢	Text
Access requirements ➢	Open
Supplemental resources ➢	Vestibular disorders: an overview of symptoms, statistics, causes, and disability **(http://www.teleport.com/~veda/overview.html#Statistics)** Vestibular rehabilitation **(http://www.teleport.com/~veda/rehab.html#What is Vestibular Rehabilitation)**
User tips ➢	See statistics for disorder
Keywords ➢	vestibular disorders rehabilitation

Video ostoscopy

http://www.li.net/~sullivan/ears.htm

Sponsor ➢	Roy F. Sullivan, Ph.D., Audiology Forum
Description ➢	Ear and hearing resource reviews
Data type ➢	Text; graphics
Access requirements ➢	Open
Supplemental resources ➢	Case study (pons1): Primary cholesteatoma in 16 month male infant **(http://www.li.net/~sullivan/pons1.htm)**
User tips ➢	Check homepage for reviews
Keywords ➢	ostoscopy

Vocal health

http://www2.shc.uiowa.edu/ncvs_home.html

Sponsor ➢	National Center for Voice and Speech (NCVS)
Description ➢	Research and resources regarding voice and speech
Data type ➢	Text; images
Access requirements ➢	Open
Supplemental resources ➢	Tips to keep you talkin' **(http://ncvs.shc.uiowa.edu/hygiene/tips.html)** Research information **(http://www2.shc.uiowa.edu/ncvs_home.html)**
User tips ➢	Check NCVS homepage for additional voice and speech sites
Keywords ➢	voice research

Pediatrics

Children with sickle cell anemia
http://www.nlm.nih.gov/databases/alerts/sickle97.html

Sponsor ➢	National Library of Medicine (NLM)
Description ➢	Full text report of Stroke Prevention Trial in Sickle Cell Anemia in Children (STOP)
Data type ➢	Text
Access requirements ➢	Open; search available
Supplemental resources ➢	Perinatal and women's health **(http://os.dhhs.gov/hrsa/mchb/mchb.htm)**
User tips ➢	See Medical Informatics category for additional databases for pediatric disorders
Keywords ➢	sickle cell anemia

Early childhood intervention
http://www.rand.org/publications/MR/MR898/

Sponsor ➢ RAND Corporation

Description ➢ Publication, *Investing in Our Children*, costs and benefits of early childhood intervention

Data type ➢ Online text

Access requirements ➢ Open

Supplemental resources ➢ RAND homepage
(http://www.rand.org/)
Hot topics in RAND research
(http://www.rand.org/HOT/index.html)

User tips ➢ Check homepage for links to RAND research areas

Keywords ➢ early childhood

Employment opportunities in pediatric anesthesia
http://www.uams.edu/spa/spajob.htm

Sponsor ➢ Society for Pediatric Anesthesia

Description ➢ Information, including jobs line, for pediatric anesthesia providers

Data type ➢ Text

Access requirements ➢ Open

Supplemental resources ➢ Society for Pediatric Anesthesia homepage
(http://www.uams.edu/spa/spa.htm)
Pediatric Database (PedBase)
(http://icondata.com/health/pedbase/pedlynx.htm)

User tips ➢ Jobs list updated regularly

Keywords ➢ pediatric anesthesiology
employment

The Future of Pediatric Education II Project

http://www.aap.org/profed/fope1.htm

Sponsor ➢ American Academy of Pediatrics (AAP)

Description ➢ Outline of future pediatric health and workforce needs

Data type ➢ Text

Access requirements ➢ Open; search enabled

Supplemental resources ➢ Child immunizations in developing countries, InfoManage International, Inc.
(http://infomanage.com/conflictresolution/medicine/birthimmune.html)
Pediatrics related links
(http://www.aapca2.org/Links/)

User tips ➢ Downloads available for Netscape and Microsoft Internet Explorer

Keywords ➢ pediatric education
preventive health

Guidelines for death scene investigation of sudden infant death syndrome (SIDS)

http://www.cdc.gov/epo/mmwr/preview/rr4510.html

Sponsor ➢ Centers for Disease Control and Prevention (CDC)

Description ➢ Recommendations of the Interagency Panel on SIDS

Data type ➢ Text

Access requirements ➢ Open

Supplemental resources ➢ American Sudden Infant Death Syndrome (SIDS) Institute
(http://www.sids.org/)
SIDS research
(http://sids-network.org/rsrch3.htm)

User tips ➢ Check SIDS site for annual SIDS data services

Keywords ➢ SIDS
infant mortality

Indicators for tracking children's well-being

http://www.nsf.gov/pubs/1997/pr9748/pr9748.txt

Sponsor ➢ National Science Foundation (NSF)

Description ➢ Report summarizing data on indicators tracking children's well being

Data type ➢ Text

Access requirements ➢ Open

Supplemental resources ➢ NSF homepage **(http://www.nsf.gov/)**
Transcripts from the Child Health 2000, 2nd World Congress **(http://edie.cprost.sfu.ca/gcnet/ch2000_2/ch2000mn.html)**

User tips ➢ Full indicator report available from National Center for Health Statistics

Keywords ➢ children

Infant cry archive

http://www.siu.edu/departments/coe/comdis/cryhome.html

Sponsor ➢ Communications Disorders and Sciences Program, Southern Illinois University at Carbondale (SIU-C)

Description ➢ Scientific repository and data links for cry research, analysis techniques, and other areas

Data type ➢ Text; audiotapes

Access requirements ➢ Open

Supplemental resources ➢ Dictionary of newborn infant cry terms and analyses **(http://www.siu.edu/departments/coe/comdis/terms.html)**
Infant cry recording **(http://www.siu.edu/departments/coe/comdis/record1.html)**

User tips ➢ Check special features link of archive for how to read sonograms of baby cries

Keywords ➢ infant cry analysis

Infectious Diseases in Children
http://www.slackinc.com/child/idc/idchome.htm

Sponsor ➢ Slack Inc.

Description ➢ Covers new drugs and procedures for diagnosing and testing pediatric infectious diseases

Data type ➢ Articles from *Infectious Diseases in Children*

Access requirements ➢ Open

Supplemental resources ➢ Directory of online articles **(http://www.slackinc.com/child/idc/idchome.htm)**

User tips ➢ See Internet pediatric infectious diseases resource

Keywords ➢ pediatric infectious diseases

Maternal and Child Health Bureau (MCHB)
http://www.os.dhhs.gov/hrsa/mchb/

Sponsor ➢ Health Resources and Services Administration (HRSA), Department of Health and Human Services (DHHS)

Description ➢ Program description; newsletters for child and adolescent health programs; health and safety in child care

Data type ➢ Text; some graphics

Access requirements ➢ Open

Supplemental resources ➢ MCH-NetLink Project, guide for instructional videoconferencing **(http://www.ichp.edu/mchb/netlink/tips/ivc.html)**
Current MCHB *Federal Register* notices **(http://www.os.dhhs.gov/hrsa/mchb/fedreg.htm)**

User tips ➢ Check link for State Children's Health Insurance Program

Keywords ➢ child health
maternal care

MedWeb pediatric Internet resources

http://www.gen.emory.edu/medweb/medweb.pediatric.html

Sponsor ➢ MedWeb, Emory University

Description ➢ Megasite resource list of Internet pediatric sources categorized by topics including child advocacy, developmental disabilities, environmental health, pediatric facilities, research

Data type ➢ Hyperlinked listing

Access requirements ➢ Open

Supplemental resources ➢ Pediatric database **(http://www.icondata.com/health/pedbase/pedlynx.htm)**

User tips ➢ Good resource for professionals and consumers

Keywords ➢ pediatric resource

Paediapedia: An Imaging Encyclopedia of Pediatric Disease

http://indy.radiology.uiowa.edu/Providers/TeachingFiles/PAP/PAPHome.html

Sponsor ➢ Michael P. D'Alessandro, M.D., Children's Hospital of Iowa

Description ➢ Text of pediatric radiology and techniques related to neonatal chest, cardiovascular, and other areas

Data type ➢ Text; images

Access requirements ➢ Open; search enabled

Supplemental resources ➢ Pediatric neurosurgery **(http://cpmcnet.columbia.edu/dept/nsg/PNS/Welcome.html)**

User tips ➢ Includes clinical/radiographic presentations

Keywords ➢ radiology

Parental control of Internet access

http://www.uab.edu/pedinfo/Control.html

Sponsor ➢	PEDINFO: A pediatrics Web Server
Description ➢	Source list of software, publications, and vendors for parental guidance of Internet access, rating system, and lock-out system for children
Data type ➢	Text; some downloadable demos
Access requirements ➢	Open for consumers and professionals
Supplemental resources ➢	Pediatric software for medical professionals **(http://www.uab.edu/pedinfo/Software.html)**
User tips ➢	List includes free and commercial demos
Keywords ➢	Internet control medical software

Pediatric cardiac arrest

http://weber.u.washington.edu/~asaccp/poca/overview.htm

Sponsor ➢	Pediatric Perioperative Cardiac Arrest (POCA), American Academy of Pediatrics' Section on Anesthesiology
Description ➢	Registry of investigations of cardiac arrests and deaths of pediatric patients related to anesthesia
Data type ➢	Text
Access requirements ➢	Text file open; registry participants restricted to pediatric health care institutions
Supplemental resources ➢	American Society of Anesthesiologists Closed Claims Projects (investigations of closed anesthesia malpractice claims) **(http://weber.u.washington.edu/~asaccp/descrip1.htm)**
User tips ➢	Bibliographies available from both organizations
Keywords ➢	pediatric anesthesia

Pediatric consumer ophthalmology
http://med-aapos.bu.edu/aapos/pedires.html

Sponsor ➢ Madelyn Hall, Southwest Washington Medical Center, Vancouver, WA

Description ➢ Consumer resource file of pediatric ophthalmologic resources including organizations; bibliographies; catalogs; for topics on diseases, eye care, albinism; cataract, and other subjects

Data type ➢ Text; topic search enabled

Access requirements ➢ Open

Supplemental resources ➢ Bibliography of Spanish ophthalmology documents **(http://med.aapos.bu.edu/PediRef/spanish_ophthalmology.html)**

User tips ➢ Citations can also be requested from organizations listed

Keywords ➢ ophthalmology

Pediatric trauma
http://www.pedi/peditrauma.html

Sponsor ➢ University of Texas Health Science Center

Description ➢ Descriptions of pediatric trauma relief methodology

Data type ➢ Text; graphics

Access requirements ➢ Open

Supplemental resources ➢ National Parent Network on Disabilities **(http://www.npnd.org/)**
National Child Care Information Center **(http://ericps.crc.uiuc.edu/nccic/nccichome.html)**

User tips ➢ See rehabilitation medicine for additional information

Keywords ➢ pediatrics

Pediatrics interactive education

http://www.medconnect.com/index.htm

Sponsor ➢ Medical Network, Inc.

Description ➢ Pediatric case studies; ambulatory pediatrics; continuing medical education (CME) in emergency medicine; pediatric electrocardiogram (ECG) casebook

Data type ➢ Text; search enabled

Access requirements ➢ Free registration and password required

Supplemental resources ➢ Jobs online according to state; free registration **(http://www.medconnect.com/newjobs/states5.htm)**

User tips ➢ See link for pediatric news

Keywords ➢ medical education
employment

Profile of children in the States: 1998 data

http://www.childrensdefense.org/states/data.html

Sponsor ➢ Children's Defense Fund (CDF)

Description ➢ Data profile of children in the United States, according to state

Data type ➢ Text

Access requirements ➢ Open

Supplemental resources ➢ CDF homepage
(http://www.childrensdefense.org/)
Key facts about uninsured children
(http://www.childrensdefense.org/health_keyfacts.html)

User tips ➢ Check CDF home page for parent resource network

Keywords ➢ uninsured children
profile, children

Spina bifida and other neural tube defects

http://www.cdc.gov/nceh/programs/in...d_prev.htm#Epidemiologic Assistance

Sponsor ➢ National Center for Environmental Health (NCEH), CDC

Description ➢ Public health recommendations regarding spina bifida

Data type ➢ Text

Access requirements ➢ Open

Supplemental resources ➢ Birth defects **(http://www.cdc.gov/nceh/programs/infants/brthdfct/prevent/ntd_prev.htm)**

User tips ➢ Check link for description of birth defects surveillance systems

Keywords ➢ birth defects
spina bifida

Pharmacology

Antibiotic utilization guidelines, 1997
http://www.intmed.mcw.edu/AntibioticGuide.html)

Sponsor ➢	Medical College of Wisconsin and Froedtert Memorial Lutheran Hospital
Description ➢	Educational tool for antimicrobial agents; costs; treatments for common infections; and surgical prophylaxis
Data type ➢	Text for professionals
Access requirements ➢	Open; password required for clinical information systems
Supplemental resources ➢	Treatment recommendations for common infections **(http://www.intmed.mcw.edu/drug/InfectionRx.html)** Antimicrobial agents, costs, and indications **(http://www.intmed.mcw.edu/AntibioticGuide.html)**
User tips ➢	See recommendations for surgical prophylaxis
Keywords ➢	antimicrobial agents

Biotechnology and drug information resources
http://pharminfo.com/phrmlink.html#assns

Sponsor ➢ PharmInfoNet

Description ➢ Links to wide range of pharmaceutical resources, namely, Biosis, Scottish, and Federal biotechnology transfer directory

Data type ➢ Hyperlinks

Access requirements ➢ Open

Supplemental resources ➢ Physicians' GenRx
(http://pharminfo.com/phrmlink.html#assns)

User tips ➢ See homepage for Virtual Library: Biotechnology

Keywords ➢ pharmacology resources

Clinical trials listing service
http://www.CenterWatch.com/

Sponsor ➢ Center Watch: Clinical trials listing service

Description ➢ Clinical trials; patient notification service; background data on clinical research; new drug therapies

Data type ➢ Text; images

Access requirements ➢ Open

Supplemental resources ➢ Listing of drug therapies approved in 1996
(http://www.centerwatch.com/drugs/DRUGLS96.HTM#Section10)
Sign-up for patient notification service about clinical trials
(http://www.CenterWatch.com/)

User tips ➢ See site for industry professional resources

Keywords ➢ clinical trials
drug therapies, approved

Drug InfoBase (Drug DB)

http://pharminfo.com/drg_mnu.html

Sponsor ➢ Pharmaceutical Information Network (PharmInfoNet)

Description ➢ Searchable databases of drug information; browse by generic or trade names

Data type ➢ Databases; some graphics

Access requirements ➢ Open

Supplemental resources ➢ Article, focus on clinical trials, October 25, 1997 **(http://pharminfo.com/pin_hp.html)**
Clinical Trials Resource Center **(http://pharminfo.com/pin_hp.html)**

User tips ➢ See homepage for disease center sites

Keywords ➢ clinical trials
megasite

FDA Medical Bulletin

http://www.fda.gov/medbull/contents.html

Sponsor ➢ U.S. Food and Drug Administration (FDA)

Description ➢ Articles related to drug treatment policy and news

Data type ➢ Text

Access requirements ➢ Open

Supplemental resources ➢ FDA alert against “Chomper” dietary supplement product, May 16, 1997 **(http://vm.cfsan.fda.gov/~lrd/hhschomp.html)**
Summary, medicinal products for human use, European Agency for Evaluation of Medicinal Products, London, October 27, 1997 **(http://www.eudra.org/frame/frameindex3.html)**

User tips ➢ FDA Bulletin updated regularly

Keywords ➢ drug alert
European drug data

Guide to taking medications
http://www.healthtouch.com/level1/leaflets/103068/103068.htm

Sponsor ➢ Healthtouch Online

Description ➢ Tips and information on medications; drug interactions; dictionary of medicine terms; non-prescription medicines

Data type ➢ Text; charts; graphics for consumers

Access requirements ➢ Open

Supplemental resources ➢ Healthtouch table of contents **(http://www.healthtouch.com/level1/hi_toc.htm)**
Tips for over-the-counter (OTC) medicines **(http://www.healthtouch.com/level1/leaflets/cfh/cfh010.htm)**

User tips ➢ Check bin for health information

Keywords ➢ over-the-counter (OTC) drugs

Internet self-assessment in pharmacology (ISAP)
http://www.cs.umn.edu/Research/GIMME/isap.html

Sponsor ➢ University of Minnesota

Description ➢ Internet self-assessment in pharmacology (ISAP), with lecture outline, drug cards, and quizzes

Data type ➢ Tutorial for students and health professionals

Access requirements ➢ Free registration; guest access available

Supplemental resources ➢ ISAP homepage **(http://www-users.cs.umn.edu/~isap/welcome.html)**

User tips ➢ Great supplement for pharmacology curriculum

Keywords ➢ pharmacology tutorial
medical education

Japanese Pharmacopoeia (JP)

http://www.mediagalaxy.co.jp/TEST/KOSEISHO/JP-HomeE.html

Sponsor > Japanese Government Ministry of Health and Welfare (MHW)

Description > Overview of Japanese pharmacopoeia

Data type > Text

Access requirements > Open

Supplemental resources > Comparison of Japan-US-EC tripolar pharmacopoeias **(http://www.mediagalaxy.co.jp/TEST/KOSEISHO/PIH/Comp/Comp-E.html)**
JP overview **(http://www.mediagalaxy.co.jp/TEST/KOSEISHO/Over/Over-E.html)**

User tips > See homepage for related JP references and sites

Keywords > pharmacopoeia, Japanese

Medical prescription of narcotics

http://www.lindesmith.org/presumm.html

Sponsor > The Lindesmith Center

Description > Swiss Heroin Prescription Report, 1997; summary of the synthesis report

Data type > Report

Access requirements > Open

Supplemental resources > Drug substitution and maintenance approaches **(http://www.lindesmith.org/premain.html)**
NIH workshop on medical utility of marijuana **(http://www.nih.gov/news/medmarijuana/MedicalMarijuana.htm#EXECUTIVE)**

User tips > Report available from the Swiss Federal Office of Public Health in Berne

Keywords > medical use of narcotics

Medicine assistance program
http://www.themedicineprogram.com/info.html

Sponsor ➢	The Medicine Program
Description ➢	Eligibility criteria for prescription medicine free-of-charge to eligible participants
Data type ➢	Text
Access requirements ➢	Open
Supplemental resources ➢	Medication information form **(http://www.themedicineprogram.com/form.html)**
User tips ➢	Send $5.00 application processing fee for each medication requested
Keywords ➢	medication assistance

MedWatch, FDA medical products reporting program
http://www.fda.gov/medwatch/

Sponsor ➢	U.S. Food and Drug Administration (FDA)
Description ➢	Program addressing drug adverse events and drug safety
Data type ➢	Text for health professionals
Access requirements ➢	Open
Supplemental resources ➢	What is a serious adverse event? **(http://pharminfo.com/medwatch/mw_ser.html)** MedWatch reporting form and instructions **(http://pharminfo.com/medwatch/mw_form.html)**
User tips ➢	See MedWatch homepage for submitting continuing education tests via Internet
Keywords ➢	medical education drug adverse events

Pharmaceutical training

http://www.aacp.org/

Sponsor ➢ American Association of Colleges of Pharmacy (AACP)

Description ➢ Pharmaceutical career information, student programs, publications, and software

Data type ➢ Text

Access requirements ➢ Open

Supplemental resources ➢ Student affairs, pharmaceutical programs **(http://www.aacp.org/aacp/student/student.html)**

User tips ➢ Download candidate's review of North American Pharmacist Licensure Examination (NAPLEX)

Keywords ➢ pharmaceutical careers

Prescription drug patient assistance programs

http://omhs.mhd.hr.state.or.us/presdrap.htm

Sponsor ➢ Pharmaceutical Research and Manufacturers of America

Description ➢ Directory of programs, contacts, products covered, and eligibility criteria of prescription assistance programs

Data type ➢ Directory

Access requirements ➢ Open

Supplemental resources ➢ Standard treatment guidelines and drugs list, South Africa **(http://www.healthlink.org.za/hst/edl/edlcover.htm)**

User tips ➢ Free directory of prescription programs available toll free number: 1-800-762-4636

Keywords ➢ medication assistance
drugs, South Africa

Rx list
http://www.rxlist.com/

Sponsor ➢ MedicationWeb.Com

Description ➢ Internet drug index of the top 200 U.S. prescriptions, 1995–1996

Data type ➢ Search enabled database

Access requirements ➢ Open

Supplemental resources ➢ Keyword search according to actions, interactions, and brands
(http://www.rxlist.com/)
Top 200 U.S. prescriptions, ranked, 1996
(http://www.rxlist.com/top200.htm)

User tips ➢ Search Rx list by imprint codes

Keywords ➢ prescription drugs

Safe medication practices
http://www.ismp.org/ISMP/Pages/about.html

Sponsor ➢ Institute for Safe Medication Practices (ISMP)

Description ➢ Medication error prevention

Data type ➢ Text

Access requirements ➢ Open

Supplemental resources ➢ ISMP medication safety alert: Beta blocker
(http://www.ismp.org/ISMP/MSAarticles/BetaBlock.html)
Article: Danger at the Drugstore
(http://www.usnews.com/usnews/issue/26phar.htm)

User tips ➢ ISMP, a free service welcomes calls from health care professionals **(e-mail: ismpinfo@ismp.org)**

Keywords ➢ medication errors

U.S. Food and Drug Administration (FDA)

http://www.fda.gov/

Sponsor ➢	U.S. Food and Drug Administration (FDA)
Description ➢	FDA information, dockets, newsletters about drugs, toxicology, food, medical devices, and electronic records
Data type ➢	Variable
Access requirements ➢	Open
Supplemental resources ➢	Regulatory guidance, Center for Drug Evaluation and Research **(http://www.fda.gov/cder/regguide.htm)** The FDA Modernization Act of 1997 **(http://www.fda.gov/opacom/backgrounders/modact.htm)**
User tips ➢	Check FDA homepage for complete listings
Keywords ➢	FDA Modernization Act, 1997 drugs

USP reference standards

http://www.usp.org/index.htm

Sponsor ➢	U.S. Pharmacopeia (USP)
Description ➢	Standards development; practitioners' reporting network; drug information
Data type ➢	Text
Access requirements ➢	Open
Supplemental resources ➢	Practitioners' reporting network for drug and devices problems, medical products, and medication errors **(http://www.usp.org/practrep/index.htm)** Healthcare Compliance Packaging Council **(http://www.unitdose.org/)**
User tips ➢	Check network for practitioners' reporting news
Keywords ➢	pharmacopoeia, U.S. medication errors

Preventive Health

Abstracts and references of prevention research
http://www.integres.org/prevres/index.html

Sponsor ➢	*The Prevention Researcher*; Integrated Research Services
Description ➢	Newsletter of prevention research and clinical topics for behavioral health care professionals
Data type ➢	Newsletter
Access requirements ➢	Open
Supplemental resources ➢	Adolescent suicide prevention, vol 3, Fall 1996 **(http://www.integres.org/prevres/v3n3abst.htm)** Drinking and drug habits of athletes **(http://www.integres.org/prevres/v3n2abst.htm)**
User tips ➢	Subscription available
Keywords ➢	prevention research general medicine

Aerobics patterns
http://www.turnstep.com/Patterns/index.html

Sponsor ➢ www.turnstep.com - The aerobics page

Description ➢ Library of aerobics patterns

Data type ➢ Variable

Access requirements ➢ Open

Supplemental resources ➢ Latest twenty-five aerobics patterns **(http://www.turnstep.com/Patterns/index.html)**
President's Council on Physical Fitness and Sports **(http://www.os.dhhs.gov/progorg/ophs/pcpfs/htm)**

User tips ➢ Add a pattern

Keywords ➢ aerobics
fitness

Batteries swallowed by young children
http://www.nisu.flinders.edu.au/pubs/shrtreps/batteries.html

Sponsor ➢ Injury Surveillance Information System (ISIS), Flinders University of South Australia

Description ➢ Report of incidence and patterns related to battery swallowing by children

Data type ➢ Text

Access requirements ➢ Open

Supplemental resources ➢ Work related injuries associated with scaffolds **(http://www.nisu.flinders.edu.au/pubs/shrtreps/scaffold.html)**
Atlas of injury death in Australia, 1990–1992 **(http://www.nisu.flinders.edu.au/data/atlas.html)**

User tips ➢ See links for additional reports and datasets

Keywords ➢ battery swallowing
scaffold accidents

Chronic disease prevention and health promotion

http://www.cdc.gov/nccdphp/

Sponsor ➢ National Center for Chronic Disease Prevention and Health Promotion (NCCDPHP), CDC

Description ➢ Site for identification, surveillance, and prevention of major chronic diseases, risk behaviors

Data type ➢ Variable

Access requirements ➢ Open; search enabled

Supplemental resources ➢ Specific populations, minority and ethnic groups **(http://www.cdc.gov/nccdphp/populati.htm)**
Report, prostate cancer, 1997 **(http://www.cdc.gov/nccdphp/dcpc/prostate/prostate.htm)**

User tips ➢ Prostate cancer file, very large

Keywords ➢ prostate cancer
ethnic health issues

Crash Analysis and Reporting Environment (CARE)

http://care.cs.ua.edu/care/introduction.html

Sponsor ➢ University of Alabama

Description ➢ Online data analysis and reporting system of traffic accidents

Data type ➢ Database and analysis

Access requirements ➢ Open; for traffic safety professionals

Supplemental resources ➢ System overview and user guide **(http://care.cs.ua.edu/htdocs/docum.htm)**

User tips ➢ First time users should review documentation guide

Keywords ➢ traffic accidents

Fitness program: Choosing a cardiovascular program
http://www.fitnesslink.com/program/cardio.htm

Sponsor ➢ Fitness Link

Description ➢ Tips for choosing a cardiovascular fitness program

Data type ➢ Newsletter

Access requirements ➢ Open

Supplemental resources ➢ Fitness Link homepage
(http://www.fitnesslink.com/index.html)
Developing a cardiovascular program
(http://www.fitnesslink.com/program/foot.htm)

User tips ➢ Site updated regularly

Keywords ➢ cardiovascular fitness
cardiovascular medicine

Injury control and violence prevention
http://www.sph.unc.edu/vincentweb/

Sponsor ➢ University of North Carolina (UNC) Vincent Web

Description ➢ Course materials from videoconference, "Getting Started in Injury Control and Violence Prevention"

Data type ➢ Report; professional resource

Access requirements ➢ Open

Supplemental resources ➢ Downloadable copy of the course workbook (PDF format)
(http://www.sph.unc.edu/vincentweb/)
MedWeb preventive medicine (megasite)
(http://www.gen.emory.edu/medweb/medweb/prevmed.html)

User tips ➢ Continuing education units offered by the Centers for Disease Control and Prevention and/or the Society of Public Health Education

Keywords ➢ injury control
medical education

1997 Manufacturer investigation files

http://www.cpsc.gov/library/foia/foia97/compliance/compliance.html

Sponsor ➢ U.S. Consumer Product Safety Commission (CPSC)

Description ➢ Commission investigation files of various products

Data type ➢ Hyperlinked text of compliance files

Access requirements ➢ Open

Supplemental resources ➢ CPSC homepage
(http://www.cpsc.gov/)
1997 Freedom of Information Act information related to CPSC data
(http://www.cpsc.gov/library/foia/foia97/foia97.html)

User tips ➢ Report unsafe products to CPSC

Keywords ➢ product safety

Prevention guidelines

http://www.cdc.gov/ncipc/pub-res/prevguid.htm

Sponsor ➢ National Center for Injury Prevention and Control (NCIPC), Centers for Disease Control and Prevention (CDC)

Description ➢ Prevention guidelines include subject and source

Data type ➢ Table

Access requirements ➢ Open

Supplemental resources ➢ NCIPC homepage
(http://www.cdc.gov/ncipc/)
Learning not to burn
(http://www.cdc.gov/ncipc/whatsnew/benton.htm)

User tips ➢ Check homepage for link to injury programs that work

Keywords ➢ injury prevention, control
violence prevention

Prototype preventive care guidelines, 1991
http://hiru.mcmaster.ca/prevent/pvcpg_00.htm

Sponsor ➢	Health Information Research Unit, Johns Hopkins University and other institutions
Description ➢	Guidelines on history, comparison, and implementation of preventive care strategies
Data type ➢	Text; tables
Access requirements ➢	Open
Supplemental resources ➢	Users' guides to medical literature on evidence-based medicine, primary studies, and other topics **(http://hiru.mcmaster.ca/ebm/userguid/userguid.htm)** Evidence-based medicine (EBM): requirements, overcoming the barriers, outcomes **(http://hiru.mcmaster.ca/ebm/userguid/overview.htm)**
User tips ➢	Check EBM quick links
Keywords ➢	evidence-based medicine medical education

Sports medicine resource
http://www.callemx.com/html/sportmed.html

Sponsor ➢	EMX, Universal Health Card
Description ➢	Sports and fitness medicine links
Data type ➢	Variable
Access requirements ➢	Open
Supplemental resources ➢	Athletic training/physical therapy links **(http://www.callemx.com/html/sportmed.html)** Falk Library's new books on sports medicine **(http://www.callemx.com/html/sportmed.html)**
User tips ➢	Consumer oriented site
Keywords ➢	fitness and health

Statistical and computing resources for injury prevention

http://www.albany.edu/sph/injr_007.html

Sponsor ➢ Center for the Advanced Study of Public Safety, University at Albany

Description ➢ Databases for National Center for Statistics, CARE, statistics and probability resources, epidemiology, and injury prevention

Data type ➢ Databases

Access requirements ➢ Open

Supplemental resources ➢ Prevention of Major Industrial Accidents Convention, 1993 **(http://turva.me.tut/fi/cis/ilo_standards/c174.htm)**

User tips ➢ Download available for WordPerfect Internet Publisher

Keywords ➢ industrial accidents

What Is preventive medicine?

http://www.acpm.org/whatis.htm

Sponsor ➢ American College of Preventive Medicine (ACPM)

Description ➢ Report defining preventive medicine

Data type ➢ Text; photos

Access requirements ➢ Open

Supplemental resources ➢ ACPM homepage, careers in preventive medicine **(http://www.acpm.org/)**
What's new in preventive medicine **(http://www.acpm.org/whatsnew.htm#frank)**

User tips ➢ Check ACPM homepage for Prevention '98

Keywords ➢ preventive medicine

Radiology

The Basics of MRI

http://www.cis.rit.edu/htbooks/mri/

Sponsor ➢	Joseph P. Hornak, Ph.D., Rochester Institute of Technology
Description ➢	Online reference covering mathematics of NMR, spin physics, NMR spectroscopy, and other topics
Data type ➢	Online text
Access requirements ➢	Open
Supplemental resources ➢	Contents **(http://www.cis.rit.edu/htbooks/mri/contents.htm)** Magnetic resonance imaging (MRI) resources **(http://www.ibd.nrc.ca/~cisti/mri.html)**
User tips ➢	Check MR resource site for image files
Keywords ➢	magnetic resonance imaging (MRI) images

Body image teaching files
http://www.uhrad.com/ctarc.htm

Sponsor ➢ Case Western Reserve University

Description ➢ Body case files include computed tomography (CT), ultrasound (US), magnetic resonance imaging (MRI), angiography and plain films

Data type ➢ Text; images

Access requirements ➢ Open

Supplemental resources ➢ Case image file, ulcer penetrating atheromatous (PAU)
(http://www.uhrad.com/ctarc/ct078.htm)
Index, musculoskeletal imaging archives
(http://www.uhrad.com/msiarc.htm)

User tips ➢ Check pediatric, positive emission tomography (PET), nuclear teaching files

Keywords ➢ imaging teaching files
diagnostic imaging

CHORUS Collaborative hypertext of radiology
http://chorus.rad.mcw.edu/

Sponsor ➢ Medical College of Wisconsin

Description ➢ Quick reference of over 1,000 documents of diseases, differential diagnosis, radiologic finding lists for neuroendocrine, cardiovascular, genito-urinary, and other systems

Data type ➢ Text; images

Access requirements ➢ For physicians and medical students

Supplemental resources ➢ Kidney index
(http://chorus.rad.mcw.edu/index/53.html)
About CHORUS
(http://chorus.rad.mcw.edu/about/CHORUS.html)

User tips ➢ Search enabled site

Keywords ➢ radiology

Clinical nuclear medicine teaching file
http://count51.med.harvard.edu/JPNM/TF.html

Sponsor ➢ Joint Program in Nuclear Medicine (JPNM), Harvard Medical School

Description ➢ Web-based nuclear medicine; teaching cases in anatomic area and imaging technique; and meeting notes and reports

Data type ➢ Multimedia

Access requirements ➢ Open

Supplemental resources ➢ Objectives for Web-based nuclear medicine **(http://count51.med.harvard.edu/JPNM/Lectures/WebBasedNucMed/Methods.html)**
Cases
(http://www.med.harvard.edu/JPNM/InterestingImages/Case1ii/Case1ii.html)

User tips ➢ See homepage for report of JPNM Internet Focus Group

Keywords ➢ nuclear medicine
medical education

Interactive tutorial on normal radiology
http://www.med.ufl.edu/medinfo/rademo/raintro.html

Sponsor ➢ University of Florida

Description ➢ Demonstration site covering human body and major imaging modalities

Data type ➢ Multimedia demo

Access requirements ➢ Open

Supplemental resources ➢ Radiologic anatomy index **(http://www.med.ufl.edu/medinfo/rademo/raindex.html)**
American Healthcare Radiology Administrators **(http://www.ahra.com/main.html)**

User tips ➢ Color monitor preferred for viewing interactive tutorial

Keywords ➢ radiology
medical education

Magnetic resonance microscopy
http://wwwcivm.mc.duke.edu/

Sponsor ➢ The Center for In Vivo Microscopy, Duke University

Description ➢ Discussion, samples of images, and movie on magnetic resonance microscopy

Data type ➢ Text; image and movie gallery

Access requirements ➢ Open

Supplemental resources ➢ What is MRI?
(http://wwwcivm.mc.duke.edu/civmMRI/MRI.html)
MRI of embryos
(http://embryo.mc.duke.edu/animal/home.html)

User tips ➢ Check MRI embryo page for related links

Keywords ➢ magnetic resonance imaging

Nuclear medicine teaching files
http://gamma.wustl.edu/home.html

Sponsor ➢ Mallinckrodt Institute of Radiology (MIR), Washington University Medical Center

Description ➢ Nuclear medicine cases, definition, and teaching files

Data type ➢ Case studies

Access requirements ➢ Open

Supplemental resources ➢ Nuclear medicine cases by study type, without diagnoses shown
(http://gamma.wustl.edu/allunknown.html)
MIR homepage
(http://gamma.wustl.edu/index.html)

User tips ➢ Check link for Society of Nuclear Medicine Web site

Keywords ➢ nuclear medicine
medical education

Physiological imaging

http://everest.radiology.uiowa.edu/

Sponsor ➢ Department of Radiology, University of Iowa College of Medicine

Description ➢ Database of physiologic imaging resources

Data type ➢ Multimedia; search enabled

Access requirements ➢ Open

Supplemental resources ➢ Hardin Meta directory of radiology and imaging Internet resources **(http://www.arcade.uiowa.edu/hardin-www/md-rad.html)**
Auditory/noise effects **(http://kanal.arad.upmc.edu/safety/auditory.html)**

User tips ➢ See physiological imaging page for link to 3D gallery

Keywords ➢ physiological imaging
MR safety

Radiology court decisions

http://www.acr.org/departments/legal/culpeper_decision.html

Sponsor ➢ American College of Radiology (ACR)

Description ➢ Radiology legal issues

Data type ➢ Text

Access requirements ➢ Open

Supplemental resources ➢ Executive issue summaries including antitrust reform, Medicaid, teleradiology, and radiation **(http://www.acr.org/departments/govt_rel/exec_summ/index.html)**
Abstract, effectiveness of radiology multimedia text versus standard lecture **(http://vh.radiology.uiowa.edu/Welco...ers/InstructionalEffectiveness.html)**

User tips ➢ Summaries are revised periodically

Keywords ➢ radiology legal issues
legal medicine

Radiology Internet teaching resources
http://www.mamc.amedd.army.mil/williams/index1.htm

Sponsor ➢ Department of Radiology, Madigan Army Medical Center

Description ➢ Textbooks on chest and cardiac radiology and genitourinary radiology; teaching files; and cases

Data type ➢ Text; images

Access requirements ➢ Open

Supplemental resources ➢ General nuclear medicine instrumentation **(http://www.mamc.amedd.army.mil/williams/NucMed/GNUC.HTM#RTFToC3)**
Interesting cases: Angiography **(http://www.mamc.amedd.army.mil/williams/TF/Angio/Unknown1/Unkn1c.html)**

User tips ➢ See table of contents for nuclear medicine text

Keywords ➢ angiography
medical education

Radiology teaching library
http://www.embbs.com/xray/xr.html#abdomen

Sponsor ➢ EMBBS Emergency Medicine and Primary Care

Description ➢ Library of hundreds of radiology images, CT scan collections, and medical photographs

Data type ➢ Images; text

Access requirements ➢ Open; for health professionals

Supplemental resources ➢ EMBBS homepage **(http://www.embbs.com/)**
Electrocardiogram of the month and EKG file room **(http://www.embbs.com/)**

User tips ➢ Download and use materials

Keywords ➢ radiology

Rehabilitative Medicine

Acute care and rehabilitation in the United States
http://www.cdc.gov/ncipc/dacrrdp/dacrrdp.htm

Sponsor ➢	National Center for Prevention and Control, Centers for Disease Control and Prevention (CDC)
Description ➢	Overview of U.S. statistical data on acute care, rehabilitation, disability prevention, and costs
Data type ➢	Text
Access requirements ➢	Open
Supplemental resources ➢	Archimedes Project FAQ **(http://www-csli.stanford.edu/arch/faq97.html)** Return-to-work programs, Research and Oversight Council on Workers Compensation, Texas **(http://www.roc.capnet.state.tx.us/rtwprog.htm)**
User tips ➢	Check data regarding acute care in the United States
Keywords ➢	acute care

Cardiac rehabilitation clinical care guidelines

http://www.a1.com/sportsmed/cardiac.htm

Sponsor ➢ American College of Sports Medicine (ACSM)

Description ➢ Recent guidelines

Data type ➢ Text

Access requirements ➢ Open

Supplemental resources ➢ ACSM homepage
(http://www.a1.com/sportsmed/)

User tips ➢ Click homepage for Healthy People 2010 objectives (comments sought)

Keywords ➢ sports medicine
cardiovascular

COACH: Transportation for riders with disabilities

http://www.dssc.org/

Sponsor ➢ Disabilities Studies and Services Center (DSSC), Academy for Educational Development (AED)

Description ➢ Searchable database of transportation training programs

Data type ➢ Text

Access requirements ➢ Open

Supplemental resources ➢ DSSC homepage
(http://www.dssc.org/)
Pocket guide to federal resources for disabilities
(gopher://gopher.gsa.gov:70/00/staff/pa/cic/fed_prog/other/fedhelp.txt)

User tips ➢ Check DSSC's searchable database

Keywords ➢ disabilities
transportation, disabled

Disabilities statutes, regulations
http://janweb.icdi.wvu.edu/kinder/index.htm

Sponsor ➢ Americans with Disabilities Act Document Center

Description ➢ Disabilities documents, federally reviewed tech sheets, and other assistance documents

Data type ➢ Text

Access requirements ➢ Open

Supplemental resources ➢ Overview, American with Disabilities Act **(http://janweb.icdi.wvu.edu/kinder/overview.htm)**
List of American Disabilities Act documents **(http://janweb.icdi.wvu.edu/kinder/document.htm)**

User tips ➢ Review document disclaimer

Keywords ➢ disabilities legislation

Disability and rehabilitation research
http://www.ed.gov/offices/OSERS/NIDRR/index.html

Sponsor ➢ National Institute on Disability and Rehabilitation Research (NIDRR)

Description ➢ NIDRR research, publications, and other disability resources

Data type ➢ Text

Access requirements ➢ Open

Supplemental resources ➢ NIDRR funded projects on the Internet **(http://www.ncddr.org/URLlist.htm#RRTC)**
Projects about women, psychiatric disability, and peer support **(http://www.psych.uic.edu/~rtc/nrtc.htm#HIV+ Experiences)**

User tips ➢ Hit link for NIDRR publications

Keywords ➢ mental health
women

Disability tables
http://web.icdi.wvu.edu/disability/tables.html

Sponsor ➢	International Center for Disability Information (ICDI)
Description ➢	Statistical tables on disabilities, employment, earnings; according to state
Data type ➢	Tables
Access requirements ➢	Open
Supplemental resources ➢	World table of new diphtheria cases, 1992–1994 **(http://web.icdi.wvu.edu/disability/world2.html)** Vocational rehabilitation employment **(http://web.icdi.wvu.edu/disability/stable3.html)**
User tips ➢	Tables data collected from multiple sources
Keywords ➢	disability employment statistics

Disability-related clearinghouses in collaboration
http://nichcy.org/clc.htm

Sponsor ➢	National Information Center for Children and Youth with Disabilities (NICHCY), Department of Education
Description ➢	Consortium of clearinghouses for disability-related data; includes URLs and e-mail addresses
Data type ➢	Directory
Access requirements ➢	Open
Supplemental resources ➢	Search engine for NICHCY's database of organizations **(http://askeric.org/plweb-cgi/fastweb?searchform+nichcy1)**
User tips ➢	Toll free number for NICHCY's database: 1-800-695-0285
Keywords ➢	disabilities

FDA approved electronic hand controller
http://www.disability.com/whatshot.shtml

Sponsor ➢ Solutions @disability.com

Description ➢ Description of surgically implanted electronic hand controller for quadriplegics

Data type ➢ Text; photos

Access requirements ➢ Open

Supplemental resources ➢ Freehand system
(http://www.neurocontrol.com/Freehand.HTM)
Rehabilitation devices research, Archimedes Project
(http://www-csli.stanford.edu/arch/faq97.html)

User tips ➢ See Vocare system for restoring bladder and bowel control resulting from spinal cord injury

Keywords ➢ electronic hand control
adaptive devices

Federal Register Notices of medical devices
http://www.fda.gov/cdrh/fedregin.html

Sponsor ➢ Center for Devices and Radiological Health (CDRH), FDA

Description ➢ Full text of regulations for medical devices

Data type ➢ Text

Access requirements ➢ Open

Supplemental resources ➢ CDRH homepage
(http://www.fda.gov/cdrh/)
Requirements of laws and regulations for medical devices
(http://www.fda.gov/cdrh/other.html)

User tips ➢ See Government Accounting Office (GAO) reports for additional information

Keywords ➢ medical devices
legal medicine

Florida Spinal Cord Injury
http://www.gbdi.com/fscirc/home.html

Sponsor ➢	Florida Spinal Cord Injury World Wide Web Resources Center (FSCIWWWRC)
Description ➢	Consumer site of news and features for the spinal cord injuried
Data type ➢	Text
Access requirements ➢	Open
Supplemental resources ➢	National Spinal Cord Injury Association **(http://www.spinalcord.org/)**
User tips ➢	Florida site is consumer oriented
Keywords ➢	rehabilitation resources spinal cord

Job Accommodation Network (JAN)
http://janweb.icdi.wvu.edu/

Sponsor ➢	West Virginia Rehabilitation Research and Training Center
Description ➢	International, toll-free consultant service providing job accommodations information
Data type ➢	Network database
Access requirements ➢	Open
Supplemental resources ➢	Points of interest, employment, disability resources **(http://janweb.icdi.wvu.edu/links/)** Web sites with resources for multiple disabilities **(http://janweb.icdi.wvu.edu/links/disres.htm)**
User tips ➢	JAN is not a job placement service
Keywords ➢	multiple disabilities disabled employment

Managed care approach to traumatic brain injury

http://www.neuro.pmr.vcu.edu/special.htm

Sponsor ➢ National Resource Center for Traumatic Brain Injury (TBI)

Description ➢ Pros and cons of treating TBI

Data type ➢ Report

Access requirements ➢ Open

Supplemental resources ➢ Videos and other materials available through National Resource Center **(http://www.neuro.pmr.vcu.edu/material/material.htm)**

User tips ➢ See materials for list of instructional videotapes on family perspective on brain injury

Keywords ➢ brain injury
managed care

Model for post-acute rehabilitation for traumatic brain injury (TBI)

http://www.ccs-rehab.com/outcomes/outmenu.htm

Sponsor ➢ Traumatic Brain and Spinal Cord Injury Projects

Description ➢ Program model for measurement of disability and rehabilitation outcomes

Data type ➢ Text

Access requirements ➢ Open

Supplemental resources ➢ Projects' homepage **(http://members.aol.com/TBISCIProj/TBISCIProj.html)**
Overview of functional independence measure (FIM) and functional assessment measure (FAM) **(http://members.aol.com/KHallVMC/OVFAM.html)**

User tips ➢ See list of TBI projects

Keywords ➢ neurology
spinal cord injury

Physical therapy
http://www.apta.org/

Sponsor ➢ American Physical Therapy Association (APTA)

Description ➢ Overview of APTA initiatives

Data type ➢ Text

Access requirements ➢ Open

Supplemental resources ➢ News: Non-coverage decision on electrical stimulation
(http://www.apta.org/public_relations/HCFAWIN.html)
Legal decisions regarding chiropractors
(http://www.apta.org/public_relations/prevail_in_PA_MI.html)

User tips ➢ Site regularly updated

Keywords ➢ rehabilitation
physical therapy

Rehabilitation Clearinghouse
http://www.cais.com/naric/

Sponsor ➢ National Rehabilitation Information Center (NARIC), National Institute on Disability and Rehabilitation Research (NIDRR)

Description ➢ Library and information center on disability and rehabilitation

Data type ➢ Text; graphics

Access requirements ➢ Open

Supplemental resources ➢ NARIC's bookmarks: Disability and rehabilitation resources
(http://www.naric.com/naric/bookmark/index.html)
NARIC resource guide for stroke survivors and their families
(http://www.rehabnet.com/archives/rehabftp/cvaguide.txt)

User tips ➢ Search by telephone (1-800-346-2742)

Keywords ➢ rehabilitation
disabilities

Rehabilitation files library

http://www.rehabnet.com/archives/rehabftp.htm

Sponsor ➢ rehabNET, Northeast Rehabilitation Network

Description ➢ Rehabilitation articles, manuals, directories, monographs in addition to freeware and shareware software

Data type ➢ Directory

Access requirements ➢ Open

Supplemental resources ➢ rehabNet homepage
(http://www.rehabnet.com/index.html)
Bobby, free Web based service to make web pages accessible to people with disabilities
(http://www.cast.org/bobby/)

User tips ➢ Check homepage for "Nerve Blocks" for limb dystonia and spasticity

Keywords ➢ rehabilitation resources
medical software

Research overview of psychiatric rehabilitation outcomes

http://web.bu.edu/SARPSYCH/wwwresinfo2.html#3

Sponsor ➢ National Clearinghouse of Rehabilitation Training Materials (NCRTM)

Description ➢ Research involving rehabilitation, treatment, quality of life, and cost outcomes of psychiatric rehabilitation

Data type ➢ Text

Access requirements ➢ Open

Supplemental resources ➢ NCRTM homepage
(http://www.nchrtm.okstate.edu/indextxt.htm)

User tips ➢ NCRTM toll free number (1-800-223-5219)

Keywords ➢ rehabilitation training materials
mental health

Voice recognition via computer
http://wata.org/watapubs/voicerec.htm

Sponsor ➢ Washington Assistive Technology Alliance (WATA)

Description ➢ Pros and cons of voice recognition

Data type ➢ Article

Access requirements ➢ Open

Supplemental resources ➢ 1997 Amendments to Individuals with Disabilities Education Act (IDEA), WATA homepage **(http://wata.org/)**

User tips ➢ Check homepage for upcoming WATA events

Keywords ➢ assistive technology

Reproductive Health

Abortion pro- and anti-choice resources
http://www.caral.org/7.docs.html#docs

Sponsor ➢	California Abortion and Reproductive Rights Action League (CARAL)
Description ➢	Web sites accessing both abortion pro- and anti-choice organizations
Data type ➢	Hyperlinked text
Access requirements ➢	Open
Supplemental resources ➢	Abortion pro-choice **(http://www.caral.org/abortion.html#pro)** Abortion anti-choice organizations **(http://www.caral.org/7.anti.html#anti)**
User tips ➢	Check CARAL homepage to access reproduction legislation
Keywords ➢	pro-abortion anti-abortion

Alternatives to female genital mutilation
http://www.path.org/html/modern_rites_of_passage.htm

Sponsor ➢ Program for Appropriate Technology in Health (PATH)

Description ➢ Modern rights of passage as alternative to genital mutilation

Data type ➢ Text

Access requirements ➢ Open

Supplemental resources ➢ PATH homepage **(http://www.path.org/)**
United Nations Population Fund (UNFPA) African Forum on Adolescent Reproductive Health recommendations **(http://www.cedpa.org/addrecs.html)**

User tips ➢ Check case studies

Keywords ➢ women's health
female genital mutilation

Assisted Reproductive Technologies (ART)
http://www.centerforhumanreprod.com/art/art.html

Sponsor ➢ Center for Human Reproduction (CHR)

Description ➢ Reports on infertility technologies, including intracytoplasmic sperm injection, in vitro fertilization, and assisted hatching

Data type ➢ Text

Access requirements ➢ Open

Supplemental resources ➢ Articles, *Journal of Assisted Reproduction and Genetics* **(http://www.centerforhumanreprod.com/chr.journals/toc_14_02.html)**
Fertility Weekly **(http://www.homepage.holowww.com/1f.htm)**

User tips ➢ Journal sites consist of full text and abstracts of recent articles

Keywords ➢ genetics
infertility

Condom breakage and slippage rates
gopher://gopher.undp.org:70/00/ungo...n/popis/journals/ifpp/v20n2/STEINER

Sponsor ➢ United Nations Population Information Network (POPIN)

Description ➢ Report of condom breakage incidence in eight countries

Data type ➢ Text (gopher menu)

Access requirements ➢ Open

Supplemental resources ➢ POPIN homepage
(http://www.undp.org/popin/)
POPIN electronic library of bibliographies and databases
(http://www.undp.org/popin/infoserv.htm)

User tips ➢ See POPIN homepage for *Worldwide Directory of Population Institutions*

Keywords ➢ contraception
family planning

Contraceptive use among women
http://www.agi-usa.org/pubs/journals/2314897.html

Sponsor ➢ Alan Guttmacher Institute

Description ➢ Article: Intended contraceptive use among women without an unmet need

Data type ➢ Text

Access requirements ➢ Open

Supplemental resources ➢ Alan Guttmacher Institute homepage
(http://www.agi-usa.org/home.html)
Teenage contraceptive health savings
(http://www.agi-usa.org/new/newsrelease29061.html)

User tips ➢ Check homepage for link to what's new

Keywords ➢ adolescent pregnancy
contraception

Emergency contraception

http://opr.princeton.edu/ec/ec.html

Sponsor ➢ Office of Population Research (OPR), Princeton University

Description ➢ Emergency contraception methods, instruction, utility, and bibliography

Data type ➢ Text

Access requirements ➢ Open

Supplemental resources ➢ OPR datasets archive
(http://opr.princeton.edu/archive/)
Contraception and reproductive health
(http://opr.princeton.edu/ec/contrac.html)

User tips ➢ Spanish translation available

Keywords ➢ contraception, emergency
HIV/AIDS

Evaluation of family planning services

http://www.cpc.unc.edu/projects.evaluation/papers/wp-o-08.html

Sponsor ➢ The Evaluation Project

Description ➢ Summaries and working papers on measurement of quality of family planning services, evaluation impact, and experimental design for program evaluation

Data type ➢ Text

Access requirements ➢ Open

Supplemental resources ➢ Project paper series
(http://www.cpc.unc.edu/projects/evaluation/papers/papers.html)
Measurement of family planning service quality
(http://www.cpc.unc.edu/projects/evaluation/papers/wp-o-02.html)

User tips ➢ Full text copies of working papers can be ordered

Keywords ➢ family planning
evaluation

Family planning and adolescent pregnancy
http://www.hhs.gov/progorg/opa/

Sponsor ➢	Office of Population Affairs (OPA), U.S. Department of Health and Human Services (DHHS)
Description ➢	Data regarding adolescent pregnancy and childbearing trends, sexuality legislation, and demonstration projects
Data type ➢	Text; graphics
Access requirements ➢	Open
Supplemental resources ➢	OPA Clearinghouse **(http://www.hhs.gov/progorg/opa/clearing.html)** Trends in adolescent pregnancy and childbearing **(http://www.hhs.gov/progorg/opa/pregtrnd.html)**
User tips ➢	Check homepage for OPA legislation
Keywords ➢	adolescent pregnancy family planning

Family planning in preventing abortions
http://www.info.usaid.gov/pop_health/

Sponsor ➢	U.S. Agency for International Development (USAID)
Description ➢	Report detailing abortion as indicator of unmet need for contraceptive use in other countries
Data type ➢	Text
Access requirements ➢	Open
Supplemental resources ➢	Process evaluation of AIDS technical support project **(http://www.info.usaid.gov/pop_health/hiv_aids/program.htm)** USAID population, health, and nutrition (PHN) **(http://www.info.usaid.gov/pop_health/)**
User tips ➢	Check USAID's HIV/AIDS activities
Keywords ➢	HIV/AIDS demographics

Gender determination
http://www.childbirth.org/articles/boyorgirl.html

Sponsor ➢ Childbirth.org

Description ➢ Online interactive test for gender determination

Data type ➢ Interactive text

Access requirements ➢ Complete and submit form

Supplemental resources ➢ Episiotomy page
(http://www.childbirth.org/articles/epis.html)
Use of episiotomy
(http://www.childbirth.org/articles/indications.html)

User tips ➢ Site for expectant parents

Keywords ➢ obstetrics
episiotomy

National summary and fertility clinic reports
http://www.cdc.gov/nccdphp/drh/arts/index.htm

Sponsor ➢ Division of Reproductive Health, Centers for Disease Control and Prevention (CDC)

Description ➢ Reports of assisted reproductive technology (ART) success rates at fertility clinics, according to national and state data

Data type ➢ Report

Access requirements ➢ Open

Supplemental resources ➢ 1995 National summary of pregnancy success rates
(http://www2.cdc.gov:81/nccdphp/invitro/Nation.asp)
1995 National report of assisted reproductive technology
(http://www.cdc.gov/nccdphp/drh/arts/national.htm)

User tips ➢ See homepage for ART glossary

Keywords ➢ fertility clinics
assisted reproductive technology

1996 World Population Overview

http://www.populationinstitute.org/overview96.html

Sponsor ➢ The Population Institute

Description ➢ Paper on the impact of the world population problem

Data type ➢ Text

Access requirements ➢ Open

Supplemental resources ➢ Overpopulation, deforestation, water scarcity, and famine
(http://www.populationinstitute.org/issue.html)
The Population Institute homepage
(http://www.populationinstitute.org/)

User tips ➢ Check homepage PopAction alert

Keywords ➢ demographics
population

No-scalpel vasectomy

http://www.avsc.org/avsc/workpap/wp3/wp_3.html

Sponsor ➢ Access to Voluntary and Safe Contraception (AVSC) International

Description ➢ Working paper: Introduction of no-scalpel vasectomy in the United States (1988–1992)

Data type ➢ Text

Access requirements ➢ Open

Supplemental resources ➢ Men as partners in reproductive health
(http://www.avsc.org/avsc/)
AVSC homepage
(http://www.avsc.org/avsc/)

User tips ➢ Hit homepage link for contraceptive options

Keywords ➢ contraception, male
reproduction

POPLINE (Population Information Online) abstracts

http://www/charm.net~ccp/popwel.html

Sponsor ➢ Johns Hopkins School of Public Health

Description ➢ Megasite of bibliographic population database in family planning technology, programs, demography, and fertility

Data type ➢ Text

Access requirements ➢ Open

Supplemental resources ➢ Sources of European population statistics **(http://www.nidi.nl/links/nidi6js.html)**

User tips ➢ POPLINE updated monthly

Keywords ➢ population
family planning

PopNet source for global population information

http://www.popnet.org/

Sponsor ➢ Population Reference Bureau (PRB)

Description ➢ Clickable world map for searching population data by keyword, organization, or topic

Data type ➢ Interactive text

Access requirements ➢ Open

Supplemental resources ➢ Catalog of *PRB Population Bulletins*, 1991–1997 **(http://www.prb.org/prb/pubs/bulletin.htm)**
Eurostat, European statistics **(http://www.popnet.org/maps/europe.htm)**

User tips ➢ View PRB homepage for 1997 World Population Data Sheet

Keywords ➢ demographics
international population data

Population and reproductive health data
http://www.pitt.edu/HOME/GHNet/poprepro.htm

Sponsor ➢ University of Pittsburgh

Description ➢ Database resources on contraception; family planning; fertility; population research; and other topics

Data type ➢ Variable

Access requirements ➢ Open

Supplemental resources ➢ Erectile dysfunction therapy **(http://www.pslgroup.com/dg/3d396.htm)**
Viagra press releases **(http://pharmacology.tqn.com/library/newdr98/b10327b.htm)**

User tips ➢ Population homepage available in Spanish and Japanese

Keywords ➢ family planning
impotence, male

Report 1997: The Right to Choose
http://www.unfpa.org/SWP/SWPMAIN.HTM

Sponsor ➢ United Nations Population Fund (UNFPA)

Description ➢ Report: Reproductive rights and sexual health

Data type ➢ Text

Access requirements ➢ Open

Supplemental resources ➢ Release: Shortfalls in population assistance **(http://www.unfpa.org/NEWS/RELEASES/RESO-REL.HTM)**

User tips ➢ Available in English, French, and Spanish

Keywords ➢ pregnancy
reproduction rights

Report: U.N. International Conference on Population (ICPD)
http://www.ppfa.org/ppfa/unconf-1.html

Sponsor ➢ Planned Parenthood Federation of America, Inc. (PPFA)

Description ➢ Report of 1994 conference on population and development

Data type ➢ Open

Access requirements ➢ Open

Supplemental resources ➢ History of Smith global gag rule
(http://www.ppfa.org/ppfa/intlgag.html)
Internet resources for family planning, population, reproductive health, HIV/AIDS, Family Health International (FHI)
(http://www.fhi.org/general/urlsrch.html#anchor37518)

User tips ➢ Check homepage link for Family Planning International Assistance

Keywords ➢ HIV/AIDS
international family planning

Research regarding impact of family planning
http://www.fhi.org/wsp/wsinfo/wsrsrit.html

Sponsor ➢ Family Health International (FHI)

Description ➢ Results of childbearing on women's earnings, quality of life; labor force participation; marital disruption

Data type ➢ Text

Access requirements ➢ Open

Supplemental resources ➢ FHI homepage
(http://www.fhi.org/fhi1.html)
Abstracts of Women's Studies Projects
(http://www.fhi.org/wsp/wsinfo/wsabs.html)

User tips ➢ FHI site available in French, Spanish, and Russian

Keywords ➢ family planning
childbearing research

School based sexuality education programs

http://www.siecus.org/progs/prog0002.html

Sponsor ➢ Sexuality Information and Education Council of the United States (SIECUS)

Description ➢ Descriptions of programs emphasizing HIV/AIDS prevention education

Data type ➢ Text

Access requirements ➢ Open

Supplemental resources ➢ SIECUS homepage
(http://www.siecus.org/siecus/)
Guidelines for comprehensive sexuality education
(http://www.siecus.org/progs/prog0003.html)

User tips ➢ Check SIECUS research fellowship program

Keywords ➢ HIV/AIDS
adolescent sexuality

Sexual side effects of antidepressants

http://www.pathfinder.com/money/latest/press/PW/1997Dec02/1787.html

Sponsor ➢ PR Newswire

Description ➢ Survey of sexual side effects related to antidepressants

Data type ➢ Text

Access requirements ➢ Open

Supplemental resources ➢ Review of sexual behavior in the United States (abstract)
(http://www.ncf.carleton.ca/ip/social.services/ppo/info/sexstat/sex/stat)
Impotence, NIH Consensus Statement
(http://text.nlm.nih.gov/nih/cdc/www/91txt.html#Head3)

User tips ➢ Full text of impotence statement available

Keywords ➢ sexuality

Sexually transmitted diseases (STDs)

http://www.aomc.org/HOD2/general/general-SEXUALLY.html#Heading53

Sponsor ➢ Arnot Ogden Medical Center

Description ➢ STDs in women, symptoms, risk factors, and prevention

Data type ➢ Text; graphics

Access requirements ➢ Open

Supplemental resources ➢ 1993 STDs treatment guidelines, CDC **(http://wonder.cdc.gov/wonder/STD/Title3301.html)**
Chlamydial infection **(http://www.aomc.org/chlamydia2.html)**

User tips ➢ Check data on twenty-five STDs that affect women

Keywords ➢ sexually transmitted disease (STD)
STD treatment guidelines

Viagra questions and answers

http://www.fda.gov/cder/consumerinfo/viagra/viagrafaq.htm

Sponsor ➢ Center for Drug Evaluation and Research (CDER), U.S. Food and Drug Administration (FDA)

Description ➢ Frequently asked questions concerning Viagra

Data type ➢ Text

Access requirements ➢ Open

Supplemental resources ➢ Drug information for Fen-Phen, Viagra, anticoagulants **(http://www.fda.gov/cder/drug.htm)**
Consumer information about Viagra **(http://www.fda.gov/cder/consumerinfo/viagra/viagra_consumer.htm)**

User tips ➢ Contact FDA Drug Information Branch, 301-827-4573, for additional Viagra information

Keywords ➢ Viagra
pharmacology

World fertility survey
http://opr.princeton.edu/archive/wfs.html

Sponsor >	Center for Human Reproduction (CHR)
Description >	World fertility survey of forty-one participating countries, classified by region
Data type >	Text
Access requirements >	Open
Supplemental resources >	Surrogacy **(http://actag.canberra.edu.au:80/actag/Reports/Other/Rep5/Rep5-1.html)**
User tips >	Survey data archived in zip files
Keywords >	fertility surrogacy

Respiratory Health

Anti-tuberculosis drug resistance in the world

http://www.who.ch/programmes/gtb/dritw/index.html

Sponsor ➢	World Health Organization (WHO) Tuberculosis Programme, Geneva
Description ➢	Background, summary on global anti-tuberculosis drug resistance
Data type ➢	Report
Access requirements ➢	Open
Supplemental resources ➢	Report foreword **(http://www.who.ch/programmes/gtb/dritw/foreword.html)** Bibliography: Statistics on allergic and lung diseases **(http://www.njc.org/Library/Lung_Stat_Bibl.html)**
User tips ➢	Bibliography cites estimates of U.S. prevalence of chronic obstructive pulmonary disease and asthma
Keywords ➢	tuberculosis pulmonary disease

Ask the expert: Antihistamine

http://www.aadmc.org/ate/antihistamine.html

Sponsor ➢	Asthma and Allergy Disease Management Center (AADMC)
Description ➢	Antihistamine questions and answers
Data type ➢	Text
Access requirements ➢	Open
Supplemental resources ➢	Anaphylaxis: Treatment and prevention **(http://www.sma.org/medbytes/allergy.htm#Pathophysiology)** New aproaches to treating asthma **(http://www.ama-assn.org/insight/spec_con/asthma/treat.htm)**
User tips ➢	See links for sinusitis pathophysiology, diagnosis, treatment, and prevention
Keywords ➢	anaphylaxis antihistamines

Asthma Information Center

http://www.mdnet.de/asthma/asthma.htm

Sponsor ➢	Rhone-Poulenc Rorer
Description ➢	Data source for asthma studies, latest development, and other topics
Data type ➢	Text for health professionals
Access requirements ➢	Open
Supplemental resources ➢	Asthma studies **(http://www.mdnet.de/asthma/physdb/asthmast.htm)** American Association of Respiratory Care (AARC) online **(http://www.aarc.org/index.html)**
User tips ➢	See AARC for latest news regarding respiratory health
Keywords ➢	asthma

Cockroach allergen as related to asthma
http://www.aaaai.org/news/acadnews/96-10/96-10-02.html

Sponsor ➢	*Academy News*, American Academy of Allergy, Asthma and Immunology (AAAAI)
Description ➢	Article, cockroach allergen as a factor in asthma severity
Data type ➢	Text
Access requirements ➢	Open
Supplemental resources ➢	Global Initiative for Asthma (GINA) **(http://www.mdnet.de/asthma/gina/index.html)** Food allergies, The Online Allergy Center **(http://www.sig.net/~allergy/food.html)**
User tips ➢	Check recent AAAAI studies
Keywords ➢	asthma food allergies

Definition of allergy and asthma specialist
http://www.aaaai.org/referral/whatis/whatis.html

Sponsor ➢	American Academy of Allergy, Asthma and Immunology (AAAAI)
Description ➢	Training and role distinctions for asthma and allergy specialists
Data type ➢	Article
Access requirements ➢	Open
Supplemental resources ➢	Asthma allergy educational materials **(http://www.aafa.org/educat.html)** Health policy education network (HPEN) articles on Medicare, health reform **(http://www.aaaai.org/watch/hpen/hpen.html)**
User tips ➢	Physician referral and information, 24-hour, line (1-800-822-2762)
Keywords ➢	asthma allergy materials

The Diagnosis of Diffuse Lung Disease

http://indy.radiology.uiowa.edu/Pr...books/DiffuseLung/DiffuseLung.html

Sponsor ➢ Jeffrey R. Galvin, M.D. and Michael P. D'Alessandro, M.D., University of Iowa College of Medicine

Description ➢ Basics of diffuse lung disease including overview, clinical workup, imaging protocol, and specific diseases

Data type ➢ Reference; images

Access requirements ➢ Open

Supplemental resources ➢ Clinical workup of diffuse lung disease **(http://indy.radiology.uiowa.edu/Pr...ffuseLung/Text/ClinicalWorkup.html)**
Information by organ system: Pulmonary **(http://indy.radiology.uiowa.edu/Pr...rs/ProviderOrgSys/OsPulmonary.html)**

User tips ➢ Health care provider data include multimedia textbooks, teaching files, patient simulations, and lectures

Keywords ➢ diffuse lung disease
pulmonary disease

Helping smokers quit

http://www.ahcpr.gov/clinic/smokepcc.htm

Sponsor ➢ Agency for Health Care Policy and Research (AHCPR)

Description ➢ Step-by-step smoking cessation guide for primary care clinicians

Data type ➢ Text

Access requirements ➢ Open

Supplemental resources ➢ Secondhand smoke, Mayo Health Oasis **(http://www.mayohealth.org/mayo/9708/htm/2nd_hand.htm)**
Smoking research, medical self-care, and naturopathic medicine **(http://www.healthy.net/clinic/dandc/smoking/)**

User tips ➢ Check AHCPR smoking resource center for consumers

Keywords ➢ second-hand smoke
smoking cessation

Prevention and treatment of influenza and the common cold

http://www.lungusa.org/noframes/learn/lung/lungcolds_flu.html

Sponsor ➢ American Lung Association and American Thoracic Society

Description ➢ Symptoms, complications, and prevention guidelines for colds and the flu

Data type ➢ Text; some graphics

Access requirements ➢ Open

Supplemental resources ➢ Homepage **(http://www.lungusa.org/index.html)**
The flu **(http://www.lungusa.org/noframes/learn/lung/flu.html#transmit)**

User tips ➢ See homepage for bin, "When you can't breathe, nothing else matters"

Keywords ➢ influenza
common cold

Respiratory problems during sleep
http://www.u-net.com/priory/cmol/STRAD.HTM

Sponsor > Chest Medicine On-Line

Description > Breathing disorders during sleep

Data type > Report

Access requirements > Open

Supplemental resources > Chest Medicine homepage **(http://www.priory.com/chest.htm)**

User tips > Read article: "Is snoring just a joke?"

Keywords > respiratory problems
sleep disorders

Reviews of respiratory tract diseases
http://www.auhs.edu/library/resource/reviews/pulm.htm

Sponsor > Health Reviews on the Internet, University of Arizona

Description > Critical care reviews for primary care providers on obstructive lung diseases; pleural effusions; critical care

Data type > Bibliography

Access requirements > Open; data for health providers

Supplemental resources > Health reviews for primary care providers **(http://www.auhs.edu/library/resource/reviews/revw_ind.htm#occup_ind)**
Respiratory links page **(http://www.xmission.com/%7Egastown/herpmed/respi.htm)**

User tips > CEUs data available for respiratory links page

Keywords > medical education
lung diseases

Sample online respiratory care examination

http://www.nbrc.org/Interactive.htm

Sponsor ➢ National Board for Respiratory Care (NBRC)

Description ➢ Sample questions from the online respiratory care examination

Data type ➢ Interactive test

Access requirements ➢ Open

Supplemental resources ➢ NBRC homepage
(http://www.nbrc.org/)
Respiratory Care Journal
(http://www.rcjournal.com/)

User tips ➢ NBRC seeks institutions for examination validation studies

Keywords ➢ allied health
respiratory examination

Substance Abuse

Access to methadone treatment for heroin addiction
http://mhnet.org/articles/nih2.htm

Sponsor ➢	Mental Health Net
Description ➢	Article describing NIH recommendation for expanding access to methadone
Data type ➢	Article
Access requirements ➢	Open
Supplemental resources ➢	National Library of Medicine (NLM) current bibliography: Effective medical treatment of heroin addiction **(http://www.nlm.nih.gov/pubs/cbm/ heroin_addiction.html#1)** Discharge from treatment for drug use **(http://www.methadone.org/discharg.html)**
User tips ➢	Check Mental Health Net for additional articles
Keywords ➢	drug treatment methadone

Action to control tobacco

http://www.tobaccofreekids.org/html/consensus_statement.html

Sponsor ➢ Effective National Action to Control Tobacco (ENACT)

Description ➢ Consensus statement of ENACT

Data type ➢ Text

Access requirements ➢ Open

Supplemental resources ➢ Campaign for Tobacco-Free Kids
(http://www.tobaccofreekids.org/)
NCADI-FDA tobacco litigation proposed resolution, June 1997
(http://www.health.org/pubs/tobres.htm)

User tips ➢ See advertiser survey on effectiveness of tobacco ads

Keywords ➢ tobacco and children
smoking

Clinical research findings on alcohol and drugs

http://www.ria.org/findings/index.html

Sponsor ➢ Research Institute on Addictions (RIA)

Description ➢ Findings on drinking and substance abuse problems among drivers, youth, and the family

Data type ➢ Text; graphics

Access requirements ➢ Open

Supplemental resources ➢ Index of RIA site and links contents
(http://www.ria.org/contents.html)
Summary, substance use and the family
(http://www.ria.org/findings/family.html)

User tips ➢ Check homepage for Minority Research Development Program (MRDP)

Keywords ➢ substance abuse
minority research program

Directory of Substance Abuse Professionals (SAP)

http://www.detnet.com/datalink/sap/index.htm

Sponsor ➢ DataLink of Onalaska, Texas

Description ➢ Directory of professionals for assessment and clinical evaluation of employee drug problems

Data type ➢ Text

Access requirements ➢ Open

Supplemental resources ➢ Who needs SAP?
(http://www.detnet.com/datalink/sap/whoneeds.htm)
World of Drug Information
(http://www.uiowa.edu/~idis/wodmar96.htm#fda1996)

User tips ➢ SAP contact number (1-800-372-4810)

Keywords ➢ directory, substance abuse professionals
drug information

Drug Abuse Warning Network (DAWN)

http://www.health.org/pubs/93dawn/93dawn.htm

Sponsor ➢ Substance Abuse and Mental Health Services Administration (SAMHSA)

Description ➢ 1993 Preliminary DAWN estimates of episodic trends in use of heroin, cocaine, and prescription drugs

Data type ➢ Text; graphics

Access requirements ➢ Open

Supplemental resources ➢ DAWN highlights
(http://www.health.org/pubs/93dawn/dw-hilit.htm)
Release: National drug use survey results, 1997
(http://www.health.org/pressrel/aug97/3.htm)

User tips ➢ See file on trends in prescription and over-the-counter (OTC) drug-related episodes

Keywords ➢ drugs
over-the-counter drug abuse

Drug and alcohol testing medical practitioners

http://www.aamro.com/

Sponsor ➢ American Association of Medical Review Officers (AAMRO)

Description ➢ Standards and certification for medical drug and alcohol testing practitioners

Data type ➢ Text

Access requirements ➢ Open

Supplemental resources ➢ AAMRO training and certification **(http://www.aamro.com/cert.html)**
1997 Registry of certified medical review officers **(http://www.aamro.com/mrolist.html)**

User tips ➢ Go to U.S. map and click a state for list of medical review officers

Keywords ➢ drug and alcohol testing services

Family approach to drug prevention

http://www.emory.edu/NFIA/

Sponsor ➢ National Families in Action

Description ➢ Drug prevention program utilizing family approach

Data type ➢ Text; some graphics

Access requirements ➢ Open

Supplemental resources ➢ Street drug information **(http://www.emory.edu/NFIA/DRUG_INFO/index.html)**
African American Family Services (AAFS) **(http://www.aafs-mn.org/content.html)**

User tips ➢ See AAFS homepage for volunteer and internship opportunities

Keywords ➢ drug prevention
street drug information

Get It Straight publication
http://www.usdoj.gov/dea/pubs/straight/cover.htm

Sponsor ➢	Drug Enforcement Administration (DEA), U.S. Department of Justice
Description ➢	Drug information for young people
Data type ➢	Text; graphics
Access requirements ➢	Open
Supplemental resources ➢	DEA homepage **(http://www.usdoj.gov/dea/)** Drug policy in the Netherlands: Hard drug "tourism" **(http://www.drugtext.nl/reports/wvc/s26.htm)**
User tips ➢	See homepage for DEA statistical data
Keywords ➢	drug policy, Netherlands drugs, adolescents

Helping patients with alcohol problems
http://www.niaaa.nih.gov/publications/physicn.htm

Sponsor ➢	National Institute on Alcohol Abuse and Alcoholism (NIAAA)
Description ➢	Physicians' guide describing screening procedures; low-risk drinking; intervention procedures
Data type ➢	Text
Access requirements ➢	Open
Supplemental resources ➢	Selected references **(http://www.niaaa.nih.gov/publications/physicn.htm)**
User tips ➢	Check link for low-risk drinking recommendations
Keywords ➢	alcohol abuse

Information about alcohol, tobacco, and other drugs

http://www.drugs.indiana.edu/radar/alerts/alerts.html

Sponsor ➢ Indiana Prevention Resource Center (IPRC), Indiana University

Description ➢ Reports and articles on drug legalization, testing issues, and fact sheets

Data type ➢ Text

Access requirements ➢ Open

Supplemental resources ➢ Alcohol Alert: Alcohol and Aging
(http://www.drugs.indiana.edu/pubs/alerts/alert2.html)
Directory of alcohol, tobacco, and other drug abbreviations
(http://www.drugs.indiana.edu/druginfo/)

User tips ➢ See *Online Dictionary of Street Drug Slang*

Keywords ➢ alcohol abuse
alcohol abuse, aging

Low-risk drinking guidelines

http://www.arf.org/lowriskEnglish.html

Sponsor ➢ Addiction Research Foundation (ARF), University of Toronto

Description ➢ Release: Low-risk guidelines balance risks and benefits

Data type ➢ Article

Access requirements ➢ Open

Supplemental resources ➢ ARF homepage
(http://www.arf.org/)
Staff publications on research studies; treatment; and prevention
(http://www.arf.org/isd/staffpub9596.html#epid)

User tips ➢ Text available in French

Keywords ➢ low risk drinking
drug-alcohol information

Methamphetamine abuse
ftp://ftp.health.org/pub/ncadi/publications/meth.txt

Sponsor ➢	Center for Substance Abuse Treatment (CSAT) and Substance Abuse and Mental Health Services Administration (SAMHSA)
Description ➢	Proceedings on the use, abuse, and sequelae of methamphetamine abuse with implications for prevention
Data type ➢	Report
Access requirements ➢	Open
Supplemental resources ➢	Tustin Police Department, descriptions of street drugs paraphernalia, symptoms, and dangers **(http://www.tustinpd.org/drugs.html)** Designer drugs, article **(http://www.thriveonline.com@@6HO1A...alth/Library/CAD/abstract16552.html)**
User tips ➢	See Tustin site for quick, easy-to-read narcotics data
Keywords ➢	drug paraphernalia designer drugs

The National Treatment Improvement Evaluation Study (NTIES)

http://www.health.org/nties97/index.htm

Sponsor ➢ Center for Substance Abuse Treatment (CSAT), Substance Abuse and Mental Health Administration, DHHS

Description ➢ NTIES highlights on drug and alcohol use; changes in criminal behavior; mental health

Data type ➢ Report

Access requirements ➢ Open

Supplemental resources ➢ CSAT block grant information **(http://www.samhsa.gov/csat/ubgas/csatintr.htm)**
Alcoholics Anonymous offices and answering services for U.S. and Canada **(http://www.alcoholics-anonymous.org/intgrp/000states.html)**

User tips ➢ See substance abuse treatment outcomes and performance pilot studies (TOPPS)

Keywords ➢ substance abuse
health funding

Needle exchange programs

http://soros.org/lindesmith/clinton/agencies.html

Sponsor ➢ The Lindesmith Center

Description ➢ Review of University of California report on needle exchange

Data type ➢ Text

Access requirements ➢ Open

Supplemental resources ➢ The Lindesmith Center homepage **(http://www.soros.org/lindesmith/tlcmain.html)**
Bibliography, public health impact of national and international needle exchange programs **(http://www.epibiostat.ucsf.edu/capsweb/publications/needleref.html)**

User tips ➢ Check Lindesmith Center homepage for publications on marijuana myths

Keywords ➢ needle exchange programs

Parent's Handbook to Substance Abuse Prevention

http://198.115.232.254/y2y/Parents_Handbook.html

Sponsor ➢ South Kingstown's Youth to Youth Web Server

Description ➢ Drug data for parents describing symptoms, myths, and deadly inhalants

Data type ➢ Text; some graphics

Access requirements ➢ Open

Supplemental resources ➢ Youth to Youth homepage
(http://198.115.232.254/y2y/default.html)
Site index
(http://198.115.232.254/y2y/substance_abuse_prevention.html)

User tips ➢ Emphasis on the facts about alcohol and drugs

Keywords ➢ parental drug education

Prevline Prevention Online

http://www.health.org/aboutn.htm

Sponsor ➢ National Clearinghouse for Alcohol and Drug Information (NCADI), Substance Abuse and Mental Health Services (SAMHSA), DHHS

Description ➢ Publications; online forums; research; statistics on alcohol and drug facts

Data type ➢ Text; graphics

Access requirements ➢ Open

Supplemental resources ➢ Research and statistics
(http://www.health.org/survey.htm)
Effects of alcohol on sexual risk behavior
(http://www.health.org/res-brf/index.htm)

User tips ➢ See dynatable of first-time substance users: in actual time

Keywords ➢ substance abuse
sexuality

Sourcebook of Criminal Justice Statistics, 24th edition, October 1997

http://www.albany.edu/sourcebook/index.html

Sponsor ➢ Bureau of Justice Statistics, U.S. Department of Justice

Description ➢ Compendium of criminal justice data in the U.S.

Data type ➢ Searchable text for viewing or downloading with Acrobat Reader

Access requirements ➢ Open

Supplemental resources ➢ Alcohol index **(http://www.albany.edu/sourcebook/1995/ind/ALCOHOL.ind.html)**
Justice Information Center, National Criminal Justice Reference Service (NCJRS) **(http://www.ncjrs.org/)**

User tips ➢ Sourcebook text is hyperlinked

Keywords ➢ criminal justice statistics

Steroid prevention with high school athletes

http://www.nida.nih.gov/NIDA_Notes/NNVol12N4/steroid.html#girls

Sponsor ➢ National Institute on Drug Abuse (NIDA)

Description ➢ Steroid prevention program with high school football players

Data type ➢ Text; graphics

Access requirements ➢ Open

Supplemental resources ➢ NIDA homepage **(http://www.nida.nih.gov/)**
Anabolic steroids **(http://www.nida.nih.gov/ResearchReports/Steroids/AnabolicSteroids1.html)**

User tips ➢ See NIDA notes for article about steroid abuse among adolescent girls

Keywords ➢ adolescent steroid use
sports medicine

Study of drug use among consumers of vocational rehabilitation services
http://www.med.wright.edu/som/sardi/epidem.html

Sponsor ➢ Rehabilitation Research and Training Center (RRTC) and Substance Abuse Intervention Programs (SARDI), Wright State University School of Medicine

Description ➢ Background and summary of study of substance use among vocational rehabilitation applicants

Data type ➢ Text

Access requirements ➢ Open

Supplemental resources ➢ SARDI
(http://www.med.wright.edu/som/sardi/about.html#Collaborative)
SARDI and RRTC homepage
(http://www.med.wright.edu/som/sardi)

User tips ➢ See homepage for substance abuse links

Keywords ➢ drugs
vocational rehabilitation

Workplace drug use
http://www.samhsa.gov/oas/wkplace/httoc.htm

Sponsor ➢ Substance Abuse and Mental Health Services Administration (SAMHSA), DHHS

Description ➢ Report of worker drug use and workplace policies and programs

Data type ➢ Report; graphics

Access requirements ➢ Open

Supplemental resources ➢ Figure, workplace access to employee assistance programs for drug problems
(http://www.samhsa.gov/oas/wkplace/workpl37.htm)

User tips ➢ See SAMHSA homepage for managed care data

Keywords ➢ workplace drug use
managed care

Veterinary Medicine

Animal diseases
http://www.mic.ki.se/Diseases/c22.html

Sponsor ➢	Karolinska Institute Library and Information Center
Description ➢	Source list of global animal disease databases
Data type ➢	Variable; megasite
Access requirements ➢	Open
Supplemental resources ➢	Vitamin-related diseases in animals **(http://www.mic.ki.se/Diseases/c22.html)** Farm animal health research, Institute for Animal Health **(http://www.mic.ki.se/Diseases/c22.html)**
User tips ➢	Interesting international sites
Keywords ➢	megasite

Animal poison control
http://www.napcc.aspca.org/

Sponsor ➢ American Society for the Prevention of Cruelty to Animals (ASPCA), National Animal Poison Control Center (NAPCC)

Description ➢ Animal poison prevention and treatment source

Data type ➢ Text

Access requirements ➢ Open

Supplemental resources ➢ Prevention of small animal poisonings **(http://www.napcc.aspca.org/smalanml.htm)**

User tips ➢ Information number: 1-800-548-2423; poison intervention assistance (fee service): 1-888-426-4435

Keywords ➢ animal poisoning

Bovine respiratory disease (BRD)
http://www.nuflor.com/free.htm

Sponsor ➢ Schering-Plough Animal Health

Description ➢ Sourcebook of BRD etiology, pathogenesis, and prevention; for veterinary professionals

Data type ➢ Reference

Access requirements ➢ Open

Supplemental resources ➢ American Association of Swine Practitioners (AASP) homepage **(http://www.aasp.org/home.html)**

User tips ➢ To receive complimentary reference hard copy, complete online survey

Keywords ➢ swine diseases
bovine respiratory disease

Canine sports medicine

http://www.cris.com/~Dovervet/csmu/

Sponsor ➢ *Canine Sports Medicine Update* (CSMU)

Description ➢ Canine health updates

Data type ➢ Newsletter

Access requirements ➢ Open

Supplemental resources ➢ Carpal hyperextension injuries **(http://www.cris.com/~Dovervet/csmu/articles/carpal_hyperext.html)**

User tips ➢ Check homepage for recent articles

Keywords ➢ canine sports medicine

Cattle disease prevention and treatment

http://www.ianr.unl.edu/pubs/animaldisease/index.htm#cattle

Sponsor ➢ University of Nebraska-Lincoln

Description ➢ Diseases of cattle, swine, sheep, poultry, horses, and livestock

Data type ➢ Text

Access requirements ➢ Open

Supplemental resources ➢ Animal diseases homepage **(http://www.ianr.unl.edu/pubs/animaldisease/index.htm#cattle)**
Blackhead disease in turkeys; symptoms and prevention **(http://www.ianr.unl.edu/pubs/animaldisease/g1226.htm)**

User tips ➢ See homepage link for general livestock diseases

Keywords ➢ agricultural animal diseases
turkey blackhead disease

Compendium of animal rabies control, 1997
http://www.avma.org/

Sponsor ➢ American Veterinary Medical Association (AVMA) Network

Description ➢ Information and data for rabies control

Data type ➢ Text; some graphics

Access requirements ➢ Open

Supplemental resources ➢ Guide to small animal poisons
(http://www.avma.org/pubhlth/poisgde.html)
Pet dermatology homepage
(http://www.vet-zone.com/special/derm.htm)

User tips ➢ Check AMVA homepage for pet bereavement information

Keywords ➢ animal poisons
rabies

Emerging animal diseases
http://www.fas.org/ahead/

Sponsor ➢ FAS Project

Description ➢ Wildlife disease; mad cow disease; fish health in the Chesapeake Bay

Data type ➢ Text

Access requirements ➢ Open

Supplemental resources ➢ Deformed frogs in Minnesota
(http://www.pca.state.mn.us/hot/frogs.html)
Wildlife disease newslettters
(http://www.fas.org/ahead/)

User tips ➢ For additional deformed frog information, check Minnesota Pollution Control Agency

Keywords ➢ animal disease
fish health

Footwarts of dairy cattle

http://sphinx.ucdavis.edu/research/footwarts/FootwartsOfDairyCattle.html

Sponsor ➢ California Veterinary Diagnostic Laboratory System (CVDLS)

Description ➢ Cattle footwarts prevalence, causes, and treatment

Data type ➢ Text

Access requirements ➢ Open

Supplemental resources ➢ Cattle and swine disease syndromes **(http://sphinx.ucdavis.edu/public/CVDLS/billing/diseases.htm)**
CVDLS homepage **(http://sphinx.ucdavis.edu/index.html)**

User tips ➢ Check homepage for link to data for diagnostic professionals

Keywords ➢ footwarts
swine disease

The Green Book

http://www.cvm.fda.gov/fda/Greenbook/greenbook.html

Sponsor ➢ Center for Veterinary Medicine (CVM), Food and Drug Administration (FDA)

Description ➢ FDA-approved animal drug list

Data type ➢ Electronic text (trial edition; subscription required later)

Access requirements ➢ Open; search enabled

Supplemental resources ➢ Animal medicinal drug use documents **(http://www.cvm.fda.gov/fda/TOCs/amducatoc.html)**
CVM online library of educational materials **(http://www.cvm.fda.gov/fda/mappgs/onlinelib.html)**

User tips ➢ Check library for medicated feed mill licensing data

Keywords ➢ animal drugs

Intestinal spirochete

http://205.221.234.10:80/spiroch/

Sponsor ➢ National Animal Disease Center, Agricultural Research Service, U.S. Department of Agriculture

Description ➢ Intestinal spirochete DNA sequences

Data type ➢ Text

Access requirements ➢ Open

Supplemental resources ➢ Unclassified intestinal spirochete DNA sequences **(http://205.221.234.10:80/spiroch/unclass.htm)**

User tips ➢ Check homepage for brachyspira aalborgi (human intestinal spirochete)

Keywords ➢ intestinal spirochete
swine disease

Laboratory animal diseases

http://www.rprc.washington.edu/aclad/index.html

Sponsor ➢ American Committee on Laboratory Animal Diseases (ACLAD)

Description ➢ Newsletters and other information regarding laboratory animal diseases

Data type ➢ Text; images

Access requirements ➢ Open

Supplemental resources ➢ What's your diagnosis? (diagnostic exercise) **(http://www.rprc.washington.edu/aclad/Whatdx.html)**
Directory of experts on laboratory animal diseases **(http://www.rprc.washington.edu/aclad/index.html)**

User tips ➢ Check homepage for specialty training contacts

Keywords ➢ laboratory animal diseases

Meat and poultry inspection under HACCP

http://www.meatami.org/haccpq&a.htm

Sponsor ➢ American Meat Institute (AMI)

Description ➢ Shifting from traditional inspection to new Hazard Analysis and Critical Control Points (HACCP) safe food system

Data type ➢ Text

Access requirements ➢ Open

Supplemental resources ➢ Humane slaughter industry guidelines **(http://www.meatami.org/FactWL01.HTM)**
Enteric diseases of cattle and swine **(http://www.nadc.ars.usda.gov/edfsru.htm)**

User tips ➢ Check homepage bin for article, "Just the facts"

Keywords ➢ meat inspection
nutrition

National poultry improvement plan

http://www.aphis.usda.gov/vs/npip/

Sponsor ➢ Animal and Plant Health Inspection Service (APHIS), U.S. Department of Agriculture

Description ➢ Progress report on eliminating poultry diseases

Data type ➢ Text

Access requirements ➢ Open

Supplemental resources ➢ Bovine tuberculosis **(gopher://gopher.aphis.usda.gov:70/00/AI.d/AHI.d/CH.d/bt.f)**
Emergency programs, USDA, APHIS Veterinary Services **(http://aphisweb.aphis.usda.gov/oa/ep-act.html)**

User tips ➢ Review APHIS foreign animal disease information

Keywords ➢ poultry diseases

Pet cancer
http://www.oncolink.upenn.edu/specialty/vet_onc/cancer.html

Sponsor ➢ OncoLink, University of Pennsylvania

Description ➢ Report on pet cancer terminology; tumor evaluation; therapy; treatment

Data type ➢ Text

Access requirements ➢ Open

Supplemental resources ➢ Veterinary oncology treatment and therapy, veterinarian resource
(http://www.oncolink.upenn.edu/specialty/vet_onc/)
Feline mammary tumors
(http://www.oncolink.upenn.edu/specialty/vet_onc/feline_mam_tumors.html)

User tips ➢ Check homepage for animal chemotherapy

Keywords ➢ animal cancer
tumors, cats

Rabies
http://www.gis.queensu.ca/RReporter/mnr.html

Sponsor ➢ Queen's University, Ontario Ministry of Natural Resources

Description ➢ Rabies reporter homepage describing rabies research and control in Ontario

Data type ➢ Newsletter

Access requirements ➢ Open

Supplemental resources ➢ Wildlife rabies control program
(http://www.gis.queensu.ca/mnrgallery.html)

User tips ➢ Check homepage for other rabies sites

Keywords ➢ rabies control

Veterinarian employment
http://www.dvmsearch.com/index.htm

Sponsor ➢	DVMSearch
Description ➢	Databank for veterinary job seekers, practice buyers, and sellers
Data type ➢	Searches available for candidates, practices for sale, positions by state or practice
Access requirements ➢	Open
Supplemental resources ➢	Search tool **(http://www.dvmsearch.com/database/search.htm)** Veterinary and animal science organizations **(http://www.avma.org/netvet/vetorg.htm)**
User tips ➢	Employment site, free
Keywords ➢	employment, veterinarian

Women's Health

Chronic pelvic pain diagnosis and management
http://www.cmegateway.com/womenshea...viders/Pelvic/pelvicpain.html#story

Sponsor ➢	Women's Health Resource Center, CME Gateway
Description ➢	Topics include chronic pain differential diagnosis, patient history, and empiric therapy; pain mapping forms included
Data type ➢	Text
Access requirements ➢	Open; for health care providers
Supplemental resources ➢	Gateway homepage **(http://www.cmegateway.com/)**
User tips ➢	Gateway is a resource for identifying online continuing medical education (CME)
Keywords ➢	medical education chronic pain management

Doctor's guide to menopause information and resources

http://www.pslgroup.com/MENOPAUSE.HTM

Sponsor ➢	PSL Consulting Group
Description ➢	Menopause news, alerts, and newsgroups
Data type ➢	Text
Access requirements ➢	Open
Supplemental resources ➢	Recruitment for Department of Agriculture live-in clinical study, postmenopausal women (compensation included) **(http://www.med.und.nodak.edu/misc/usda/pmw.htm)** Menopause medical news and alerts **(http://www.pslgroup.com/MENOPAUSE.HTM)**
User tips ➢	See e-mail instructions for notification of site updates
Keywords ➢	menopause clinical trial

Food safety, nutrition, and cosmetics

http://vm.cfsan.fda.gov/~dms/wh-toc.html

Sponsor ➢	Center for Food Safety and Applied Nutrition, U.S. Food and Drug Administration (FDA)
Description ➢	Information for women by age and health conditions; topics include cosmetics, dietary supplements, infant formula, and others
Data type ➢	Text
Access requirements ➢	Open
Supplemental resources ➢	Artificial nail remover poisoning risk **(http://vm.cfsan.fda.gov/~dms/cos-823.html)** FDA Office of Woman's Health Web site **(http://vm.cfsan.fda.gov/~dms/wh-toc.html)**
User tips ➢	See information for pregnant women
Keywords ➢	cosmetics nutrition

Gynecologic endoscopy resources
http://medweb.nus.sg/isge/resource.html

Sponsor ➢ International Society for Gynecologic Endoscopy (ISGE)

Description ➢ Worldwide resources of data on laparoscopic surgery, surgeons, hysterectomy, and related topics

Data type ➢ Multimedia

Access requirements ➢ Open

Supplemental resources ➢ Outpatient laparoscopic hysterectomy: A review of 50 patients
(http://medweb.nus.sg/isge/resource.html)
Advances in laparoscopic surgery
(http://medweb.nus.sg/isge/resource.html)

User tips ➢ See diagnostic and therapeutic endoscopy

Keywords ➢ endoscopy
gynecologic

Gynecologic oncology tutorials
http://gynoncology.obgyn.washington.edu/Tutorials/nest3.html

Sponsor ➢ Vaginal Cancer Center, University of Washington

Description ➢ Tutorials for cervical, ovarian, vulvar, gestational, and other cancers; prepared for junior and senior residents

Data type ➢ Tutorial; text; images

Access requirements ➢ Open

Supplemental resources ➢ Carcinoma, vaginal
(http://gynoncology.obgyn.washington.edu/Tutorials/Vaginalcancer.html#treat)
Tutorials index
(http://gynoncology.obgyn.washington.edu/Tutorials/Gyntut.html)

User tips ➢ Check index for pain control management

Keywords ➢ gynecologic tumors
cancer

Marching through the visible woman

http://www.crd.ge.com/cgi-bin/vw.pl

Sponsor ➢ National Library of Medicine (NLM)

Description ➢ Digital image; visible human female database includes results, conclusions, and references

Data type ➢ Digital atlas

Access requirements ➢ Open

Supplemental resources ➢ Use of visualization tool kit to create personal copy of visible woman **(http://www.crd.ge.com/cgi-bin/vw.pl)**

User tips ➢ See companion site for the visible man

Keywords ➢ anatomy

MDL 926 breast implant litigation, November 7, 1997

http://www.fjc.gov/BREIMLIT/mdl926.htm

Sponsor ➢ Federal Judicial Center

Description ➢ Dates, deadlines, and recent developments of breast implant litigation

Data type ➢ Text; images

Access requirements ➢ Open

Supplemental resources ➢ Status report on breast implant safety **(http://www.fda.gov/fdac/features/995_implants.html#known)**

User tips ➢ See images of silicone gel–filled breast implants

Keywords ➢ breast implant
legal medicine

Megasite, women's health
http://www.pitt.edu/HOME/GHNet/GHWomen.html

Sponsor ➢ Women's Health Global Health Network

Description ➢ Megasite of resources, materials on aging; cancer; domestic violence; infectious diseases

Data type ➢ Variable

Access requirements ➢ Open

Supplemental resources ➢ MedWeb gynecology and women's health **(http://www.gen.emory.edu/medweb/medweb/gynecology.html#History)**
American Medical Women's Association (AMWA), summaries of women's health projects **(http://www.amwa-doc.org/edproj.htm...anced Curriculum on Women's Health)**

User tips ➢ Contact number for AMWA: 1-800-866-0400

Keywords ➢ health training

Menopause Online
http://www.menopause-online.com/

Sponsor ➢ Menopause Online, Michael O'Reilly, M.D.

Description ➢ Menopause problems; treatments; and resources

Data type ➢ Text

Access requirements ➢ Open

Supplemental resources ➢ Menopause or PMS? **(http://www.menopause-online.com/problems.htm)**
Bladder control for women **(http://www.niddk.nih.gov/UIBCW/bcw/bcw.htm)**

User tips ➢ See homepage for natural remedies

Keywords ➢ menopause
PMS

OB-GYN medical professional data

http://www.obgyn.net/site_map/mp-map.htm

Sponsor ➢ OBGYN.net, Zeneca Pharmaceuticals

Description ➢ OB/Gyn links (about 3,000); international links; clinical books; organizations; employment; journals

Data type ➢ Text

Access requirements ➢ Open; some links restricted to physicians

Supplemental resources ➢ OB-GYN-L forum (medical professionals only) **(http://forums.obgyn.net/forums/ob-gyn-l/)**
Maternal mortality in Saudi Arabia **(http://www.kfshrc.edu.sa/annals/154/94181/94181.html)**

User tips ➢ See homepage for international OB/GYN data according to country

Keywords ➢ obstetrics
gynecology

Obstetrics and gynecology board certification

http://www.metronet.com/~rhino/FAQS.htm

Sponsor ➢ American Board of Obstetrics and Gynecology

Description ➢ OB/GYN questions and answers regarding board certification

Data type ➢ Text

Access requirements ➢ Open

Supplemental resources ➢ OB/GYN board homepage **(http://www.metronet.com/~rhino/)**

User tips ➢ Check link, what is the board?

Keywords ➢ OB/GYN certification

Oxford endometriosis gene study update

http://www.medicine.ox.ac.uk/ndog/oxegene/results.htm

Sponsor ➢ Obstetrics and Gynaecology, University of Oxford

Description ➢ Study results and publications of worldwide research study to identify genes responsible for endometriosis

Data type ➢ Text

Access requirements ➢ Open

Supplemental resources ➢ Oxford gene study homepage **(http://www.medicine.ox.ac.uk/ndog/oxegene/oxegene.htm#What)**

User tips ➢ Sign up as a study participant

Keywords ➢ endometriosis

Research of health issues among women with disabilities

http://WWW.CDC.GOV/nceh/programs/disabil/research.htm

Sponsor ➢ Office on Disability and Health, National Center for Environmental Health (NCEH)

Description ➢ Descriptions of prevention programs for women with mobility impairments; violence against women with disabilities

Data type ➢ Text

Access requirements ➢ Open

Supplemental resources ➢ Women with disabilities homepage **(http://WWW.CDC.GOV/nceh/programs/disabil/women.htm)**
International forum for women with disabilities **(http://www.wwwd.org)**

User tips ➢ See homepage for site on limb loss

Keywords ➢ women, disabilities
mobility impairment

Women's community prevention study centers

http://odp.od.nih.gov/whi/cpstopic.htm

Sponsor ➢ Women's Health Initiative (WHI), National Institutes of Health (NIH)

Description ➢ WHI funded prevention centers listed according to topics related to hysterectomy, physical fitness, and other topics

Data type ➢ Text

Access requirements ➢ Open

Supplemental resources ➢ WHI homepage **(http://odp.od.nih.gov/whi/)**
Office of Research on Women's Health (ORWH) **(http://ohrm.od.nih.gov/orwh/index.html)**

User tips ➢ See homepage updates on clinical trial and observational study

Keywords ➢ clinical trials
preventive research

Women's health "ground rounds" menu

http://lib-sh.lsumc.edu/fammed/grounds/grounds.html

Sponsor ➢ Louisiana State University Medical Center, Shreveport

Description ➢ Protocols and lecture handouts on menopause; pap smears; contraception, hormone replacement, and other women's issues

Data type ➢ Text

Access requirements ➢ Open

Supplemental resources ➢ LSU Medical Center homepage **(http://lib-sh.lsumc.edu/)**
Patient education menu **(http://lib-sh.lsumc.edu/fammed/pted/pted.html#Gyn)**

User tips ➢ Patient materials include low literacy materials

Keywords ➢ menopause
medical education

Women's health topics
http://www.medscape.com/Home/Topics/WomensHealth/womenshealth.html

Sponsor ➢	Medscape Oncology
Description ➢	Current news, peer-reviewed clinical articles about reproduction, cancer, nutrition, breast cancer, and pregnancy
Data type ➢	Text; images; search enabled
Access requirements ➢	Open
Supplemental resources ➢	OB/GYN Toolbox **(http://www.cpmc.columbia.edu/resources/obgyntools/)**
User tips ➢	Medscape site updated regularly
Keywords ➢	cancer gynecology resources

Appendix

Sponsor Representation According to Type

U.S. Federal government or related organizations

Agency for Health Care Policy and Research (AHCPR)
Agency for International Development (USAID)
Agency for Toxic Substances and Disease Registry (ATSDR)
Agriculture Research Service (ARS), Department of Agriculture (USDA)
Animal and Plant Health Inspection Service (APHIS), Department of Agriculture
Armed Forces Institute of Pathology (AFIP), Center for Advanced Pathology
Army Dental Corps
Brookhaven National Laboratory
Bureau of Health Professions, Health Resources and Services Administration
Bureau of Justice Statistics, Department of Justice
Bureau of Labor Statistics (BLS)
California Veterinary Diagnostic Laboratory System (CVDLS)
Cancer Cooperative Research
CancerNet, National Cancer Institute (NCI), National Institutes of Health (NIH)
Cansearch
Census Bureau
Center for Advanced Pathology
Center for Devices and Radiological Health (CDRH), FDA
Center for Drug Evaluation and Research, FDA
Center for Food Safety and Applied Nutrition, FDA
Center for Managed Care, Health Resources and Services Administration (HRSA)
Center for Mental Health Services (CMHS), Knowledge Exchange Network (KEN)
Center for Nutrition Policy and Promotion, Department of Agriculture (USDA)
Center for Substance Abuse Treatment (CSAT)
Center for Veterinary Medicine (CVM), Food and Drug Administration
Centers for Disease Control and Prevention (CDC)
Clinical Neurogenetics Branch, National Institute of Mental Health (NIMH)
Columbus Center for Marine Biotechnology
Computer Retrieval of Information on Scientific Projects (CRISP)
Congressional Institute
Consensus Development Program, National Institutes of Health (NIH)
Consumer Product Safety Commission (CPSC)
Department of Defense (DOD)
Department of Energy (DOE)
Department of Health and Human Services (DHHS)
Department of Labor (DOL)
Department of Legal Medicine, Armed Forces Institute of Pathology (AFIP)
Department of Radiology, Madigan Army Medical Center
Department of Veterans Affairs (VA), Veterans Health Administration
Division of Adolescent and School Health (DASH), NCCDPHP, CDC

Division of Health Care Services, Institute of Medicine
Division of Nursing, Health Resources and Services Administration (HRSA), DHHS
Division of Reproductive Health, CDC
Division of Student Assistance, Health Resources and Services Administration, DHHS
Drug Enforcement Administration (DEA)
Electric and Magnetic Fields Research and Public Information Dissemination Program (EMFRAPID), CDC
Environfacts Warehouse, Environmental Protection Agency (EPA)
Environmental Protection Agency (EPA)
Epidemiology Program Office, Centers for Disease Control and Prevention (CDC)
Federal Aviation Administration (FAA), Department of Transportation
Federal Emergency Management Agency (FEMA)
Federal Interagency Council on Statistical Policy (Fedstats)
Federal Judicial Center
Federal Office of Rural Health Policy, Health Resources Services Administration (HRSA)
FEDIX
Food and Consumer Service, Department of Agriculture
Food and Drug Administration (FDA)
Food and Nutrition Information Center (FNIC), USDA/FDA
Foodborne Illness Education Information Center, USDA/FDA
Forensics Laboratory, U.S. National Fish and Wildlife
Government Printing Office
Health Care Financing Administration (HCFA), DHHS
Healthfinder, DHHS
Health Resources and Services Administration (HRSA), DHHS
Human Developmental Anatomy Center, Armed Forces Institute of Pathology (AFIP)
Information Center for Acquired Deaf-blindness
Institute of Medicine
Institute of Neurotoxicology and Neurological Disorders (INND)
International Emergency and Refugee Health, NCEH, CDC
International Food Information Council (IFIC)
Joint United Nations Programme on HIV/AIDS (UNAIDS)
Library of Congress
Medicare Payment Advisory Commission
Mine Safety and Health Administration (MSHA), Department of Labor
National Action Plan on Breast Cancer (NAPBC)
National Ag Safety Database (NASD)
National Aging Information Center (NAIC), DHHS
National Agricultural Statistics Service, Department of Agriculture (USDA)
National Animal Disease Center, Agricultural Research Service (ARS)
National Cancer Institute (NCI), National Institutes of Health (NIH)
National Center for Chronic Disease Prevention and Health Promotion (NCCDPHP), CDC
National Center for Environmental Health (NCEH), CDC
National Center for Health Statistics (NCHS)
National Center for Health Workforce Information and Analysis, HRSA
National Center for Infectious Diseases (NCID), CDC
National Center for Injury Prevention and Control (NCIPC), CDC
National Center for Voice and Speech (NCVS)
National Center on Elder Abuse (NCEA)
National Cholesterol Education Program
National Clearinghouse for Alcohol and Drug Information (NCADI)
National Clearinghouse of Rehabilitation Training Materials (NCRTM)
National Council for Agriculture Education
National Council on the Aging (NCOA), DHHS
National Criminal Justice Reference Service (NCJRS)
National Education Center for Agricultural Safety
National Eye Institute (NEI) , NIH
National Fire Academy, Fire Administration (USFA)
National Heart, Lung, and Blood Institute (NHLBI), NIH
National Information Center for Children and Youth with Disabilities (NICHCY), Department of Education
National Information Center on Deafness (NICD), Gallaudet University

National Information Clearinghouse on Children Who are Deaf-blind (DB-Link)
National Institute for Occupational Safety and Health (NIOSH)
National Institute of Allergy and Infectious Diseases (NIAID)
National Institute of Arthritis and Musculoskeletal Diseases (NIAMD)
National Institute of Dental Research (NIDR)
National Institute of Diabetes and Digestive and Kidney Diseases (NIDDK)
National Institute of Environmental Health Sciences (NIEHS)
National Institute of Mental Health (NIMH)
National Institute of Neurological Disorders and Stroke (NINDS)
National Institute of Nursing Research (NINR)
National Institute on Aging (NIA), DHHS
National Institute on Alcohol Abuse and Alcoholism (NIAAA)
National Institute on Deafness and Other Communication Disorders (NIDCD)
National Institute on Disability and Rehabilitation Research (NIDRR)
National Institute on Drug Abuse (NIDA)
National Institutes of Health (NIH)
National Library of Medicine (NLM), NIH
National Network of Libraries of Medicine (NN/LM)
National Rehabilitation Information Center (NARIC)
National Science Foundation (NSF)
National Vital Statistics System
Nephrology Service, Walter Reed Army Medical Center (WRAMC)
Nutrient Data Laboratory, Agricultural Research Service (ARS), USDA
Occupational Safety and Health Administration (OSHA), Department of Labor (DOL)
Occupational Safety and Health Review Commission (OSHRC)
Office of Alternative Medicine (OAM), NIH
Office of Communications, NIH
Office of Disability, Aging, and Long-Term Care Policy (DALTCP)
Office of Minority Health, DHHS
Office of Population Affairs (OPA), DHHS
Office of Public Health and Science (OPHS), DHHS
Office of Rare Diseases (ORD) NIH
Office of Research on Women's Health (ORWH)
Office of the Armed Forces Medical Examiner
Office of the Inspector General, Social Security Administration (SSA)
Office of the Special Assistant for Gulf War Illnesses, Department of Defense
Office on Disability and Health, NCEH, CDC
Pan American Health Organization (PAHO)
Physician Payment Review Commission
President's Council on Physical Fitness and Sports
Rehabilitation Research and Training Center (RRTC)
Social Security Administration (SSA)
Substance Abuse and Mental Health Services Administration (SAMHSA)
Substance Abuse Intervention Programs (SARDI)
Task Force, National Health Care Reform
Telemedicine and Advanced Technology Research Center (TATRC), Department of Defense
The Combined Health Information Database (CHID)
U.S. Congress
U.S. Court of Appeals, Fourth Circuit
U.S. Patent and Trademark Office
U.S. Senate, Special Committee on Aging
United Nations Population Fund (UNFPA) African Forum on Adolescent Reproductive Health
United Nations Population Information Network (POPIN)
United Nations World Food Programme (WFP)
Women, Infants, and Children (WIC) National Breastfeeding Promotion Campaign
Women's Health Initiative (WHI), National Institutes of Health (NIH)
WONDER
World Bank Group
World Health Organization (WHO)
World Health Organization (WHO) Nursing Board
World Health Organization (WHO) Tuberculosis Programme, Geneva

State, local, academic, and other public or related medical institutions

Academy for the Advancement of Diabetes Research and Treatment

AIDS Knowledge Base, University of California, and St. General Hospital
Alabama Department of Mental Health and Mental Retardation
Alfred Adler Institute
American Academy of Anti-Aging Medicine
Anders Nattestad, DDS, PhD, University of Copenhagen, Denmark
Angiographic Anatomy at Syracuse Neurosurgery (SUNY-HSC)
Archival Data Online Repository, University of Wisconsin-Madison
Arnot Ogden Medical Center
Bankslab, Guided Navigation and Infant Vision Laboratory, University of California at Berkeley
Baylor College of Dentistry
Biotechnology Information Institute
Bone and Joint Center, University of Washington
Boston Children's Hospital
Boston University Alzheimer's Disease Center
British Library for Development Studies
Bureau of Primary Care and Rural Health Systems, Utah Department of Health
Case Western Reserve University
Catfish Institute
Center for AIDS Prevention Studies (CAPS), University of California, San Francisco
Center for Health and the Global Environment, Harvard Medical School
Center for In Vivo Microscopy, Duke University
Center for the Advanced Study of Public Safety, University of Albany
Center for the Health Professions, University of California, San Francisco
Children's Hospital of Iowa
Clinical Trials Resource Center
CliniWeb, Oregon Health Sciences University
College of Osteopathic Medicine and Telecommunications Center, Ohio University
Columbia University, Columbia-Presbyterian Medical Center
Commonwealth of Massachusetts, Division of Registration
Communications Disorders and Sciences Program, Southern Illinois University at Carbondale Community Outreach Health Information System (COHIS), Boston University Medical Center
Computer Vision
Cornell Theory Center (CTC), Cornell University Medical College
CUErgo: Cornell Ergonomics Web
Dartmouth Medical College
Department of Anesthesiology, University of Virginia
Department of Clinical and Applied Psychology, U Bonn, Germany
Department of Neurosurgery, University of Southern California (USC)
Department of Radiology, University of Iowa College of Medicine
Digestive Disease Center
Documents Center, University of Michigan
Drugs and Devices Information Line, Harvard School of Public Health
Duke University Medical Center
Early Psychosis Prevention and Intervention Centre (EPPIC)
Emory University
Emory University Health Sciences Center Library
Eugene Loke and the National University of Singapore
Falk Library, University of Pittsburgh
Franklin Institute Science Museum
Friedrich-Alexander-University of Erlangen-Nurnberg, School of Medicine
Gait Analysis Laboratories
GASNet, Yale University School of Medicine
Georgetown University School of Nursing
Georgia Board of Nursing
GHDNet, Ehime University School of Medicine
Gottingen University
Hamline University
Harborview Medical Center, University of Washington
Harvard AIDS Institute
Harvard Medical School
Health Information Research Unit, John Hopkins University and other institutions
Indiana Prevention Resource Center (IPRC), Indiana University
Injury Surveillance Information System (ISIS), Flinders University of South Australia
Institute for Traditional Medicine (ITM) Online
Integrated Public Use Microdata Series (IPUMS)
Iowa State University
Johns Hopkins Bayview Medical Center

Johns Hopkins Hospital
Johns Hopkins School of Public Health
Joint Program in Nuclear Medicine (JPNM), Harvard Medical School
Karolinska Institute Library and Information Center
Laboratory of Neuroinformatics, Wake Forest University
Legal Information Institute, Cornell Law School
Louisiana State University Medical Center
MacArthur Research Network on Mental Health and the Law
MacLean Center for Clinical Medical Ethics, University of Chicago
Madelyn Hall, Southwest Washington Medical Center, Vancouver, WA
Mallinckrodt Institute of Radiology (MIR), Washington University Medical Center
Marshall University School of Medicine
Massachusetts General Hospital
Mayo Medical Center
Medical College of Wisconsin
Medistat
Minimally Invasive Surgery Center, The Cleveland Clinic Foundation (CCF)
Minnesota Historical Census Projects, University of Minnesota
National Forensic Hospital Data Network
National Pediatric and Family HIV Resource Center and NJ Medical School
National University of Singapore, Centre for Medical Informatics and Biostatistics
Natural Hazards Research and Applications Information Center, University of Colorado, Boulder
Netherlands Institute of Gerontology (NIG)
New York Online Access to Health (NOAH)
New York State Department of Health
New York University (NYU), Department of Neurosurgery
North Carolina Industrial Commission
Obstetrics and Gynaecology, University of Oxford
Office of Medical Informatics, University of Florida
Office of Population Research (OPR), Princeton University
Office of Psychological Services, Bartow County School System
OncoLink, University of Pennsylvania Cancer Center Resource
Pharmaceutical Information Network (PharmInfoNet) gastroenterological resources
Public Health Law Project, University of Missouri at Kansas City
Robotics and Intelligent Machines Laboratory, University of California at Berkeley
Rochester Institute of Technology
Rollins School of Public Health, Emory University
Rosenthal Center for Complementary and Alternative Medicine
Royal College of Surgeons of England
Shrine of North America
South Kingstown's Youth to Youth Web Server
Stanford Arthritis and Rheumatology Research
Stanford Division of General Internal Medicine
Syracuse Neurosurgery (SUNY-HSC)
The Center for the Health Professions, University of California, San Francisco
Toxicology Treatment Program (TTP), University of Pittsburgh
TraumAID Project, University of Pennsylvania and Allegheny University
Tulane Medical Library
Tustin Police Department
University of Alabama
University of Arizona College of Medicine
University of California-Davis, Oregon State, Michigan State University, and Cornell University
University of Calgary
University of California, Irvine
University of Chicago Hospital
University of Copenhagen, Denmark
University of Edinburgh
University of Geneva School of Dentistry
University of Genova, Italy
University of Iowa College of Medicine
University of Kentucky
University of Michigan-Dearborn
University of Minnesota
University of Nebraska-Lincoln
University of North Carolina, Division of Neurosurgery
University of Oklahoma Health Sciences Center
University of Pittsburgh
University of Sheffield
University of Texas Health Science Center

University of Washington, Department of Health Sciences
University of Washington, Department of Radiology
University of Wisconsin—Madison
Villanova Center for Information Law and Policy
West Virginia Rehabilitation Research and Training Center
Wilmer Eye Institute

Professional trade organizations

Academy for the Advancement of Diabetes Research and Treatment
Accreditation Council for Graduate Medical Education (ACGME)
Aerospace Medical Association
American Academy of Allergy, Asthma and Immunology
American Academy of Allergy, Asthma and Immunology (AAAAI) Allied Health Professionals Committee
American Academy of Anti-Aging Medicine
American Academy of Audiology
American Academy of Child and Adolescent Psychiatry (AACAP)
American Academy of Dermatology
American Academy of Experts in Traumatic Stress
American Academy of Hospice and Palliative Medicine
American Academy of Neurology (AAN)
American Academy of Ophthalmology (AAO)
American Academy of Orthopaedic Surgeons (AAOS)
American Academy of Otolaryngology-Head and Neck Surgery, Inc.
American Academy of Pain Management (AAPM)
American Academy of Pediatrics (AAP)
American Academy of Physician Assistants (AAPA)
American Academy of Psychiatry and the Law
American Academy of Wound Management
American Association for Chronic Fatigue Syndrome (AACFS)
American Association for Medical Transcription (AAMT)
American Association for Pediatric Ophthalmology and Strabismus (AAPOS)
American Association for the Study of Liver Diseases (AASLD)
American Association of Clinical Endocrinologists (AACE) and American College of Endocrinology (ACE)
American Association of Colleges of Nursing (AACN)
American Association of Colleges of Osteopathic Medicine (AACOM)
American Association of Colleges of Pharmacy (AACP)
American Association of Critical-Care Nurses (AACN)
American Association of Dental Schools (AADS)
American Association of Immunologists (AAI)
American Association of Medical Assistants (AAMA)
American Association of Medical Review Officers (AAMRO)
American Association of Nurse Anesthetists (AANA)
American Association of Occupational Health Nurses, Inc. (AAOHN)
American Association of Oral and Maxillofacial Surgery (AAOMS)
American Association of Oral Biologists (AAOB)
American Association of Psychiatric Technicians, Inc. (AAPT)
American Association of Respiratory Care (AARC)
American Association of Spinal Cord Injury Nurses (AASCIN)
American Association of Swine Practitioners homepage (AASP)
American Board of Forensic Odontology, Inc. (ABFO)
American Board of Obstetrics and Gynecology
American Board of Psychiatry and Neurology, Inc. (ABPN)
American College of Cardiology (ACC)
American College of Emergency Physicians (ACEP)
American College of Gastroenterology (ACG)
American College of Healthcare Executives (ACHE)
American College of Nurse Practitioners (ACNP)
American College of Occupational and Environmental Medicine (ACOEM)
American College of Physicians (ACP)
American College of Preventive Medicine (ACPM)

APPENDIX: SPONSOR REPRESENTATION ACCORDING TO TYPE

American College of Radiology (ACR)
American College of Rheumatology (ACR)
American College of Sports Medicine (ACSM)
American Committee on Laboratory Animal Diseases (ACLAD)
American Dental Assistants Association (ADAA)
American Dental Association (ADA)
American Dental Hygienists Association (ADHA)
American Dietetic Association (ADA)
American Egg Board
American Gastroenterological Association (AGA)
American Health Information Management Association (AHIMA)
American Hospital Association (AHA)
American Industrial Hygiene Association
American Lung Association and American Thoracic Society
American Meat Institute (AMI)
American Medical Association (AMA)
American Medical Informatics Association (AMIA)
American Medical Students Association
American Medical Technologists (AMT)
American Medical Women's Association (AMWA)
American Nurses Association (ANA)
American Optometric Association (AOA)
American Organization of Nurse Executives (AONE)
American Orthopaedic Society for Sports Medicine (AOSSM)
American Physical Therapy Association (APTA)
American Psychiatric Association (APA)
American Psychological Association (APA)
American Public Health Association (APHA)
American Society for Aesthetic Plastic Surgery
American Society for Clinical Oncology (ASCO)
American Society for Dermatologic Surgery
American Society for Gastrointestinal Endoscopy (ASGE)
American Society of Anesthesiologists
American Society of Cataract and Refractive Surgery and American Society of Ophthalmic Administrators
American Society of Parasitologists
American Society of Plastic and Reconstructive Surgeons (ASPR)
American Society of Radiologic Technologists (ASRT)
American Speech-Language-Hearing Association (ASHA)
American Urological Association (AUA)
American Veterinary Medical Association (AVMA) Network
Association of American Indian Physicians (AAIP)
Association of American Medical Colleges (AAMC)
Association of Educators in Radiological Sciences, Inc. (AERS)
Association of Ohio Philanthropic Home Administration (AOPHA)
Association of Operating Room Nurses, Inc. (AORN)
Association of Schools of Allied Health Professions
British Medical Association (BMA) Foundation for AIDS
Canadian Cardiovascular Society (CCS)
Carpet and Rug Association
Chlorine Chemistry Council (CCC)
Educational Commission for Foreign Medical Graduates (ECFMG)
FDI World Dental Federation
Forensic Science Society
Healthcare Compliance Packaging Council
Hispanic Nurses Association
HIV/AIDS Information Center, *Journal of the American Medical Association* (JAMA)
Home Care Aide Association of America, (HCAAA)
International Society for Gynecologic Endoscopy
International Society for Magnetic Resonance in Medicine (ISMRM)
International Society of Dermal Therapists
Joint Commission on Accreditation of Healthcare Organizations (JCAHO) and National Committee for Quality Assurance (NCQA)
Joint Commission on Allied Health Personnel in Ophthalmology (JCAHPO)
Joint Review Committee—Athletic Training (JRC-AT)
Joint Review Committee on Education in Radiologic Technology (JRCERT)
Marin AIDS Project (MAP)
Massachusetts Medical Society
National Association for Home Care (NAHC)
National Association of Medical Examiners (NAME)

National Association of Physicians for the Environment (NAPE)
National Black Nurses Association (NBNA)
National Board for Respiratory Care (NBRC)
National Hospice Organization (NHO)
National League for Nursing (NLN)
National Organization for Associate Degree Nursing (N-OADN)
National Society of Genetic Counselors
National Student Nurses' Association (NSNA)
Nursing Ethics Network (NEN)
Nursing Informatics Working Group, AMIA
OB/GYN Board
Pediatric Perioperative Cardiac Arrest (POCA)
Pharmaceutical Research and Manufacturers of America
Plastic Surgery Educational Foundation (PSEF)
PsychNet APA
Public Health Foundation
Society for Pediatric Anesthesia
Society of American Gastrointestinal Endoscopic Surgeons (SAGES)
Texas Academy of Family Physicians
Visiting Nurse Associations of America (VNAA)
World Resource Institute

Health organizations, publishers, conferences

Academy for Educational Development (AED)
Access to Voluntary and Safe Contraception (AVSC) International
Accreditation Council for Graduate Medical Education (ACGME)
Action on Smoking and Health (ASH)
Addiction Research Foundation (ARF)
African American Family Services (AAFS)
Alan Guttmacher Institute
Alcoholics Anonymous
Alzheimer Research Forum
Alzheimer's Association
Alzheimer's Disease Online Learning Center
American Academy of Experts in Traumatic Stress
American Anorexia/Bulimia Association, Inc. (AABA)
American Association for Chronic Fatigue Syndrome (AACFS)
American Association of Medical Review Officers (AAMRO)
American Association of Retired Persons (AARP)
American Cancer Society (ACS)
American Council for Headache Education (ACHE)
American Heart Association (AHA)
American Journal of Nursing (AJN)
American Juvenile Arthritis Organization, Arthritis Foundation
American Liver Foundation (ALF)
American Lung Association and American Thoracic Society
American Lyme Disease Foundation, Inc. (ALDF)
American Red Cross
American Sudden Infant Death Syndrome (SIDS) Institute
American Telemedicine Association (ATA)
Americans with Disabilities Act Document Center
Antiviral Agents Bulletin
Anxiety Disorders Association of America (ADAA)
Arthritis Foundation
Asthma and Allergy Foundation of America
Behavior OnLine
BioLib Project, Bioinformatics Library
Body Health Resources Corp. and Bristol-Myers, Roxane, Chiron, Ortho Biotech
Brain Injury Association, Inc.
Brain Tumor Society
Burn Survivors Online
California Abortion and Reproductive Rights Action League (CARAL)
Canine Sports Medicine Update (CSMU)
Cardiology Compass
Cedros Network
The Center: Post-Traumatic and Dissociative Disorders Program
Center for Health Care Strategies (CHCS)
Center for Human Reproduction (CHR)
Center for Workplace Health
Center Watch
CFIDS Association of America
Childhood Brain Tumor Foundation
Children's Cancer Group (CCG)
Children's Defense Fund (CDF)
Children's Motility Disorder Foundation
CHORUS
Continence Specialists Registry
Continence Worldwide, Continence Foundation
Coronary Club
Critical Path AIDS Project

Delmar Publishers
Derweb
Direct Information on Research and Treatment
Disabilities Studies and Services Center (DSSC)
Doctors Without Borders USA, Inc.
Educational Commission for Foreign Medical Graduates (ECFMG)
Effective National Action to Control Tobacco (ENACT)
Electronic Journal of Wound Management Practice
EMBBS Emergency Medicine and Primary Care
Emergency Nursing World
Emergency Preparedness Information Exchange
Epilepsy Foundation of America (EFA)
Eurotransplant Foundation, The Netherlands
Family Health International (FHI)
Far West Laboratory for Educational Research and Development and Southwest Regional Laboratory
Federal Telemedicine Gateway, Joint Working Group on Telemedicine (JWGT) Inventory
Fitness Link
Fletcher Allen Health Care (FAHC)
Florida Spinal Cord Injury World Wide Web Resources Center
Foundation for Ichthyosis and Related Skin Types (FIRST)
Gait Analysis Laboratory, Alfred I. duPont Institute
Garlic Information Centre
Gay Men's Health Committee (GMHC)
General Practice On-Line
GERD Information Resource Center, Astra Merck Inc.
Global Emergency Medicine Archives (GEMA)
Global Micronutrient Network
Global Telemedicine Technologies II
Gynecologic oncology group (GOG/CHTN) ovarian tissue bank
Hardin Meta directory of radiology and imaging Internet resources
Health Care Liability Alliance (HCLA)
Health Effects Institute (HEI)
Health On the Net Foundation (HON)
Health Opps
Healthtouch Online
Healthweb Nursing
HIV/AIDS Information Center
HIV/AIDS Treatment Information Service (ATIS)
HIV Positive Resources and Assistance
Incontinence Center
Institute for Safe Medication Practices (ISMP)
Integrated Research Services
International Association for the Study of Pain (IASP)
International Association of Physicians and AIDS (IAPAC)
International Bone Marrow Transplant Registry (IBMTR)
International Center for Disability Information (ICDI)
International Council for Control of Iodine Deficiency Disorders
International Council of Medical Acupuncture and Related Techniques (ICMART)
International Foundation for Functional Gastrointestinal Disorders (IFFGD)
International Medical Corps
International Foundation for Helicobacter and Intestinal Immunology
Internet Mental Health
Kids Foundation Research Institute
Leukemia Information Center
Lindesmith Center
Lippincott Nursing Center
Longevity Institute International
MacArthur Research Network
Managed Health Care Improvement Task Force
Marin AIDS Project
Martindale Virtual Medical Center
Medic Alert
Medical Treatment Effectiveness Program (MEDTEP)
Medical World Search
MedicationWeb.Com
Medicine On-Line
Medscape Oncology
Menopause Online
Mental Health Net
Merck & Company, Inc.
Model Performance Evaluation Program (MPEP)
Mosby Consumer Health
Muscular Dystrophy Association (MDA)
Musella Foundation for Brain Tumor Research and Information
Myopia Control Network Service (MCNS)

National AIDS Fund
National Center for Emergency Medicine Informatics (NCEMI)
National Center for Homeopathy
National Center for Nutrition and Dietetics
National Childhood Cancer Foundation (NCCF)
National Coalition for the Homeless
National Council of State Boards of Nursing
National Depressive and Manic-Depressive Association (DMDA)
National Families in Action
National Fraud Information Center
National Gulf War Resource Center
National Health Care for the Homeless Council
National Multiple Sclerosis Society (MS)
National Neurofibromatosis Foundation, Inc.
National Organization for Rare Disorders, Inc. (NORD)
National Osteoporosis Foundation (NOF)
National Parent Network on Disabilities
National Policy and Resource Center on Women and Aging
National Pressure Ulcer Advisory Panel (NPUAP)
National Program of Cancer Registries (CDC)
National Psoriasis Foundation (NPF)
National Registry for Ichthyosis and Related Disorders
National Resource Center for Traumatic Brain Injury (TBI)
National Safety Council (NSC)
National Skin Centre
National Spinal Cord Injury Association
National Stroke Association (NSA)
Netherlands Leprosy Relief Association (NSL)
Nursing Ethics Network (NEN)
Nursing Informatics Working Group (AMIA)
OB/GYN Toolbox
Occupational Safety and Health Net (OSHNET)
Ontario Health Care Evaluation Network (OHCEN)
Ophthalmic Photographers' Society, Inc.
Oral Cancer Information Center
Organizing Committee of the XI International Conference on AIDS
Osteoporosis and Related Bone Disease~National Resource Center (ORBD~NRC)
Patho.Wat.ch
Pediatric Critical Care Medicine (PedsCCM)
Pediatric Dentistry, "just for kidds"
Pediatric Toxicology (PedTox) Registry
Pharmaceutical Information Network (PharmInfoNet)
PharmInfoNet's Digestive Disease Center
Physician's News Digest
Physicians' GenRx
Planned Parenthood Federation of America, Inc. (PPFA)
Population Institute
Population Reference Bureau (PRB)
Program for Appropriate Technology in Health (PATH)
Psychiatric Society for Informatics (PSI)
Public Health Foundation (PHF)
Rad Sci Online
RAND Corporation
Rehabilitation Research and Training Center (RRTC)
rehabNET, Northeast Rehabilitation Network
Research Institute on Addictions (RIA)
Respiratory Care Online
Restoration of Appearance and Function Trust (RAFT)
Robert Wood Johnson Foundation
Rocky Mountain Herbal Institute
Rural Center for AIDS/STD Prevention (RCAP)
Society for Academic Emergency Medicine (SAEM) emergency medicine research database project
Second European Interdisciplinary Meeting, Germany, 1995
Second International Gastric Cancer Congress
Sense, the National Deafblind and Rubella Association
Sexuality Information and Education Council of the U.S. (SIECUS)
Slack Inc.
Substance Abuse Intervention Programs (SARDI)
Sudden Arrhythmia Death Syndromes (SADS) Foundation
Suicide Awareness Voices of Education (SAVE)
Thomson Publishing
TransWeb
TraumAID Project
Traumatic Brain and Spinal Cord Injury Projects

Travel Health Information and Referral Service
Tumor Board
21st Annual Convening of Crisis Intervention Personnel
Twin-to-Twin Transfusion Syndrome (TTTS) Foundation
UK, Psychiatry On-Line
University of North Carolina (UNC), Vincent Web
U.S. Pharmacopeia (USP)
Virtual Nursing Center, Martindale's Health Science Guide
Washington Assistive Technology Alliance (WATA)
Washington Publishing Company
Web Vision
Whole Nurse
Women's Health Global Health Network
Women's Health Resource Center, CME Gateway
World of Drug Information
Worldwide Nurse, Internet Nursing Index

Foreign government or related organizations

Asian Disaster Preparedness Center (ADPC)
BioMechanics
British Library for Development Studies
Cedros Network
DGV of the Commission of the European Communities
Electronic Development and Environment Information System (ELDIS)
Europath
European Agency for Evaluation of Medicinal Products
European Commission and Pfizer Pharmaceutical Group
Eurotransplant Foundation, The Netherlands
International Occupational Safety and Health Information Centre (CIS), International Labour Office (ILO)
Japanese Government Ministry of Health and Welfare (MHW)
National Skin Centre (NSC), Singapore
Netherlands Cancer Institute
Novartis Foundation Leprosy Fund
Ontario Health Care Evaluation Network (OHCEN)
Occupational Safety and Health Web (OSHWEB)
Philippine Cities Disaster Mitigation Project
Public Health Division, Department of Human Services, Victoria, Australia
Queen's University Ontario Ministry of Natural Resources
Special Senate Committee on Euthanasia and Assisted Suicide, Canada
The National Board of Health and Welfare, Sweden

Private sector, individuals, and commercial sponsors

Access Excellence
Achoo Healthcare Online
Acupuncture.com
American Society for the Prevention of Cruelty to Animals (ASPCA)
Anspach, Instrument Makar, Inc.
Anthony R. Torkelson, Ph.D.
Aquaculture Network Information Center (AquaNIC)
Arent Fox
ASCRS Ophthalmic Services Corp.
BioMechanics Desk Reference, 1997
Carolyn Crowson and Noel Crowson
Childbirth.org
Colgate–Palmolive Company
CoMed Communications Internet Health Forum (CCIHF)
DataLink of Onalaska, Texas
Dr. Carl Stewart
Dr. Philip Cumpston
DVMSearch
EMX, Universal Health Card
Eric H. Chudler, Ph.D.
Family Internet
FAS Project
Fosmire Solka Stenton
Galaxy
Geocities
Greenstone Healthcare Solutions
Health Care Communication Group
Health Insurance Association of America (HIAA)
Health On the Net Foundation (HON)
Health Opps
Health Reviews on the Internet
Home Health Care In Depth, Olsten Health Services
Informative Graphics Corp.
Internet Medical Education, Inc.
Internet Pathology Laboratory
James Norman, M.D.
Jerome Z. Litt, M.D.
Jim Martindale

Judith M. Kuster, certified speech-language pathologist
MedAccess Corporation
MedExplorer
Medical Multimedia Group
Medical Network, Inc.
Medical World Search
MediQual Systems, Inc.
Mental Health Net
Mental Health Infosource (MHi)
National Animal Poison Control Center (NAPCC)
Nerd World Media
Nurses Protection Group (NPG) and Allied Health Providers
O. Arthur Stiennon, M.D.
Olsten Health Services
P/S/L/ Consulting Group Inc.
PEDINFO
Pfizer Corporate Philanthropy Program
PR Newswire
PSL Consulting Group
Rhone-Poulenc Rorer
Robert Whalen
Roger G. Worthington, P.C.
Roy F. Sullivan, PhD.
Schering-Plough Animal Health
Silver Platter Information, Inc. and Physicians' homepage
SleepDocs Online
Solutions@disability.com
Sympatico
Telenursing Resources
The Virtual Medical Center
UNC-TV
WebDoctor
www.turnstep.com—The aerobics page
Zeneca Pharmaceuticals

Glossary

Acrobat reader: a computer accessory allowing clear camera-ready document viewing and copying; Acrobat, PDF, and other file readers can be downloaded through the Internet.

baud: the rate per second at which data can be transmitted over a modem and telephone or other communication system; baud rates range from the slower 2,600 to the fastest current rate of 128 baud; download speed varies according to the remote computer.

browsers: a software program allowing navigation and viewing of Web sites. Internet Explorer, Mosaic, and Netscape Navigator are a few popular browsers. The *Directory* entries note several sites for downloading these and other browsers. Browsers are typically large files.

CD-ROM: abbreviation for compact disc, read-only-memory.

computer hardware: describes any part of a computer system that can be physically touched, including the keyboard, mouse, **disk drives,** printer, power case, and monitor.

computer system: refers to the hardware which includes the system unit, keyboard, monitor, and accessories such as the mouse, printer, accessory boards (which allow options for added memory, sound, games, etc.), and modem.

computer virus: programs designed to replicate or repeat and spread throughout computer files and hardware; computer viruses spread like infections; if unrepaired, viruses cause data deletion as well as computer malfunctioning; antivirus software reduces possibilities of virus infections.

crash: total breakdown of computer functions caused by malfunctions such as hard disk failure, virus contamination, or inappropriate hardware or software; manuals generally indicate types of conditions considered fatal to computers; crash is likely to erase programs and files.

database: a collection of related information; a useful manager for organizing or categorizing data.

desktop computer: sometimes referred to as *microcomputer;* typically contains a microprocessor with input-output devices and storage capacity; usually contained in one unit; a complete computer system designed to fit on top of a desk.

disk drive: a device that reads data from a magnetic disk and is stored in the computer's memory. Examples of disk drives are **hard disk, floppy disk,** or **CD-ROM.**

document: any data created with an application; data may be typed, edited, viewed, and saved; a document may be a report, picture, or letter and is stored as a **file** on a disk.

download: process of transferring programs from a remote site, i.e., the Internet or a remote computer program via a modem and a telephone line; for example, reports, publications, and other materials from online services can be transferred or downloaded to desktop computers; downloaded files may be viewed, printed, or saved; download time depends on modem speed and size of the downloaded program; see *upload.*

electronic transactions: transfer of data by computer modem.

e-mail: the ability to send and receive data messages around the world in seconds at nominal telephone costs; a great application for Internet correspondence; both sender and receiver must have e-mail addresses, (e.g., an Internet e-mail address, i.e., jones567@hotmail com); free Internet e-mail is available through Hotmail and Yahoo.

file: a collection of information that has been given a name and is stored on a disk; may be a document or an application in text or other multimedia formats; files contain one or more documents.

file format: method used to electronically store data in a file. Depending on computer capability, files can be stored in text, image, or multimedia formats.

file transfer: movement of a file between a personal computer and remote computer; see **upload** and **download.**

floppy disk: a disk that can be inserted in and removed from a floppy disk drive; disks or diskettes are 3½″ or 5¼″ with variable capacities.

graphics: electronic pictures or images in monochrome or full color.

hard disk: sometimes called *fixed disk,* the hard disk is permanently mounted in the computer power case and holds any saved files.

homepage: the first page of a sponsor's **web site;** in addition to the sponsor, homepages provide **links** to the site content.

hyperlinks: anything on a Web page that goes to another page or entry by clicking.

HTML (Hypertext Markup Language): language used to create and design Web pages.

keyword: a word or phrase used to find specific data.

link: an electronic connection or direct access from one Web page to another that can be activated by a simple mouse click. In addition to links designated by name, some are distinguished by different colors or underlining.

modem: a device for transmitting and receiving computer data over telephone lines.

MPEG: graphic or multimedia viewing format; also includes TIFF, GIF, and others.

multimedia: a system capable of displaying information in various media forms such as sound, graphics, animation, text, and video; requires **CD-ROM** and other drives such as sound, etc.

password: personalized secret word required to access computer files.

PDF: format following exact reproduction of original text.

personal computer: abbreviated as *pc;* a moderately priced microcomputer system intended for personal or business use; see **desktop computer.**

software: set of instructions that make computer hardware perform tasks; programs, operating systems, device drivers, and applications are all examples of software; Internet software is required to view and retrieve Internet data.

software developers: companies and individuals that invent or develop software packages.

software piracy: illegal purchase or use of copied or counterfeit software.

storage: retaining copies of data files on hard, floppy, or backup drives.

text file: a file consisting entirely of ASCII (regular alphabet) or characters typed on a regular keyboard.

Uniform Resource Locator: see **URL.**

upload: to copy or send a file from user's computer to a remote computer.

URL: Uniform Resource Locator, the electronic home address of the Internet World Wide Web or WWW information site. URLs generally, not always, begin with "http://."

video screen: shows images similar to a television screen; also referred to as display monitor.

Web site: the compiled destination of an Internet homepage and supporting pages of text and graphics.

Quickie Search Spreadsheet

Primary Topic	URL	Page
Aging		
Aging bibliographic and database reference system	http://www.ageinfo.org/bibinfo.html	1
Alcohol and aging	http://www.drug.indiana.edu/pubs/alerts/alert2.html	2
Alzheimer's Disease Education and Referral (ADEAR) Center	http://www.cais.com/adear/	2
Alzheimer's disease	http://med-amsa.bu.edu/Alzheimer/home.html	3
Alzheimer's disease Web sites for lay persons	http://www.alzforum.org/public/layperson_sites.html	3
Clearinghouse on Abuse and Neglect of the Elderly (CANE)	http://interinc.com/NCEA/main.html	4
Elder abuse diagnosis and services	http://www.ianet.org/nyeac/	4
European Alzheimer Projects	http://www.alzheimer-europe.org/	5
Geriatric topics	http://www.mayo.edu/geriatrics-rst/2.GeriPage.html	5
International comparisons of care for aging	http://aspe.os.dhhs.gov/daltcp/home/internat.htm#INDICATORS	6
Nursing home costs, hospital admissions, and hospice use	http://www.elder-law.com/elder/1996/issue344.html	6
Services for seniors over age 50	http://www.aarp.org/	7
Services for the elderly	http://www.ncoa.org/	8
Skilled nursing facilities under Medicare	http://www.hcfa.gov/medicare/snfs.htm	8
Task force report: Long-term care reform in the States, 1997	http://www.ncsl.org/ihpp/ltc/report.htm	9
III European Congress of Gerontology	http://www.nig.nl/congres/3rdeuropeancongress1995/ttp-abs.html	9
Women and aging	http://www.brandeis.edu/heller/national/index.html	10

Primary Topic	URL	Page
Allied Health		
Accreditation of allied health programs for athletic training	http://www.cewl.com/cewl/jrc-at/jrcfaq.html	11
Allied health professions registration in Massachusetts	http://www.magnet.state.ma.us/reg/ah.htm	12
Allied health resources	http://www.delmaralliedhealth.com	12
Allied health resources—genetic counselors	http://www.kumc.edu/GEC/prof/nsgc.html	13
Allied health travel grants	http://www.aaaai.org/profinfo/membserv/allied/abstrav/abstravl.html	13
Evaluation of health professions schools	http://futurehealth.ucsf.edu/ccph/exsumm.html#IV_FIND	14
Health care assisting resources	http://www.delmaralliedhealth.com/hca/index.html	14
Home health services reimbursement, Ohio	http://aopha.org/pphhr.htm	15
Magnetic resonance technologist training	http://www.t2star.com/smrt/curr_guide.html	15
Medical assistants certification and licensure	http://www.aama-ntl.org/ed/cerlic.html	16
Medical technologists	http://www.amt1.com/mt.html	16
Medical transcription careers	http://www.aamt.org/aamt/carfaq.htm	17
National Health Care Skill Standards Project (NHCSSP)	http://www.fwl.org/nhcssp/health.htm	17
Ophthalmic medical assisting	http://www.jcahpo.com/index.html#top	18
Physician assistants (PAs) and emergency medicine	http://www.aapa.org/gandp/emerg.htm	18
Profiles of allied health top industry employers	http://www.healthopps.com/healthopps/health3.html	19
Psychiatric technicians	http://www.aapt.com/whatis.htm	19
Radiologic technologists	http://www.asrt.org/	20
Rural physicians and physician assistants loan repayment program	http://hlunix.hl.state.ut.us/primary_care/elrp.html	20
Standards for hair removal	http://www.isdt.org/p19.htm	21
Vision 2006	http://www.ahima.org/visin/vision.overview.html	21
Alternative Medicine		
Adverse events of some Chinese herbal medicines	http://www.Acupuncture.com/Herbology/Toxic.htm	22
Alternative medical courses at U.S. medical schools	http://cpmcnet.columbia.edu/dept/rosenthal/guide.html	23
Alternative medicine bibliography	http://www.pitt.edu/~cbw/refe.html	23
American Indian ethnobotany database	http://www.umd.umich.edu/cgi-bin/herb/	24
Environmental links to breast cancer	http://www.wri.org/health/slidntro.htm	24
Ethnobotany	http://www.gene.com/ae/RC/Ethnobotany/index.html	25
Garlic and pregnancy	http://www.mistral.co.uk/garlic/preg.htm	25
Herbage ethnobotanical monographs	http://www.herbweb.com/pix/A.htm	26
Homeopathy: Natural medicine for the 21st century	http://www.homeopathic.org/index1.htm	26
Medical acupuncture	http://www.med.auth.gr/~karanik/english/main.htm	27
Medicinal and poisonous plant databases	http://www.inform.umd.edu/EdRes/Col..._biology/Medicinals/medicinals.html	27

Primary Topic	URL	Page
Medicinal biological researchers	http://walden.mo.net/~tonytork/resindex.html	28
Medicines from the sea	http://www.columbuscenter.org/~judy/scitalk/	28
Office of Alternative Medicine (OAM) Clearinghouse	http://altmed.od.nih.gov/oam/clearinghouse/#access	29
Phytochemical and ethnobotanical databases	http://www.ars-grin.gov/~ngrisb/	29
Practitioner Reference Guide	http://www.europa.com/~itm/pract.htm	30
Resources for herbalists	http://www.ronan.net/%7Ermhi/a/g.favoritwebs.html	30
Cancer		
Bone Marrow Transplants—A Book of Basics for Patients	http://www.oncolink.upenn.edu/specialty/chemo/bmt/bmt_1.html#chapter_1	31
Bone marrow transplant for multiple myeloma	http://www.oncolink.upenn.edu/classroom/bmtmm/intro.html	32
Breast Cancer Information Clearinghouse	http://nysernet.org/bcic/	32
Cancer research and programs	http://www.cancer.org/main.html	33
CCG Protocol: D9602 for low-risk rhabdomyosarcoma	http:www.nccf.org/nccf/protocol/d9602.htm	33
Clinical trials information for physicians	http://cancer.med.upenn.edu/pdq_html/3/engl/303901.html	34
Clinical trials information, National Cancer Institute (NCI)	http://cancer.med.upenn.edu/clinical_trials/	34
Ethnic-oriented cancer information	http://cancernet.nci.nih.gov/ethnic/ethnic_health.htm	35
Gastrointestinal cancers	http://www.oncolink.com/disease/gastro1/	35
Health professionals—global resources	http://cancernet.nci.nih.gov/global/glo_hp.htm	36
International bone marrow transplant registry	http://www.social.com/health/nhic/data/hr1400/hr1495.html	36
Leukemia information	http://www.meds.com/leukemia/leukemia.html	37
National Action Plan on Breast Cancer (NAPBC)	http://www.napbc.org/	37
NCI/PDQ treatment and prevention statements	http://www.oncolink.upenn.edu/pdq_html/	38
Nonsteroidal antiandrogens treatment, advanced prostate cancer	http://www.comed.com/Prostate/advanced/antiandrogens.html	39
Online medical dictionary—cancer	http://www.graylab.ac.uk/omd/index.html	39
Oral cancer	http://www.oralcancer.org/	40
START oncology reference	http://www.oncoweb.com/	40
Supercomputers in medical diagnosis	http://www.tc.cornell.edu/er96/ff03summer/ff04lungs.html	41
Surveillance, epidemiology, and end results (SEER)	http://www-seer.ims.nci.nih.gov/	41
Telematics for health professionals	http://telescan.nki.nl/action/action.htm	42
Tumor Board	http://www.tumorboard.com/	42
Cardiovascular Medicine		
Cardiac rehabilitation and prevention information	http://www.jhbmc.jhu.edu/cardiology/rehab/profinfo.html	43
Cardiologists resources	http://139.137.56.94:8080/HOT_HART/Heart.htm	44
Cardiovascular information	http://www.nhlbi.nih.gov/nhlbi/cardio/cardio.htm	44

Primary Topic	URL	Page
Congestive heart failure	http://web.bu.edu/COHIS/cardvasc/heart/chf.htm	45
Coronary artery examination	http://www.afip.mil/homes/cardio/grosub_4.htm	45
Coronary Club Heartline	http://www.heartline-news.org/	46
Electrocardiographic rhythms	http://www.med-edu.com/patient/arrhythmia/rhythms-5.html#S_ARREST	46
Facts about heart/lung transplants	gopher://fido.nhlbi.nih.gov:70/00/educprog/other/gppubs/hrtlung.txt	47
Heart attack survival calculator	http://www.mediqual.com/library/amicalc/heart.htm	47
The human heart	http://www.sln.fi.edu/biosci/	48
Hypertension in African-Americans	http://www.wramc.amedd.army.mil/de...rology/lectures.nathxhtn/index.htm	48
Inherited long QT syndrome	http://www.sads.org/overview.html	49
Institutional resources for congenital heart defects	http://www.ohsu.edu/cliniweb/C14/C14.240.400.html	49
Introduction to expert computer systems in medicine	http://wailer.uokhsc.edu/acc95-expert-systems.html	50
Medical/scientific statements	http://www.americanheart.org/pubs/scipub/statements/	50
Regulations regarding physician supervision of diagnostic tests	http://www.acc.org/healthpol/supervision.html	51
Standards for adult nuclear cardiology training	http://www.ccs.ca/consensus/standards/norm5/	51
"White coat" hypertension in black female population	http://www.cityscape.co.uk/users/ad88/med/whiteco1.htm	52
Dental Health		
ADA dental newsline	http://www.ada.org/consumer/radio/radio.html	53
Computer applications in dental training	http://cpmcnet.columbia.edu/dept/de...cs/AOFC_Course/AOFC_Objectives.html	54
Computer based learning materials in dentistry	http://www.derweb.ac.uk/tm1.html	54
Curriculum guidelines for oral biology	http://www2.musc.edu/AAOB/GradOBCurr.html	55
Dental hygienist	http://www.adha.org/homepage.htm	55
Dental legislation testimony	http://www.aads.jhu.edu/kennedy.htm	56
Dental scholarships	http://www.colgate.com/Pro/continuing_education/scholarships.html	56
Dental telecommunication network (DenTelNet)	http://biz.onramp.net/Den-Tel-Net/	57
Dental Trauma Server	http://www.unige.ch/smd/orthotr.html	57
Dentistry resources	http://www.pitt.edu/~cbw/dental.html	58
Detecting oral cancer	http://www.tambcd.edu/oralexam/nidroc00.htm	58
Endodontic, resident case reports	http://www.tambcd.edu/endo/index.html	59
Financial aid for dental students	http://www.dencom.army.mil/recruit.dir/index.html	59
Job report for dental assistants	http://www.exchangenet.com/howto/career/R0381.html	60
National Oral Health Information Clearinghouse (NOHIC)	http://www.aerie.com/nohicweb/ohmap.html	60
Oral health booklets	http://blake.oit.unc.edu/health/english/booklets/index.html	61
Pediatric dentistry	http://www.flash.net/~dkennel/index.htm	61
Systemic antibiotic therapy in oral surgery	http://www.odont.ku.dk/antibiotics/main.html	62

Primary Topic	URL	Page
Tempomandibular tutorial	http://www.rad.washington.edu/Anatomy/TMJ/TMJISMAP.html	62
Training for oral and maxillofacial surgeons	http://www.aaoms.org/resreach.html	63
Dermatology		
Annual report, 1996: Pressure sore prevention and other topics	http://www.raft.ac.uk/reports/96ar05.htm	64
Botulinum toxin wrinkle treatment	http://medweb.nus.sg/nsc/commskin/botox.html	65
Cutaneous drug reaction database	gopher://gopher.Dartmouth.EDU.70/00/Research/BioSci/CDRD/README	65
Dermatology and other medical journals	http://www.webmedlit.com/	66
Dermatology Online Atlas (DOIA) Erlangen	http://www.derma.med.uni-erlangen.de/bilddb/diagnose/englisch/dg_c.htm	66
Derminfo-Net	http://www.derm-infonet.com/	67
DermPath Tutor: Tutorial in Diagnosis	http://tray.dermatology.uiowa.edu/DPT/DPTutor.htm	67
FDA hearing on autologous cells	http://www.fda.gov/search97cgi/vtop...ResultStart%3D1%26ResultCount%3D25&	68
Ichthyosis reference	http://www.libertynet.org/~ichthyos/referenc.htm#107	68
National Arthritis and Musculoskeletal and Skin Diseases Information Clearinghouse (NAMSDIC)	http://chid.nih.gov/subfile/contribs/ar.html	69
Patient education on popular treatments	http://www.asds-net.org/poptreatments.html#Overview of Popular Treatments	69
Plastic surgery information service	http://www.plasticsurgery.org/	70
Psoriasis drug alert	http://www.psoriasis.org/pressrel/skin-cap.html	70
Types and severity of burns	http://www.alpha-tek.com/burn/type.htm	71
Update on Ultrasound lipoplasty	http://www.surgery.org/enhanced/media/position/update/update.html	71
Emergency Medicine		
Asian Urban Disaster Mitigation Program (AUDMP)	http://hoshi.cic.sfu.ca/adpc/audmp/audmp.html	72
Concept for the Global Health Disaster Network (GHDNet)	http://hypnos.m.ehime-u.ac.jp/GHDNet/concept	73
Database of injury mechanisms and diagnoses	http://www.cis.upenn.edu/~traumaid/mjd/html/	73
Disaster relief services	http://www.crosssnet.org/what.html	74
Doctors Without Borders USA, Inc.	http://www.dwb.org/voluntr.htm	74
Drug dosages in medical emergencies	http://www.priory.co.uk/journals/emerg.htm	75
Emergency assistance: Refugees and displaced persons	http://www.cdc.gov/nceh/programs/internat/ierh/ierh.htm	75
Emergency management of spider bites	http://gema.library.ucsf.edu:8081/Originals/Tamkin/recluse.html	76
Emergency medicine and primary care	http://www.embbs.com/	76
Expert witness guidelines in emergency medicine	http://www.acep.org/POLICY/PO004114.HTM	77
Global Emergency Management System (GEMS) resources	http://www.fema.gov/cgi-shl/dbml.ex...on=query&template=/gems/g_index.dbm	77
Guide to medical abbreviations	http://ncemi.org/tla/index.htm	78
Medical education software archive	http://sun3.lib.uci.edu/~sclancy/med-ed/	78

Primary Topic	URL	Page
Oklahoma bombing: Mental health response	http://www.aaets.org/arts/art5.htm	79
Radiological Emergency Preparedness (REP) Program	http://www.fema.gov/pte/rep/	79
Self-study course for emergency response to terrorism	http://www.usfa.fema.gov/nfa/tr_ertss.htm	79
Wound care specialization trend	http://members.aol.com/woundnet/trend.htm	80
Wound healing using color digital image processing	http://www.smtl.co.uk/World-Wide-Wounds/1997/july/Berris/Berris.html	80
Environmental Health		
Carpet emissions and indoor air quality	http://www.carpet-rug.com/carpet.html	81
Electric and magnetic fields (EMF) research	http://www.niehs.nih.gov/emfrapid/home.htm	82
Environmental Health Clearinghouse	http://infoventures.com/e-hlth/about-eh.html	82
Glossary of environmental health terms	http://www.health.state.ny.us/nysdoh/consumer/environ/toxglos.htm	83
Hazards literature database (HazLit)	http://www.Colorado.EDU/hazards/litbase/litindex.htm	83
Lead screening guidelines	http://WWW.CDC.GOV/nceh/programs/lead/guide/1997/docs/backgr.htm	84
Medical surveillance during Operations Desert Shield/Desert Storm	http://www.gulflink.osd.mil/nfl/	84
Mesothelioma treatment options	http://www.mesothel.com/pages/mesopage.htm	85
National Toxicology Program	http://ntp-server.niehs.nih.gov/	85
Pesticide Information Profiles (PIPs)	http://ace.ace/orst.edu/info/extoxnet/pips/ghindex.html	86
Pollution database	http://www.webdirectory.com/Pollution/	86
Public health assessments, 1995–1996	http://atsdr1.atsdr.cdc.gov:8080/HAC/PHA/	87
Public policy challenges facing chlorine chemistry	http://www.c3.org/library/cth2.html	87
Role of climate in selected diseases in the United States	http://www.med.harvard.edu/chge/EID/more_disease.html	88
Smoking and health	HTTP://ASH.ORG	88
Strategic Plan for Health Effects of Air Pollution (1997–2000)	http://www.healtheffects.org/strategy.htm	89
Summary of proceedings of National Conference on Air Pollution Impacts on Body Organs	http://www.intr.net/napenet/airsum.html#Droller	89
Teaching resources in occupational and environmental health	http://www.med.ed.ac.uk/hew/alpha.html	90
Epidemiology		
Allergy and infectious diseases funding opportunities	http://web.fie.com/htbin/wfSearch	91
Bird flu influenza outbreak	http://www.accessv.com/~mhfung/flu.htm	92
The Blue Book	http://hna.ffh.vic.gov.au/phb/hprot/inf_dis/bluebook/index.htm	92
Comprehensive Epidemiologic Data Resource (CEDR)	http://cedr.lbl.gov/catalog/catalog1.html	93
Ebola vaccine candidate	http://www.gene.com/ae/WN/SU/ebola198.html	93
Emerging Infectious Diseases (EID)	http://www.cdc.gov/ncidod/EID/access.htm	94
Epi Info programs for epidemiologic analysis	http://www.cdc.gov/epo/epi/epiinfo.htm	94

Primary Topic	URL	Page
Eurosurveillance Weekly	http://www.eurosurv.org/	95
Evaluating disease management interventions	http://www.sapien.net/dmw/aud/transcripts/96_09_25.htm	95
Guidelines for epidemiology practices for drug, device, and vaccine research in the United States	http://www.hsph.harvard.edu/Organizations/DDIL/gep.html	96
Healthy travel	http://www.travelhealth.com/genguide.htm	96
Hepatitis A to E	http://www.cdc.gov/ncidod/diseases/hepatitis/slideset/hep00025.htm	97
Homeowner's guide to ecology and environment management of Lyme disease	http://www.w2.com/docs2/d5/lyme1.html)	97
Leprosy management projects	http://foundation.novartis.com/leproj.htm	98
Parasitic diseases	http://www.mic.ki.se/Diseases/c3.html	98
Rare diseases clinical research database	http://rarediseases.info.nih.gov/ord/wwwprot/index.shtml	99
Rare disorders database	http://www.nord-rdb.com/~orphan/rdb/rd0057.htm	99
Sanitation inspections of international cruise ships, Green Sheet	http://www.cdc.gov/nceh/programs/sanit/vsp/scores/scores.htm	100
Search results for immunization and infectious diseases	http://www.healthfinder.gov/htmlge...MUNIZATION+AND+INFECTIOUS+DISEASES	100
Toxicology Internet resources	http://www.pitt.edu/~martint/welcome.htm#mothp	101
Weekly Epidemiological Record (WER)	http://www.who.ch/wer/wer_home.htm	101
Yellow Book Online: Health information for international travel, 1996-1997	wysiwyg://119/http://www.cdc.gov/travel/yellowbk/home.htm	102
Gastroenterology		
Acute stress ulceration	http://gasbone.herston.uq.edu.au/te...hvc_stul/stressul.html#Pathogenesis	103
Adenocarcinoma of the esophago-gastric junction	http://nt1.chir.med.tu-muenchen.de/slides/igcc/classificat/epi/sld019.htm	104
Approach to patient with acute hepatitis	http://uhs.bsd.uchicago.edu/uhs/topics/hepatitis.html	104
Diabetes Research International Network (DRI NET)	http://drinet.med.miami.edu/	105
Electrogastrography	http://www.ee.ualberta.ca/~mintchev/www.html	105
Fundoplication	http://www.motility.org/fundo.htm	106
Gastroenterology training	http://www.gastrojournal.org/policy/v110n4p1266.html	106
GastroLinks	http://pharminfo.com/disease/gastro/gastrolinks.html#body	107
Hans Popper Society: Histopathological cases	http://hepar-sfgh.ucsf.edu/popper.htm	107
Helicobacter pylori	http://www.helico.com/	108
Incontinence and irritable bowel syndrome research	http://www.execpc.com/iffgd/research.html	108
Introduction to gastroesophageal reflux disease (GERD)	http://www.gerd.com/intro/home.htm	109
Laparoscopic surgery during pregnancy	http://www.sages.org/sg_pub23.html	109
Legislative action: Colorectal cancer screening	http://www.asge.org/doc/85	110
The Longitudinal Muscle in Esophageal Disease	http://www.inxpress.net/~oastiennon/	110

Primary Topic	URL	Page
Minimally invasive surgery for heartburn	http://www.ccf.org/pc/misc/nfnissen.htm	111
National Digestive Diseases Information Clearinghouse (NDDIC)	http://www.niddk.nih.gov/Brochures/NDDIC.htm	111
Overview of UK national groin hernia outcomes project	http://www.rcseng.ac.uk/res&aud/audit/hernia/	112
Pressure ulcer research	http://www.npuap.org/prevmon.html	112
Prevention and treatment of complications of diabetes	http://www.cdc.gov/nccdphp/ddt/ddt/brn_tx2.htm	113
Research agenda on liver and related diseases	http://gi.ucsf.edu/alf/alf/alfpubpol.html	113
Treatment of reflux esophagitis	http://pharminfo.com/meeting/ACG/acg_ehlb12.html	114
General Medicine		
Adolescent health, state of the nation	http://www.cdc.gov/nccdphp/dash/ahson/ahson/htm	115
Adolescent suicide prevention	http://hiru.mcmaster.ca/ohcen/groups/hthu/95-12.htm	116
African-American crisis in health care	http://www.unctv.org/localpro/local01/bifserie/bif00g.htm	116
AMA Physician Select (online doctor finder)	http://www.ama-assn.org/aps/amahg.htm	117
Ambulatory research with family physicians	http://www.tafp.com/starnet.htm	117
Annals clinical extracts	http://www.acponline.org/index.htm	118
Anti-aging data sources	http://worldhealth.net/	118
Certification of foreign medical graduates	http://www.ecfmg.org/	119
EthnoMed: Ethnic Medicine Guide	http://www.hslib.washington.edu/clinical/ethnomed/	119
European pancreas transplant activities	http://www.transplant.org/eur/WWW/Organs/Pancreas/rechts.html	120
Family health	http://www.tcom.ohiou.edu/family-health.html	120
Generalist Physician Initiative (GPI)	http://charlotte.hsc.missouri.edu/	121
Guidelines for Adolescent Preventive Services (GAPS)	http://www.ama-assn.org/adolhlth/recomend/monogrf1.htm#immunizations	121
Health care quality registers in Sweden	http://www.sos.se/mars/kva040/kva040.htm#why	122
Healthy People 2000 fact sheet	http://nhic-nt.health.org/nmp/hp2kpage/hp2kfct1.htm	122
High blood cholesterol in adults	http://dragon.labmed.umn.edu/~relson/atp_home.html	123
Hospice fact sheet	http://www.nho.org/facts.htm	123
Information for providers	http://www.health.state.ny.us/nysdoh/provider/provider.htm	124
Information overload of physicians	http://ahcpr.gov/research/physprac.htm	124
The interactive patient	http://medicus.marshall.edu/medicus.htm	125
Medic Alert purpose	http://www.medicalert.org/Pages/Pages/b_atrisk/b_risk01.html	125
Medical palmtop PCs	http://med-amsa.bu.edu/AMSA/palmtop/writing.html#Article 1	126
Medical robotics	http://robotics.eecs.berkeley.edu/~mcenk/medical#vr	126
Minority Health Resource Center	http://www.omhrc.gov/welcome.htm#TOC	127
Multimedia clinical examination	http://www.crc.nus.sg/CH/students/mce.html	127
National Pain Data Bank	http://www.AAPAINMANAGE.org/npdb/graphs.html	128

Primary Topic	URL	Page
National Resident Matching Program (NRMP)	http://www.aamc.org/about/progemph/nrmp/start.htm	128
Policies for graduate medical education review	http://www.acgme.org/acgme/polprod/MPCONTS.htm	129
Post-traumatic stress disorder and aircraft incidents	http://www.gretmar.com/webdoctor/aviation.html	129
Poverty reduction and the World Bank, 1996 and 1997	http://www.worldbank.org/html/extdr/pov_red/default.htm	130
Primary care baseline	http://www.med.ufl.edu/medinfo/baseline/index.html	130
Rural health services	http://www.nal.usda.gov/ric/richs/	131
Transformation of the U.S. health care market	http://www.rwjf.org/health/dec95.htm	131
Transplantation resources on the Internet	http://www.transweb.org/resources_index.html	132
Twin-to-twin transfusion	http://www.tttsfoundation.org/	132
Health Funding Policy		
Acronym dictionary	http://www.wpc-edi.com/AcronymDictionary/Dictionary.html	133
Advocacy papers: Improving Medicare and Medicaid	http://www.aha.org/AdvPapers.html	134
AHCPR data and surveys	http://www.ahcpr.gov/data/	134
AMA releases on physician assisted suicide	http://www.ama-assn.org/ad-com/releases/1996/tr329.htm	135
Assisted suicide in Canada	http://www.parl.gc.ca/english/senate/com-e/euth-e/rep-e/lad-tc-e.htm	135
Assisted suicide statement	http://www.aahpm.org/main.shtml	136
Congressional Medicare testimony, 1997	http://www.PPRC.GOV/congtest.htm	136
Death and dying	http://www.nap.edu/readingroom/books/approaching/	137
Federal research and education funding opportunities	http://www.rams-fie.com/opportunity.htm	137
Funding opportunities database	http://cos.gdb.org/repos/fund/	138
Health care for the homeless	http://www.nashville.net/~hch/index.html	138
Managed care	http://www.hrsa.dhhs.gov/hrsa/mngdcare/cmc.htm	139
Medicaid consumer information	http://www.hcfa.gov/medicaid/mcaicnsm.htm	139
Medicaid managed care	http://www.chcs.org/mmcp.htm	140
Medicare-Medicaid public use data files	http://www.hcfa.gov/stats/stats.htm	140
Medicine and public health	http://www.nyam.org/pubhlth/medpub1.html	141
National and international standards for healthcare codes	http://www.mcis.duke.edu/standards/HL7/termcode/codehome.htm	141
National Health Security Plan	http://sunsite.unc.edu:80/nhs/NHS-T-o-C.html	142
National Institutes of Health (NIH) consensus and technology reports	http://text.nlm.nih.gov/ftrs/pick?c...nih&cc=1&oldK=48264&t+884114739	142
National Practitioner Data Bank (NPDB)	http://www.hrsa.dhhs.gov/bhpr/dqa/factshts/fsreport.htm	143
New Supplemental Security Income (SSI) childhood disability legislation	http://www.ssa.gov/policy/child.htm	143
Pfizer venture philanthropy	http://www.pfizer.com/pfizerinc/philanthropy/grant/grant.html	144
Prevailing healthcare charges system (PHCS)	http://www.hiaa.org/healthcare/index.html	144

Primary Topic	URL	Page
Privatization and public health	http://www.phf.org/priv_execsumm.htm	145
U.S. medical insurance coverage, 1992–1993	http://www.census.gov/hhes/www/hlth9293.html	145
HIV/AIDS		
Abstracts, XI International Conference on AIDS	http://sis.nlm.nih.gov/aidsabs.htm	146
AIDS health fraud	http://www.applicom.com/tcrs/Fraud.htm	147
AIDS patent database	http://patents.cnidr.org/welcome.html	147
AIDS prevention strategies	http://www.epibiostat.ucsf.edu/capsweb/index.html	148
The body: A multimedia AIDS and HIV information resource	http://www.thebody.com/cgi-bin/body.cgi	148
Drug development and approval process in the '90s	http://www.critpath.org/research/process.htm	149
Framework for antiretroviral therapy	http://www.bmaids.demon.co.uk/pubs/antiret.htm	149
Guidelines for antiretroviral agents for HIV in adults and adolescents	http:/207.226.163.175/hiv/nihreport/guide/	150
HIV/AIDS and health care workers	http://aepo-xdv-www.epo.cdc.gov/wonder/prevguid/p0000344/p0000344.htm	150
HIV/AIDS drug assistance programs	http://www.hivpositive.com/f-Resour...-16-PharmDrugPgms/PharmCoPgrms.html	151
HIV/AIDS treatment information	http://www.hivatis.org/	151
HIV/AIDS treatment	http://www.ama-assn.org/special/hiv/treatmnt/treatmnt.htm	152
HIV/STD prevention in rural America	http://www.indiana.edu/~aids/news/news7.html	152
Inmates' HIV prevention needs	http://www.epibiostat.ucsf.edu/capsweb/inmatetext.html	153
National AIDS Clearinghouse	http://www.cdcnac.org/nacdb.html	153
1997 National Conference on Women and HIV (NCWH)	http://www.iapac.org/clinmgt/ncwh/index.html	154
Nutrition in pediatric HIV infection	http://www.hivpositive.com/f-Nutrition/f-3-PediatricNeut/n-Zafonte.html	154
Pediatric AIDS Clinical Trials Group (PACTG)	http://pactg.s-3.com/pinfo.htm	155
Skin diseases in patients with HIV infection	http://www.mediconsult.com/noframes...rgies/shareware/allergies/9736.html	155
State of the art: HIV vaccines	http://www.critpath.org/aric/dirt/10/index.htm	156
Strategic United Nations plan for AIDS (1996–2000)	http://www.us.unaids.org/highband/projects/strat_plan.html#what	156
Textbook on HIV Disease, 2nd edition	http://hivinsite.ucsf.edu/akb/1994/index.html	157
Legal Medicine		
Declaration of Helsinki	http://www.ams.med.uni-goettingen.de/~rhilger/dek_htv.html	158
Ethics and computerization of medicine	http://ccme-mac4.bsd.uchicago.edu/CCMEdocs/Info	159
Federal health care liability reform data	http://www.wp.com/hcla/page.htm	159
Federal judicial health decisions	http://www.fjc.gov/	160
Health research and public health sites	http://weber.u.washington.edu/~hserv/hsic/resource/phlinks.html	160
Law and the physician	http://plague.law.umkc.edu/Xfiles/x_t.htm	161
Legal Medicine, Open File 97	http://www.afip.mil/legalmed/openfile97/toc97.html	161

Primary Topic	URL	Page
List of top health frauds	http://www.fda.gov/opacom/backgrounders/tophealt.html	162
Managed health care	http://www.chipp.cahwnet.gov/mctf/front.htm	162
Medicine and law	http://www.physiciansnews.com/law/dvindex.html	163
Patient confidentiality	http://www.acep.org/POLICY/PO004155.htm	163
Physician's guide to medical liability issues	http://www.afss.com/physguid.htm	164
Rare case registry: Confidentiality submission issues	http://anes01.wustl.edu/RARE/Rare_guide.html	164
Medical Informatics		
Biostatistics resources	http://www.sph.emory.edu/bios/bioslist.html	165
CDC Wonder	http://wonder.cdc.gov/Wonder/background.html	166
Combined Health Information Database (CHID)	http://chid.nih.gov/	166
Congressional megasite	wysiwyg://56/http://lcweb.loc.gov/global/legislative/mega.html	167
Doctor's Guide to the Internet	http://www.pslgroup.com/DOCGUIDE.HTM	167
Electronic Development and Environment Information System (ELDIS)	http://www.ids.ac.uk/eldis/eldis.html	168
Electronic information resources for health officers	http://www.cdc.gov/elecinfo.htm	168
Evaluating Internet medical information	http://www.fda.gov/fdac/features/596_info.html#site	169
Federal statistical databases	http://www.fedstats.gov/search.html	169
Federal Web Locator (FedWeb)	http://www.law.vill.edu/Fed-Agency/fedwebloc.html	170
Health data warehouse	http://www.cdc.gov/nchswww/nchshome.htm	170
Health/medical topics and resources	http://www.noah.cuny.edu/qksearch.html	171
Healthfinder: Medical and health information	http://www.healthfinder.gov/	171
HON Media Gallery	http://www.hon.ch/Media/media.html	172
Index of Internet medical resources	http://www.gretmar.com/webdoctor/window.html	172
Integrated public use microdata series (IPUMS)	http://www.hist.umn.edu/~ipums/	173
Internet Grateful Med	http://igm.nlm.nih.gov:80/	173
Karolinska Institute Library and Information Center	http://www.mic.ki.se/Diseases/index.html	174
Martindale's "The Reference Desk"	http://www-sci.lib.uci.edu/	174
MedAccess On-Line	http://www.medaccess.com/	175
MedExplorer health/medical Internet search engine	http://www.medexplorer.com/	175
Medical case presentations and teaching files	http://www.geocities.com/HotSprings/2255/index.html	176
Medical Encyclopedia on the Net—Diseases	http://www.mosbych1.com/mhc/index/	176
Medical journals	http://www.webmedlit.com/	177
Medical World Search	http://www.mwsearch.com/help.html	177
Medistat	http://biomed.nus.sg/MSTAT/welcome.html	178
MedWeb	http://www.gen.emory.edu/MEDWEB/medweb.html	178

Primary Topic	URL	Page
Merck Manual of Medical Information—Home edition, 1997	http://www.merck.com/!!tcfQIINcStcfRL31_X/pubs/mmanual_home/	179
Morbidity and Mortality Weekly Report (MMWR)	http://www.cdc.gov/epo/mmwr/mmwr.html)	179
Natality, morbidity, mortality statistics	http://www.lib.umich.edu/libhome/PubHealth.lib/bib/statistics.html	180
National Library of Medicine (NLM)	http://www.nlm.nih.gov/	180
New England Journal of Medicine online	http://www.nejm.org/	180
NIH Health Information Index, 1997	http://www.nih.gov/news/96index/pubincov.htm	181
Online medical journals and references	http://www-informatics.ucdmc.ucdavis.edu/informatics/MedRefs.html-ssi	181
Recommendations for clinical software systems	http://amia2.amia.org/v04n06/442.htm	182
Thomas Legislative Information on the Internet	http://thomas.loc.gov/	182
U.S. National Library of Medicine (NLM)	http://www.nlm.nih.gov/	183
United States Congress	http://www.access.gpo.gov/congress/index.html	183
World Health Organization Statistical Information System (WHOSIS)	http://www.who.ch/whosis/whosis.htm#databases	184
W3–Electronic Medical Record System (W3-EMRS)	http://www.emrs.org/medweb/	184
Medical Specialties		
Anesthesiology		
Blood, fluid, and electrolyte replacement lecture	http://www.med.virginia.edu/som-cl/anesth/education/blood.htm	185
Global Textbook of Anesthesiology	http://www.gasnet.eur.nl/gta/	186
Practice parameters for physicians	http://gasnet.med.yale.edu/mirror/asa/Practice_Parameters/prac_TOC.html	186
Endocrinology		
Clinical guidelines for endocrine conditions	http://www.aace.com/guidelines/	187
Endocrine surgery	http://endocrine-surgery.com/Welcome.html	187
Forensics		
Autopsy diagrams	http://www.afip.mil/oafme/diagrams.html	188
Forensic odontology certification	http://www.abfo.org/qualific.htm	188
Forensic protocols for human hair comparisons	http://olmec.lab.r1.fws.gov/proto/methods.htm	189
Forensic resources	http://www.hypernet.on.ca/quincy/formedic.htm	189
Landmark cases in forensic psychiatry	http://ua1vm.ua.edu/~jhooper/landmark.html	190
Medical examiner and coroner information-sharing program	http://www.cdc.gov/nceh/pubcatns/1994/cdc/brosures/me-cbro.htm	190
Qualifications for forensic psychiatry	http://www.cc.emory.ed/AAPL/abpn.htm	191
Writing cause-of-death statements	http://WWW.TheNAME.org:80/main.htm	191
Genetics		
DNA vaccine	http://www.genweb.com/Dnavax/dnavax.html	192

Primary Topic	URL	Page
Human cloning ban, U.S. House of Representatives	http://www.scienceXchange.com/aai/newsletter/November/cloning.htm	192
Human genome maps	http://www.oxmol.com/biolib/map/	193
Pathology		
Human anatomy online	http://www.innerbody.com/indexbody.html	193
Pathology mini-tutorials	http://www-medlib.med.utah.edu/WebPath/TUTORIAL/TUTORIAL.html#3	194
Visible embryo project	http://magenta.afip.mil/embryo/HomePage.html	194
Radiography		
Medical radiography homepage	http://www.aers.org	195
Medical radiography resources	http://web.wn.net/~usr/ricter/web/medradhome.html	195
Radiographic anatomy of the skeleton	http://www.scar.rad.washington.edu/RadAnatomy.html	196
Telemedicine		
European telepathologist sites	http://europath.imag.fr/vpage/V.EPS.html	196
Reimbursement of telemedicine consultations	http://206.156.10.7/scripts/esrimap.dll?name=Reporter&cmd=Report_1	197
Telemedicine and technology transfer sites	http://ourworld.compuserve.com/home.../global_telemedicine_apex/sites.htm	197
Telemedicine and the law	http://www.arentfox.com/telemedicine.html	198
Telemedicine confidentiality statements	http://www.vtmednet.org/telemedicine/privacy.htm	198
Telemedicine in action	http://www.va.gov/telemed/teleactn.htm	199
Telemedicine research	http://www.matmo.org/	199
Telepathology tips from Armed Forces Institute of Pathology (AFIP)	http://www.afip.mil/telepath/tips/tip1.html	200
Urology		
End-stage Renal disease	http://www.niddk.nih.gov/EndStageRenalDisease/EndStageRenalDisease.html	200
Laboratory regulation in urological offices	http://auanet.org/pub_pat/policies/...Laboratory regulation in urological	201
Marketing continence	http://www.continenceworldwide.com/articles/3.html	201
Urologic trauma	(http://indy.radiology.uiowa.edu/Pro...nRef/FPHandbook/Chapter01/15-1.html)	202
Mental Health		
Adolescent and child psychiatry	http://www.aacap.org/web/aacap/	203
Anorexia/bulimia	http://members.aol.com/amanbu/index.html	204
Calendar of events for mental health professionals	http://www.umdnj.edu/psyevnts/meet.FEB00.html#Date	204
Common misconceptions about suicide	http://www.save.org/	205
Computerized measurement of health and thermal pain perception	http://www.psychologie.uni-bonn.de/kap/for/bio/com.htm	205
Consumer's guide to treatment of anxiety disorders	http://www.adaa.org/4_info/4a_cgt/4a_02.htm	206
Crisis intervention	http://www.uic.edu/orgs/convening/Proceed21.htm	206

Primary Topic	URL	Page
Crisis intervention resource manual	http://www.bartow.k12.ga.us/psych/crisis/crisis.htm	207
Disorders and treatments index	http://www.cmhc.com/selfhelp.htm	207
Dissociative disorders	http://www.voiceofwomen.com/VOW2_11950/centerarticle.html	208
Early diagnosis and management of psychosis	http://home.vicnet.net.au/~eppic/intervene.html#anchor436997	208
Electroconvulsive therapy (ECT)	http://www.mentalhealth.com/book/p45-ect1.html	209
European-American descriptions of disorders	http://www.mentalhealth.com/main.html	209
Gestalt therapy	http://www.behavior.net/mhn/bolfor...th=8&detail=description&lastread=5	210
Index of reports on disorders	http://www.mhsource.com/disorders/	210
Insanity defense	http://www.psych.org/public_info/INSANI~1.HTM	211
Interactive testing in psychiatry (ITP)	http://www.med.nyu.edu/Psych/ITP/gpm2.html	211
Managed care and mental health program funding	http://mimh.edu/TM/T3780	212
Mental disorders	http://www.nimh.nih.gov/hotsci/hotsci.htm	212
Mental health bill of rights	http://helping.apa.org/rights.html	213
Mental health research, volunteer opportunities	http://www.nimh.nih.gov/~cng/volnteer.htm	213
Mental health services databases	http://www.mentalhealth.org/mhorgsdb/index.htm	214
Mental health statistics	http://www.mentalhealth.org/mhstats/index.htm	214
Multimedia library courses	http://www.mhsource.com/edu/hmstudy/all2.html#disorders	215
Overview of depressive illness and symptoms	http://www.ndmda.org/depover.htm	215
Personality disorders	http://www.ns.sympatico.ca/Contents/Health/LISTS/B4-C03-06_all1.html	216
Psychiatry and the Web	http://www.psych.med.umich.edu/web/psytimes/psychwww.htm	216
Schizophrenia	http://www.cityscape.co.uk/users.ad88/schizo.htm	217
Violence risk assessment study	http://ness.sys.virginia.edu/macarthur/violence.html	217
Musculoskeletal Health		
Acute low back problems in adults	http://text.nlm.nih.gov/ftrs/tocview	218
Aquatic therapy	http://www.biomech.com/archive/1997/bdr97/aquatxt.html	219
Arthritis and lupus clinical trials	http://preferences.stanford.edu/arthritis/recruit.htm	219
Arthritis sites for consumers	http://www.nerdworld.com/cgi-bin/vdata.cgi?783	220
Clinical guidelines for prevention of postmenopausal osteoporosis	http://www.aace.com/guidelines/osteoporosis.html	220
Computers and arthritis	http://weber.u.washington.edu/~dboo...subjects/arthritis/xzzzzzzd3_1.html	221
Cutting Edge Reports on osteoporosis	http://www.nof.org/cutedg3.html	221
Gait lab case presentations	http://gait.aidi.udel.edu/res695/ho...d_ortho/gait_lab/cases/casehome.htm	222
Hand and finger pain	http://www-med.stanford.edu/school/DGIM/Teaching/Modules/handfinger.html	222
Interactive test for knee injury	http://www.med.und.nodak.edu:80/depts/fpc/knee/knee.htm	223
Lumbar laminectomy	http://familyinternet.com/mhc/scr/002973sc.htm	223

Primary Topic	URL	Page
Lupus	http://www.hamline.edu/lupus/	224
Muscular dystrophy research updates	http://www.mdausa.org/research/updates.html	224
Orthopedic outcomes assessment	http://www.aaos.org/wordhtml/outcomes.htm	225
Osteopathic medicine	http://www.aacom.org/what.htm	225
Osteoporosis and men	http://www.osteo.org/osteoinmen.html	226
Pediatric rheumatology	http://www.arthritis.org/ajao/athreya/athreya_part_1.shtml	226
Rheumatology megasite	http://www.gen.emory.edu/medweb/medweb.rheumatology.html	227
Rheumatology resources	http://www.rheumatology.org/patient/factsheet.html	227
Wheeless' Textbook of Orthopaedics	http://www.medmedia.com/med.htm	228
Neurology		
ANGEL Neurosurgical Information Resource	http://www.usc.edu/hsc/neurosurgery/Neurosurgeons/angindx.html	229
Brain tumor noteworthy treatments	http://www.virtualtrials.com/noteworth.html	230
Brain tumor online resources	http://www.tbts.org/onlinere.htm	230
Childhood Cancer Ombudsman Program	http://www.mnsinc.com/cbtf/ombuds.html	231
Chronic fatigue and immune dysfunction syndrome (CFIDS)	http://www.cfids.org/cfids.html	231
Chronic fatigue syndrome (CFS)	http://weber.u.washington.edu/~dedra/aacfs1.html	232
Chronic fatigue syndrome (CFS) treatments and studies	http://www.cdc.gov/ncidod/diseases/cfs/cfshome.htm	232
Costs and causes of traumatic brain injury	http://www.biausa.org/costsand.htm	233
Dictionary of pain terms	http://weber.u.washington.edu/~crc/IASP/dict.html#RTFToC11	233
Headache causes	http://www.achenet.org/whatcause.htm	234
Human brain project	http://www-hbp.scripps.edu/Home.html	234
Huntington's disease latest news	http://www.angelfire.com/al/leonc/	235
Multiple sclerosis	http://www.nmss.org/home.html	235
Neurofibromatosis	http://www.nf.org/	236
Neurological clinical trials	http://www.innd.org/trials.htm	236
Neuroscience for kids	http://weber.u.washington.edu/~chudler/neurok.html	237
Online neurosurgery resident's handbook	http://sunsite.unc.edu/Neuro/handbook/handbook.html	237
Patient information guide for neurology	http://www.aan.com/public/pig.html	238
Sleep medicine online	http://www.users.cloud9.net/~thorpy/sleepdoc.html	238
Spike Train Analysis Graphical Environment (Stranger) package	http://biogfx.neuro.wfu.edu/stranger/analysis.html	239
Spine disorders	http://mcns10.med.nyu.edu/cases/spine.html	239
Stroke emergency evaluation and treatment	http://www.stroke.org/First_Few_Hours.html	240
Stroke treatment in children	http://www.ninds.nih.gov/HEALINFO/D...ke%20proceedings/chd-resp.htm#Treat	240
Traumatic brain injury (TBI) in the United States	http://www.cdc.gov/ncipc/dacrrdp/tbi.htm	241

Primary Topic	URL	Page
Whole brain atlas	http://www.med.harvard.edu/AANLIB/home.html	241
Women with epilepsy	http://www.efa.org/what/wei/wei.html	242
Nursing and Home Health Care		
American Association of Colleges of Nursing	http://www.aacn.nche.edu/	243
American Association of Critical-Care Nurses (AACN)	http://www.aacn.org/	244
Continence program in long-term care settings	http://www.ahcpr.gov/clinic/uidon.htm	244
Graduate education in nursing informatics	http://www.gl.umbc.edu/~abbott/NIprogram.htm	245
Health care workers with bloodborne disease, HIV	http://www.aorn.org/nsgtoday/hiv.htm	245
Home care aide	http://www.nahc.org/HCA/home.html	246
Home care online	http://www.nahc.org/	246
Home health care classification: Nursing diagnoses, interventions	http://www.dml.georgetown.edu/research/hhcc/	247
Hospital to home care for nurses	http://www.okqchomehealth.com/indepth/hospital.htm	247
Influencing Congress: Ten commandments	http://www.nurse.org/acnp/leg/10com.shtml	248
Language for an interstate model of nursing regulation	http://www.ncsbn.org/files/newsreleases/nr971216.html	248
Legislative position statement on job protection	http://www.aana.com/notices/notice10.htm	249
MedExplorer Internet nursing resources	http://www.medexplorer.com/m-nurse.htm	249
Nursing and midwifery	http://www.who.ch/programmes/nur/wha455en.htm	250
Nursing education and practice, U.S.	http://www.bibl-u-szeged.hu/bibl/afit/nursingw.html	250
Nursing ethical conflict in the workplace	http://www.bc.edu/bc_org/avp/son/ethics/research.html	251
Nursing informatics, enhancing patient care	http://www.nih.gov/ninr/vol4/index.html	251
Nursing malpractice	http://www.npg.com/npg/whocan.htm#0	252
Nursing personnel in schools	http://www.aap.org/policy/01584.html	252
Nursing role in the new marketplace	http://www.nursingcenter.com/career/guide97/articles/g7baer.html	253
Pharmacotherapeutics for advanced practice nurses in rural Georgia	http://www2.gasou.edu/nursing/pharm/#Program Driectors and Faculty	253
Prescriptive privileges for nurse practitioners	http://www.nln.org/pr050104.htm	254
Private duty nursing services	http://www.cancer.org/rig/rigduty.html	254
State licensure guide	http://www.nursingcenter.com/career/guide/Licensure.cfm	255
Telephone or triage nursing	http://www.katsden.com/telenurse/triage.html	255
Using anesthesia bags	http://www.hooked.net/~gtrimble/using_anesthesia_bags.html	256
Visiting Nurse Associations of America (VNAA)	http://www.vnaa.org/body_default.html	256
Nutrition		
Annual reports on family expenditures	http://www.usda.gov/fcs/cnpp.htm	257
Aquaculture	http://www.ansc.purdue.edu/aquanic/home.htm	258

Primary Topic	URL	Page
The Bad Bug Book	http://vm.cfsan.fda.gov/~mow/intro.html	258
Catfish production teaching plan	http://www.catfishinstitute.com/home.html	259
Closing the gap on food safety standards	http://ificinfo.health.org/insight/ih-cgof.htm	259
Crop production data	http://www.usda.gov/nass/aggraphs/graphics.htm	260
Egg nutrition	http://www.aeb.org/	260
Food and drug law history	http://www.fda.gov/opacom/backgrounders/miles.html	261
Foodborne illness education	http://www.nal.usda.gov/fnic/foodborne/foodborn.htm	261
Hazard Analysis Critical Control Points (HACCP) training	http://www.nal.usda.gov/fnic/foodborne/haccp/index.shtml	262
Insects for food	http://www.ent.iastate.edu/Misc/InsectsAsFood.html	262
Iodine deficiency disorders (IDD) database	http://www.idrc.ca/mi/idddocs/iddindex.htm	263
Nutrition library catalog	http://www.geocities.com/HotSprings/2455/tableofcont.html	263
Poverty and nutrition in welfare societies	http://www.edv.agrar.tu-muenchen.de...es/9510-Poverty-Nutrition/agev1.htm	264
Protein Data Bank (PDB)	http://www.pdb.bnl.gov/	264
USDA Food Composition Databases	http://www.nal.usda.gov/fnic/foodcomp/	265
Vegetarian diets	http://www.fortran.com/%7Ernepomuc/heal/ada.htm#authors	265
Weight-control Information Network (WIN)	http://www.niddk.nih.gov/Gastric/Gastsurg.html/	266
Women, Infants, and Children (WIC) Nutrition Program	http://www.usda.gov/fcs/wic/wicfac~2.htm	266
World food emergency weekly reports	http://www.vita.org/disaster/wfp/	267
Occupational Health		
Accident causes and prevention	http://www.cdc.gov/niosh/nasd/video/av00400.html	268
Census of occupational injuries, fatalities, and illnesses	http://stats.bls.gov/oshhome.htm	269
Cumulative trauma disorder (CTD)	http://ctdnews.com/	269
Dust sampling results (metal and nonmetal mines)	http://www.msha.gov/STATS/SAMPLING/MAINPGE.htm	270
Ergonomics	http://ergo.human.cornell.edu/	270
Ergonomics—statistics	http://www.osha-slc.gov/ergo/Statistics.html	271
Experiences of Texas workers denied spinal surgery	http://www.roc.capnet.state.tx.us/spinal.htm	271
Index of occupational safety and health files	http://osh.net/	272
1997 Decisions of the Occupational Safety and Health Review (OSHRC)	http://www.oshrc.gov/comm97.html	272
Nursing home occupational injuries	http://www.osha-selc.gov/SLTC/NursingHome/index.html	273
Occupational health issues	http://www.aiha.org:80/govt.html	273
Occupational safety and health databases	http://turva.me.tut.fi/cis/occupational_safety_databases2.htm	274
OSHA statistics and data	http://www.osha.gov/oshstats/index.html	274
Plain facts about farmer health	http://www.nsc.org/necas/aghealth.htm	275
State profiles of occupational safety and health	http://ftp.cdc.gov/niosh/ia.html	275

Primary Topic	URL	Page
Trigger finger disorder	http://www.sechrest.com/mmg/ctd/trigger.html	276
Workers compensation law materials	http://www.law.cornell.edu/topics/workers_compensation.html#menu	276
Ophthalmology		
Collaborative ocular melanoma study (COMS)	http://webeye.ophth.uiowa.edu/coms/	277
Computer vision	http://www.cs.cmu/edu/~cil/vision.html	278
Current eye research	http://www.wilmer.jhu.edu/research.htm	278
Eye Net	http://www.eyenet.org/member/visit_aao/fax_on_demand.html#seminars	279
Free eyeglasses for kids	http://www.tdl.com/~kids/FreeEyeglasses.html	279
National eye-health related organizations	http://www.nei.nih.gov/publications/sel-org.htm	280
Ophthalmic photography	http://webeye.ophth.uiowa.edu/ops/index.htm	280
Ophthalmology multimedia theater	http://www.eyeworld.org/October/theater.html	281
Optometry career guidance	http://www.aoanet.org/career-guidance.html	281
Orbital and eye lesions	http://patho.wat.ch:80/ophthalmo	282
Pediatric ophthalmology and strabismus	http://med-aapos.bu.edu/default.html	282
Photoreceptors	http://insight.med.utah.edu/Webvision/photo1.html	283
Spatially guided navigation and infant vision	http://john.berkeley.edu/Features/demos.html	283
Vision research WWW servers	http://www.socsci.uci.edu:80/cogsci/vision.html	284
Otolaryngology		
Acoustic emissions from dysfunctional temporomandibular joints (TMJs)	http://www.geocities.com/CapeCanaveral/8462/index.html	285
Clinical and special services for the deaf and hard of hearing	http://www.gallaudet.edu/~nicd/health.html	286
Deaf-blind children	http://www.tr.wou.edu/dblink/data/index.htm	286
Deafness and Communication Disorders Information Clearinghouse	http://www.aerie.com/nihdb/nidcd/dctest.html	287
Ear, Nose, and Throat Information Center	http://www.netdoor.com/entinfo/index.html	287
Materials for acquired deaf-blindness	http://www.dbcent.dk/uk/materials.htm#faktatop	288
Meeting the needs of the deaf-blind	http://www.vois.org.uk/vois-bin/chapter/sense?2	288
Net connections for communication disorders and sciences	http://www.mankato.msus.edu/dept/comdis/kuster2/welcome.html	289
Technology 2000: Clinical applications for speech-language pathology	http://www.asha.org/professionals/tech_resources/tech2000/5.htm	289
Vestibular rehabilitation	http://www.mayo.edu/vest-rehab/	290
Video ostoscopy	http://www.li.net/~sullivan/ears.htm	290
Vocal health	http://www2.shc.uiowa.edu/ncvs_home.html	291
Pediatrics		
Children with sickle cell anemia	http://www.nlm.nih.gov/databases/alerts/sickle97.html	292

Primary Topic	URL	Page
Early childhood intervention	http://www.rand.org/publications/MR/MR898/	293
Employment opportunities in pediatric anesthesia	http://www.uams.edu/spa/spajob.htm	293
The Future of Pediatric Education II Project	http://www.aap.org/profed/fope1.htm	294
Guidelines for death scene investigation of sudden infant death syndrome (SIDS)	http://www.cdc.gov/epo/mmwr/preview/rr4510.html	294
Indicator for tracking children's well-being	http://www.nsf.gov/pubs/1997/pr9748/pr9748.txt	295
Infant cry archive	http://www.siu.edu/departments/coe/comdis/cryhome.html	295
Infectious Diseases in Children	http://www.slackinc.com/child/idc/idchome.htm	296
Maternal and Child Health Bureau (MCHB)	http://www.os.dhhs.gov/hrsa/mchb/	296
MedWeb pediatric Internet resources	http://www.gen.emory.edu/medweb/medweb.pediatric.html	297
Paediapedia: An Imaging Encyclopedia of Pediatric Disease	http://indy.radiology.uiowa.edu/Providers/TeachingFiles/PAP/PAPHome.html	297
Parental control of Internet access	http://www.uab.edu/pedinfo/Control.html	298
Pediatric cardiac arrest	http://weber.u.washington.edu/~asaccp/poca/overview.htm	298
Pediatric consumer ophthalmology	http://med-aapos.bu.edu/aapos/pedires.html	299
Pediatric trauma	http://www.pedi/peditrauma.html	299
Pediatrics interactive education	http://www.medconnect.com/index.htm	300
Profile of children in the States: 1998 data	http://www.childrensdefense.org/states/data.html	300
Spina bifida and other neural tube defects	http://www.cdc.gov/nceh/programs/in...d_prev.htm#Epidemiologic Assistance	301
Pharmaceutical Medicine		
Antibiotic utilization guidelines, 1997	http://www.intmed.mcw.edu/AntibioticGuide.html)	302
Biotechnology and drug information resources	http://pharminfo.com/phrmlink.html#assns	303
Clinical trials listing service	http://www.CenterWatch.com/	303
Drug InfoBase (Drug DB)	http://pharminfo.com/drg_mnu.html	304
FDA Medical Bulletin	http://www.fda.gov/medbull/contents.html	304
Guide to taking medications	http://www.healthtouch.com/level1/leaflets/103068/103068.htm	305
Internet self-assessment in pharmacology (ISAP)	http://www.cs.umn.edu/Research/GIMME/isap.html	305
Japanese Pharmacopoeia (JP)	http://www.mediagalaxy.co.jp/TEST/KOSEISHO/JP-HomeE.html	306
Medical prescription of narcotics	http://www.lindesmith.org/presumm.html	306
Medicine assistance program	http://www.themedicineprogram.com/info.html	307
MedWatch, FDA medical products reporting program	http://www.fda.gov/medwatch/	307
Pharmaceutical training	http://www.aacp.org/	308
Prescription drug patient assistance programs	http://omhs.mhd.hr.state.or.us/presdrap.htm	308
Rx list	http://www.rxlist.com/	309
Safe medication practices	http://www.ismp.org/ISMP/Pages/about.html	309

Primary Topic	URL	Page
U.S. Food and Drug Administration (FDA)	http://www.fda.gov/	310
USP reference standards	http://www.usp.org/index.htm	310
Preventive Health		
Abstracts and references of prevention research	http://www.integres.org/prevres/index.html	311
Aerobics patterns	http://www.turnstep.com/Patterns/index.html	312
Batteries swallowed by young children	http://www.nisu.flinders.edu.au/pubs/shrtreps/batteries.html	312
Chronic disease prevention and health promotion	http://www.cdc.gov/nccdphp/	313
Crash Analysis and Reporting Environment (CARE)	http://care.cs.ua.edu/care/introduction.html	313
Fitness program: Choosing a cardiovascular program	http://www.fitnesslink.com/program/cardio.htm	314
Injury control and violence prevention	http://www.sph.unc.edu/vincentweb/	314
1997 Manufacturer investigation files	http://www.cpsc.gov/library/foia/foia97/compliance/compliance.html	315
Prevention guidelines	http://www.cdc.gov/ncipc/pub-res/prevguid.htm	315
Prototype preventive care guidelines, 1991	http://hiru.mcmaster.ca/prevent/pvcpg_00.htm	316
Sports medicine resource	http://www.callemx.com/html/sportmed.html	316
Statistical and computing resources for injury prevention	http://www.albany.edu/sph/injr_007.html	317
What is Preventive Medicine?	http://www.acpm.org/whatis.htm	317
Radiology		
The Basics of MRI	http://www.cis.rit.edu/htbooks/mri/	318
Body image teaching files	http://www.uhrad.com/ctarc.htm	319
CHORUS collaborative hypertext of radiology	http://chorus.rad.mcw.edu/	319
Clinical nuclear medicine teaching file	http://count51.med.harvard.edu/JPNM/TF.html	320
Interactive tutorial on normal radiology	http://www.med.ufl.edu/medinfo/rademo/raintro.html	320
Magnetic resonance microscopy	http://wwwcivm.mc.duke.edu/	321
Nuclear medicine teaching cases	http://gamma.wustl.edu/home.html	321
Physiological imaging	http://everest.radiology.uiowa.edu/	322
Radiology court decisions	http://www.acr.org/departments/legal/culpeper_decision.html	322
Radiology Internet teaching resources	http://www.mamc.amedd.army.mil/williams/NucMed/gnuc_toc.htm	323
Radiology teaching library	http://www.embbs.com/xray/xr.html#abdomen	323
Rehabilitation Medicine		
Acute care and rehabilitation in the United States	http://www.cdc.gov/ncipc/dacrrdp/dacrrdp.htm	324
Cardiac rehabilitation clinical care guidelines	http://www.a1.com/sportsmed/cardiac.htm	325
COACH: Transportation for riders with disabilities	http://www.dssc.org/	325

Primary Topic	URL	Page
Disabilities statutes, regulations	http://janweb.icdi.wvu.edu/kinder/index.htm	326
Disability and rehabilitation research	http://www.ed.gov/offices/OSERS/NIDRR/index.html	326
Disability tables	http://web.icdi.wvu.edu/disability/tables.html	327
Disability-related clearinghouses in collaboration	http://nichcy.org/clc.htm	327
FDA approved electronic hand controller	http://www.disability.com/whatshot.shtml	328
Federal Register Notices of medical devices	http://www.fda.gov/cdrh/fedregin.html	328
Florida Spinal Cord Injury	http://www.gbdi.com/fscirc/home.html	329
Job Accommodation Network (JAN)	http://janweb.icdi.wvu.edu/	329
Managed care approach to traumatic brain injury	http://www.neuro.pmr.vcu.edu/special.htm	330
Model for post-acute rehabilitation for traumatic brain injury (TBI)	http://www.ccs-rehab.com/outcomes/outmenu.htm	330
Physical therapy	http://www.apta.org/	331
Rehabilitation Clearinghouse	http://www.cais.com/naric/	331
Rehabilitation files library	http://www.rehabnet.com/archives/rehabftp.htm	332
Research overview of psychiatric rehabilitation outcomes	http://web.bu.edu/SARPSYCH/wwwresinfo2.html#3	332
Voice recognition via computer	http://wata.org/watapubs/voicerec.htm	333
Reproductive Health		
Abortion pro- and anti-choice resources	http://www.caral.org/7.docs.html#docs	334
Alternatives to female genital mutilation	http://www.path.org/html/modern_rites_of_passage.htm	335
Assisted Reproductive Technologies (ART)	http://www.centerforhumanreprod.com/art/art.html	335
Condom breakage and slippage rates	gopher://gopher.undp.org:70/00/ungo...n/popis/journals/ifpp/v20n2/STEINER	336
Contraceptive use among women	http://www.agi-usa.org/pubs/journals/2314897.html	336
Emergency contraception	http://opr.princeton.edu/ec/ec.html	337
Evaluation of family planning services	http://www.cpc.unc.edu/projects.evaluation/papers/wp-o-08.html	337
Family planning and adolescent pregnancy	http://www.hhs.gov/progorg/opa/	338
Family planning in preventing abortions	http://www.info.usaid.gov/pop_health/	338
Gender determination	http://www.childbirth.org/articles/boyorgirl.html	339
National summary and fertility clinic reports	http://www.cdc.gov/nccdphp/drh/arts/index.htm	339
1996 World Population Overview	http://www.populationinstitute.org/overview96.html	340
No-scalpel vasectomy	http://www.avsc.org/avsc/workpap/wp3/wp_3.html)	340
POPLINE (Population Information Online) abstracts	http://www/charm.net~ccp/popwel.html	341
PopNet source for global population information	http://www.popnet.org/	341
Population and reproductive health data	http://www.pitt.edu/HOME/GHNet/poprepro.htm	342
Report 1997: The Right to Choose	http://www.unfpa.org/SWP/SWPMAIN.HTM	342
Report: U.N. International Conference on Population (ICPD)	http://www.ppfa.org/ppfa/unconf-1.html	343

Primary Topic	URL	Page
Research regarding impact of family planning	http://www.fhi.org/wsp/wsinfo/wsrsrit.html	343
School based sexuality education programs	http://www.siecus.org/progs/prog0002.html	344
Sexual side effects of antidepressants	http://www.pathfinder.com/money/latest/press/PW/1997Dec02/1787.html	344
Sexually transmitted diseases (STDs)	http://www.aomc.org/HOD2/general/general-SEXUALLY.html#Heading53	345
Viagra questions and answers	http://www.fda.gov/cder/consumerinfo/viagra/viagrafaq.htm	345
World fertility survey	http://opr.princeton.edu/archive/wfs.html	346
Respiratory Health		
Anti–tuberculosis drug resistance in the world	http://www.who.ch/programmes/gtb/dritw/index.html	347
Ask the expert: Antihistamine	http://www.aadmc.org/ate/antihistamine.html	348
Asthma Information Center	http://www.mdnet.de/asthma/asthma.htm	348
Cockroach allergen as related to asthma	http://www.aaaai.org/news/acadnews/96-10/96-10-02.html	349
Definition of allergy and asthma specialist	http://www.aaaai.org/referral/whatis/whatis.html	349
The Diagnosis of Diffuse Lung Disease	http://indy.radiology.uiowa.edu/Pr...books/DiffuseLung/DiffuseLung.html	350
Helping smokers quit	http://www.ahcpr.gov/clinic/smokepcc.html	351
Prevention and treatment of influenza and the common cold	http://www.lungusa.org/noframes/learn/lung/lungcolds_flu.html	351
Respiratory problems during sleep	http://www.gbdi.com/fscirc/home.html	352
Reviews of respiratory tract diseases	http://www.auhs.edu/library/resource/reviews/pulm.htm	352
Sample online respiratory care examination	http://www.nbrc.org/Interactive.htm	353
Substance Abuse		
Access to methadone treatment for heroin addiction	http://mhnet.org/articles/nih2.htm	354
Action to control tobacco	http://www.tobaccofreekids.org/html/consensus_statement.html	355
Clinical research findings on alcohol and drugs	http://www.ria.org/findings/index.html	355
Directory of Substance Abuse Professionals (SAP)	http://www.detnet.com/datalink/sap/index.htm	356
Drug Abuse Warning Network (DAWN)	http://www.health.org/pubs/93dawn/93dawn.htm	356
Drug and alcohol testing medical practitioners	http://www.aamro.com/	357
Family approach to drug prevention	http://www.emory.edu/NFIA/	357
Get It Straight publication	http://www.usdoj.gov/dea/pubs/straight/cover.htm	358
Helping patients with alcohol problems	http://www.niaaa.nih.gov/publications/physicn.htm	358
Information about alcohol, tobacco, and other drugs	http://www.drugs.indiana.edu.druginfo/	359
Low-risk drinking guidelines	http://www.arf.org/lowriskEnglish.html	359
Methamphetamine abuse	ftp://ftp.health.org/pub/ncadi/publications/meth.txt	360
The National Treatment Improvement Evaluation Study (NTJES)	http://www.health.org/nties97/index.htm	360
Needle exchange programs	http://soros.org/lindesmith/clinton/agencies.html	361

Primary Topic	URL	Page
Parent's Handbook to Substance Abuse Prevention	http://198.115.232.254/y2y/Parents_Handbook.html	362
Prevline Prevention Online	http://www.health.org.aboutn.htm	362
Sourcebook of Criminal Justice Statistics, 24th edition, 1997	http://www.albany.edu/sourcebook/index.html	363
Steroid prevention with high school athletes	http://www.nida.nih.gov/NIDA_Notes/NNVol12N4/steroid.html#girls	363
Study of drug use among consumers of vocational rehabilitation services	http://www.med.wright.edu/som/sardi/epidem.html	364
Workplace drug use	http://www.samhsa.gov/oas/wkplace/httoc.htm	364
Veterinary Medicine		
Animal diseases	http://www.mic.ki.se/Diseases/c22.html	365
Animal poison control	http://www.napcc.aspca.org/	366
Bovine respiratory disease (BRD)	http://www.nuflor.com/free.htm	366
Canine sports medicine	http://www.cris.com/~Dovervet/csmu/	367
Cattle disease prevention and treatment	http://www.ianr.unl.edu/pubs/animaldisease/index.htm#cattle	367
Compendium of animal rabies control, 1997	http://www.avma.org/	368
Emerging animal diseases	http://www.fas.org/ahead/	368
Footwarts of dairy cattle	http://sphinx.ucdavis.edu/research/footwarts/FootwartsOfDairyCattle.html	369
The Green Book	http://www.cvm.fda.gov/fda/Greenbook/greenbook.html	369
Intestinal spirochete	http://205.221.234.10:80/spiroch/	370
Laboratory animal diseases	http://www.rprc.washington.edu/aclad/index.html	370
Meat and poultry inspection under HACCP	http://www.meatami.org/haccpq&a.htm	371
National poultry improvement plan	http://www.aphis.usda.gov/vs/npip/	371
Pet cancer	http://www.oncolink.upenn.edu/specialty/vet_onc/cancer.html	372
Rabies	http://www.gis.queensu.ca/RReporter/mnr.html	372
Veterinarian employment	http://www.dvmsearch.com/index.htm	373
Women's Health		
Chronic pelvic pain diagnosis and management	http://www.cmegateway.com/womenshea...viders/Pelvic/pelvicpain.html#story	374
Doctor's guide to menopause information and resources	http://www.pslgroup.com/MENOPAUSE.HTM	375
Food safety, nutrition, and cosmetics	http://vm.cfsan.fda.gov/~dms/wh-toc.html	375
Gynecologic endoscopy resources	http://medweb.nus.sg/isge/resource.html	376
Gynecologic oncology tutorials	http://gynoncology.obgyn.washington.edu/Tutorials/nest3.html	376
Marching through the visible woman	http://www.crd.ge.com/cgi-bin/vw.pl	377
MDL 926 breast implant litigation, November 7, 1997	http://www.fjc.gov/BREIMLIT/mdl926.htm	377
Megasite, women's health	http://www.pitt.edu/HOME/GHNet/GHWomen.html	378
Menopause Online	http://www.menopause-online.com/	378

Primary Topic	URL	Page
OB-GYN medical professional data	http://www.obgyn.net/site_map/mp-map.htm	379
Obstetrics and gynecology board certification	http://www.metronet.com/~rhino/FAQS.htm	379
Oxford endometriosis gene study update	http://www.medicine.ox.ac.uk/ndog/oxegene/results.htm	380
Research of health issues among women with disabilities	http://WWW.CDC.GOV/nceh/programs/disabil/research.htm	380
Women's community prevention study centers	http://odp.od.nih.gov/whi/cpstopic.htm	381
Women's health "ground rounds" menu	http://lib-sh.lsumc.edu/fammed/grounds/grounds.html)	381
Women's health topics	http://www.medscape.com/Home/Topics/WomensHealth/womenshealth.html	382

Keyword Index

B

D

F

G

H

I

J

K

L

N

O

P

Q

R

Y